MAVERICKS of MEDICINE

Contemplating the Future of Medicine with Andrew Weil, Jack Kevorkian, Bernie Siegel, Ray Kurzweil, and Others

Interviews by David Jay Brown with:

Andrew Weil
Jack Kevorkian
Bernie Siegel
Barry Sears
Larry Dossey
Ray Kurzweil
Michael West
Leonard Hayflick
Kary Mullis
Aubrey de Grey
Peter Duesberg
Raphael Mechoulam
Rick Strassman
Michael Fossel
Joseph Knoll
John Guerin
Jonathan Wright
Garry Gordon
Jacob Teitalbaum
Marios Kyriazis
Durk Pearson and Sandy Shaw

MAVERICKS of MEDICINE

Conversations on the Frontiers of Medical Research

Interviews by David Jay Brown

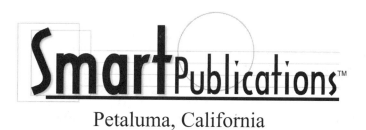

Petaluma, California

MAVERICKS OF MEDICINE
Interviews by David Jay Brown

Published by:

SmartPublications™

PO Box 4667
Petaluma, CA 94955
www.smart-publications.com

Published in the United States of America
First Edition, 2006

Library of Congress Control Number: 2006931394

ISBN: 1-890572-19-5   978-1-890572-19-8   **Softcover**

Warning—Disclaimer

More Interviews with Mavericks of Medicine!

Would you like to learn more about the latest medical research?
Simply register now for your free subscription to *Smart Publications Update!*
Smart Publications Update (A $36.00 value) provides the most blatantly-honest, valuable information on the health-enhancement and supplement industry you can find anywhere today.

You get more from David Jay Brown with occasional interviews from the Maverick thinkers of the future. Also, each issue of *Smart Publications Update* contains reviews of the latest scientific work in nutritional and anti-aging medicine. And great articles relating to health. Take care of yourself and those you love by staying in the loop on this rapidly unfolding science.

Name: _____

Company: _____

Address: _____

City/State/Zip: _____

email: _____

Title of book this card was in: _____ Mavericks of Medicine

Simply photocopy, fill out, and mail this information, and we'll rush you the latest issue...FREE!

Or call us, Toll Free, at 1-800-976-2783 to register today!

Mail to: **Smart Publications™, PO Box 4667, Petaluma, CA 94955**

TABLE of CONTENTS

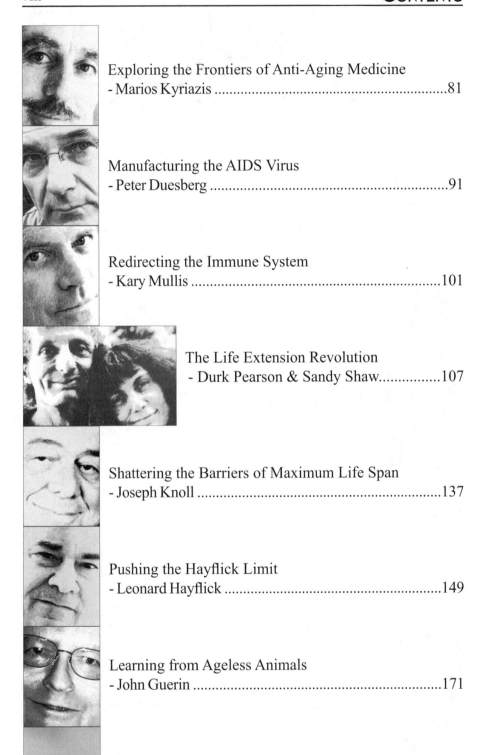

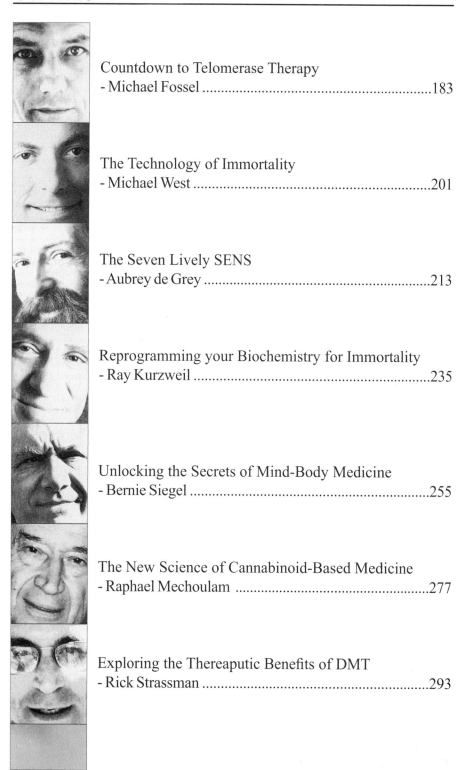

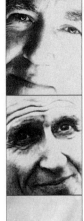

For

Robert Anton Wilson

ACKNOWLEDGEMENTS

As with most books, many people played valuable roles in its creation.

This book resulted from conversations that I had with my friend and colleague John Morgenthaler. John is responsible for coining the term "smart drugs," for writing the first books on the subject, and for much of the public's awareness about how certain drugs and nutrients can enhance cognitive performance. I met John backstage on the set for the Montel Williams Show in 1990, right after his book *Smart Drugs and Nutrients* was first published, and a large portion of what I know about these substances I initially learned from him. Learning about cognitive enhancers like hydergine and deprenyl changed my life, so I am indebted to John in numerous ways—including his valuable help as the editor and publisher of this book. So, first and foremost I would like to thank John for making this book possible.

I would also like to thank my associates at Health Freedom Nutrition, Ed Kinon and Dale Fowkes, for their encouragement and excitement about the project. Extra special thanks go to Erin Eileen Jarvis, for her invaluable biochemical expertise and generous help with the glossary, and to Louise Reitman, Joe & Suzie Wouk, Amy Barnes Excolere, Anna Damoth, Arleen Margulis, Sherry and Serena Hall, Jesse Ray Houts, Valerie Leveroni Corral, Robin Rae & Brummbaer, Clifford Pickover, Robert Anton Wilson, Deed DeBruno, Dana Bomar, Steven W. Andersen, and Carolyn Mary Kleefeld.

I would also like to thank the following individuals for their valuable help: Ruth Holmes, Mike Morganroth, Amy Powers, Brian Becker, Nancy Olmstead, Anne Genovese, Nancy Mullis, Sandy Oppenheim, Jean-Louis Husson, Richard Goldberg, Holly Morgenthaler, Carrie Scharf, Lamika Keller, Nancy Guyon, Chris Higgins, Annie Sprinkle, Denise Stow, Russel Jaffe, M.D., Randy Baker, M.D., Mimi Hill, Dana Peleg, Carole Myers, David Wayne Dunn, Robin Atwood, Emily Brown, Sherri

Paris, Mike Corral, Denis Berry, the members of WAMM and the RAW Group Mind, Senta Rose Hernandez, Lisa Marie Souza, Katherine Covell, Bethan Carter, Rupert Sheldrake, Michael Brown, Sammie and Tudie, Heather Hazen, Karen Lieberman, Bernadette Wilson, Nick Herbert, Jody Lombardo, Paula Rae Mellard, Jack Edwards, M.D., Oscar Janiger, M.D., Robin Chase, Matthew Steiner, Scott Crowley, Sylvia Thyssen, Robert Forte, Dina Meyer, Cheryle and Gene Goldstein, Linda Meyer, Arlene Istar Lev, and Shahab Geranmayeh.

I would also like to express my sincere gratitude to all the people that I interviewed for their vauable time, generous help, and thoughtful speculations.

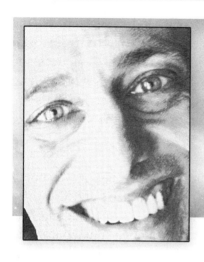

INTRODUCTION

David Jay Brown

As with science, the history of medicine reveals that knowledge often advances through the ideas of maverick thinkers—ideas that were initially greeted with disbelief or even mockery. For example, in 1847, when the Hungarian physician, Ignaz Semmelweis, started making the claim that puerperal fever was contagious, and that poor sanitation was responsible for spreading the illness from one new mother to another, his fellow physicians thought that he was crazy. "Wash your hands!" he shouted in the hospital maternity wards of Vienna, while the other doctors laughed.

Likewise, in 1628, when British physician, William Harvey, first proposed that the heart might be a pump at the center of a closed circulatory system—rather than a "heater" for the blood, as was thought at the time—he was ridiculed by his medical colleagues who thought the idea ridiculous. Then, in 1718, when Lady Mary Wortley Montagu insisted that live smallpox culture be introduced into her son's veins as an inoculation against the disease, her contemporaries thought that she was worse than nuts. Yet, with time, the ideas of these courageous individuals were vindicated, and history simply abounds with examples of how eccentric individuals—that were initially regarded as quacks—helped to advance science and medicine.

Both science and medicine are inherently conservative. Scientists and physicians are trained to always lean toward convention and to be suspicious of new ideas. This tendency to test new procedures carefully, and to make new declarations cautiously, is partially why science and medicine have been so successful and have such reliable track records. However, it is also why the conventional or mainstream core of established scientific and medical institutions—such as the American Medical Association—always advances much more slowly than the peripheral research frontiers, where eccentric individuals are experimenting with unorthodox possibilities that sometimes conflict with conventional thought.

While the right amount of skepticism can be healthy, and it's certainly necessary for science and medicine to advance, it can also stand in the way of progress. Unrestrained skepticism can mutate into neophobia—the fear of novelty—if it isn't properly balanced with open-mindedness and curiosity. Neophobia prevents the unbiased experimentation with new possibilities, and, in its more extreme forms, even causes conventional scientists and physicians to ridicule new ideas simply because they are unconventional. Having a proper balance of open-mindedness and skepticism is essential for science and medicine to properly advance.

While maverick thinkers certainly aren't always right, without these courageous individuals all scientific and medical progress would stagnate. The history of medicine reveals that during every time period in history there has been maverick thinkers who were ridiculed by their colleagues for having unconventional ideas that were later vindicated. This means that right now—in the historical epoch in which we currently find ourselves—this scenario is most likely taking place. So then, with this illuminating insight in mind, let us now consider who some of the promising maverick thinkers of our time might be, and what their ideas about medicine might mean.

Conversations on the Frontiers of Medical Research

In your hands is a collection of interdisciplinary interviews that I did with some of the most brilliant and controversial medical researchers and practitioners of our time. This collection of interviews with eminent physicians and cutting-edge researchers explores innovative work in the areas of life extension, cognitive enhancement, improved health and performance, integrative medicine, stem cell research, novel pharmacological and nutritional therapies, prosthetic implants, holistic and traditional medicines, mind-body medicine, euthanasia, and the integration of medicine with other fields of science.

As with my three previous interview books—*Mavericks of the Mind, Voices from the Edge,* and *Conversations on the Edge of the Apocalypse*—the people who I chose to interview are those creative and controversial thinkers who have stepped outside the boundaries of conventional thought and seen beyond the traditional view. I chose highly accomplished people who dare to question authority and think for themselves because it is often this capacity for independent thought that lies at the heart of their exceptional abilities and accomplishments. In questioning old belief systems, and traveling beyond the edges of the established horizons to find their answers, these unconventional thinkers have gained revolutionary insights, and they offer some unique solutions to the problems that are facing modern medicine.

Some of the questions that I will be discussing with these brilliant and courageous individuals have profound implications. What are some of the biggest problems with the way that medicine is practiced today, and what can be done to help improve the situation? What role does the mind play in the health of the body? How can people improve their cognitive or sexual performance? What are the primary causes of aging? What are currently the best ways to slow down, or reverse the aging process and extend the human life span? How long is it possible for the human life span to be extended? What are some of the new medical treatments that will be coming along in the near future? Do we have the right to die? What role does spirituality play in medicine? Speculating on these important questions can help us to understand our bodies better, improve our health, enhance our performance, and live longer happier lives. Let's take a look at some of these questions more closely.

What's Wrong With Modern Medicine and How Can We Improve It?

Almost everyone agrees that something is wrong with modern medicine. I recently attended a talk given by Andrew Weil, and when he announced his prediction that the healthcare system in America would soon collapse, everyone in the room vigorously applauded. However, although most people agree that something is wrong with modern medicine, not everyone agrees as to what it is and what to do about it.

On a most basic level, many patients simply feel that their physicians can't relate to what they're going through and that they're treated like a statistic. As a way to help remedy this situation, mind-body physician Bernie Siegel told me, "One simple suggestion would be to put every doctor into a hospital bed for a week as a patient. Put them in a hospital where they are not known, and have them admitted with a life-threatening illness as their diagnosis. Then let them stay there."

Another big problem with modern medicine is expense. The skyrocketing cost of healthcare, and the lack of healthcare insurance by many, is a serious problem. According to Larry Dossey, the author of *Space, Time, and Medicine*, "We're nearing fifty million people in this country who don't have health insurance." So what does Dr. Dossey suggest? "We need government-financed, centralized healthcare for everybody," he said.

However, not everyone that I spoke with agrees that socialized healthcare is such a good idea. When I spoke with life extension researcher Durk Pearson he said, "The most dangerous possible thing I can think of—other than having a complete police state like Nazi Germany or Soviet Russia—is to have a national medical program. Because, believe me, they are not going to be acting in your interest—they're going to be acting in their interest. There's no such thing as a free lunch. When you have a government health system, you have a bunch of bureaucrats telling you when it's time to die. The reason is very simple. They'll never collect back from you as much tax money as they spend taking care of you, so it's time for you to die. Read up on Nobel prize-winning economist James Buchanan's Public Choice Theory."

Ironically, many people also seriously question the safety of modern medicine—and for good reason. Dr. Dossey also told me that, "The death rate in American hospitals from medical mistakes, errors, and the side-effects of drugs now ranks as the third leading cause of death, behind heart disease and cancer." Although some people who have studied the statistics that Dr. Dossey is referring to disagree with these figures, they don't disagree by much, as even the most hard-nosed skeptics rank medical errors and drug side-effects as the fifth or sixth leading cause of death in American hospitals. Not a very comforting thought.

So the lack of trust that many people have toward modern medicine is understandable. However, an even greater cause for concern is that many people think that the medical establishment and the federal government are deliberately impeding medical advances that might divert profits away from pharmaceutical companies. For example, Durk Pearson—who won a landmark lawsuit against the Food and Drug Administration (FDA), charging the government agency with unconstitutionally restricting manufacturers from distributing truthful health information that could save people's lives—told me that he thought that the FDA was "the biggest barrier between life extension and people."

Pearson told me that this is simply because many people in the FDA are financially intertwined with the pharmaceutical companies. According to Pearson's partner, life extension researcher Sandy Shaw "...right now the FDA favors drug companies. There's no doubt about it. The drug companies are in bed with the FDA. The FDA is in bed with the drug companies." What this means is that the FDA generally supports patented drugs over natural dietary supplements—regardless of the scientific evidence—because the drug companies can't profit off them.

Pharmaceutical companies are seen by many as being motivated primarily by profit, and a lot of people are concerned that this motivation adversely affects their research agendas and marketing strategies. To help solve this problem, retrovirus researcher Peter Duesberg suggested that we "Generate a free market for scientific ideas in which funding depends on logic, scientific principles, and useful results, rather than on the approval...of "peer-review." Since the "peers" represent the established scientific monopolies, their self-interest demands "science" that confirms and extends the status quo rather than innovation, which threatens their considerable scientific and commercial investments."

When I spoke with natural medicine advocate Jonathan Wright he offered some insight into why the research agendas of the pharmaceutical companies might be off track to begin with. He said, "So far as medicine in general goes, our very biggest mistake...started in the early part of the twentieth century, and it continues to this day—and that is, relying on patent medicines to heal the body. This has been an enormous mistake, because the condition necessary to patent anything says that it can not occur in nature. But our bodies are made of materials that are entirely natural. ...The best it's going to do is suppress symptoms, and yet the medical profession has gone along with this for over a century."

However, Dr. Wright told me that he thought that the solution to this problem was very simple. He said, "Everything we need to do can be summed up in these two words: copy nature." For example, research has shown that when engaging in hormone replacement therapy it is essential that one use hormones that are biologically identical to those found in the human body, if one wishes to avoid the potentially deadly side-effects from taking patented synthetic hormones. The scientific evidence certainly suggests that we should avoid that which is unnatural to the body, and that an important secret to health and longevity is simply to mimic what nature does. Others point out that this is a good place to start, but that we can also significantly improve upon nature.

Our conventional medical system is entirely oriented toward the treatment of disease, illness, and injury. Little attention is given to making healthy people healthier and for improving physical, sexual, and cognitive performance. However, there are now many drugs, herbs, and nutrients available that have been shown to improve physical endurance, cognitive abilities, memory, and sexual performance. In the pages that follow, I discuss these drugs and dietary supplements with Durk Pearson and Sandy Shaw, Jonathan Wright, Ray Kurzweil, and others.

These performance-enhancing supplements appear to compensate for some of the decline in performance caused by aging. If cognitive and sexual performance can be enhanced in the elderly, then perhaps other consequences of aging can also be reversed. Understanding and reversing the aging process is another important theme in this book.

Reversing the Aging Process and Life Extension Research

Although there are some good theories of aging, and a lot of progress has been made in terms of understanding why we age, the aging process is still largely mysterious. Some of the most important theories of aging—such as the free radical and cross-linking theories—are discussed in this book, along with proposals for how we might halt and reverse the aging process.

When I spoke with Leonard Hayflick, the microbiologist who discovered that healthy somatic cells can only divide a finite number of times (now known as the "Hayflick limit"), he defined aging as " ... the random systemic loss of molecular fidelity, that—after reproductive maturity—accumulates to levels that eventually exceed repair, turnover, or maintenance capacity."

British biogerontologist, Aubrey de Grey, told me that he thinks that there are seven primary reasons why aging occurs. He said, "These are intrinsic side-effects of metabolism, of being alive in the first place, and they are things that build up throughout life. Although these side-effects are not the cause of aging, they start to become harmful once they get to a certain level of abundance. Once there's enough of them around the body starts to suffer from them and eventually it suffers seriously." Dr. de Grey believes that this process is reversible, and he has assembled a master plan for doing so that a substantial number of other life extension researchers are taking seriously. In the pages that follow, Dr. de Grey speaks with us about this.

Perhaps the most compelling reason to believe that radical life extension might be possible is because not all animals age like we do. In fact, it appears that some animals don't age at all. When I interviewed John Guerin, director of the Ageless Animals Project, he told me about rockfish caught off the coast of Alaska that were hundreds of years old, healthy, and fertile. Whales have been known to live for over two hundred years without showing any signs of aging. A male whale that was over a hundred years old was harpooned while it was in the midst of having sex. Guerin believes that by studying these types of animals we can learn why they live so long without losing vitality or fertility and then apply that knowledge to extending the life span of human beings.

Technology theorist and inventor, Ray Kurzweil, spoke to me about how nanotechnology, artificial intelligence, and robotics will eventually allow humans to live for indefinite periods of time without aging. Dr. Kurzweil thinks that "nanobots, blood cell-size devices that could go inside the body and keep us healthy from inside" will be available in about two decades. So, Dr. Kurzweil believes, if we can just stay alive for another fifteen or twenty years we'll be able to live forever.

Nanotechnology would not only allow for radical life extension, but also for a dramatic improvement in all physical capabilities—including brain functions. Dr. Kurzweil believes that the line between biology and technology is going to completely blur together in the decades to come, and that nanotechnological brain implants will substantially increase our intelligence and dramatically expand the power of the human mind. The power of the mind, and its relationship to medicine, is another important theme in this book.

Mind-Body Medicine

When I was in college during the early eighties, my maverick mentor Russel Jaffe told me that the most effective tool discovered by modern medicine was being overlooked by the majority of physicians. Dr. Jaffe was, of course, referring to the placebo effect, the power of the mind to affect the health of the body. Numerous studies have demonstrated that what we believe about a medical treatment dramatically effects how we respond to it. This is why when pharmaceutical companies develop a new drug it is always tested against inactive sugar pills—placebos—that are known to improve symptoms and facilitate cures simply because the patient and/or the physician believe that the new drug might work.

However, ironically, when I studied psychobiology at USC and NYU, I was taught by most of my professors that the placebo effect was simply something to be controlled for in experimental or clinical trials. In other words, it was like a nuisance that interfered with our understanding about the effects of a new drug or procedure, and most researchers and healthcare practitioners simply shrugged the placebo effect off as simply irrelevant. This was in the days before we really understood that what we believe not only directly impacts how we feel, but it measurably affects our physiology as well. We now know that the mind and body are simply two parts of the same inseparable system, and each dramatically affects the other.

Candace Pert, the neuroscience researcher who discovered the opiate receptor in the brain (and who I interviewed for my previous book *Conversations on the Edge of the Apocalypse*), brought about a paradigm shift in modern medicine by pioneering research that revealed an intimate relationship between the mind and body. Her interdisciplinary research into the relationship between the nervous system and the immune system demonstrated a body-wide communication system mediated by peptide molecules and their receptors. Dr. Pert believes this to be the biochemical basis of emotion and the potential key to understanding many challenging diseases. Dr. Pert's research provides a basis for understanding why cancer patients can measurably reduce tumor growth through the process of visualization, and why placebos can cause measurable physiological changes.

In his practice as a general and pediatric surgeon, Bernie Siegel began recognizing common personality characteristics in those patients who did well and those who didn't. In his bestselling book *Love, Medicine, and Miracles*, Dr. Siegel describes how exceptional cancer patients survive because of their attitude and beliefs. When I spoke with Dr. Siegel he told me, "You can't separate thoughts and beliefs from your body. In other words, what you think, and what you believe, literally changes your body chemistry."

Studies confirm Dr. Siegel's observations. For example, a PET scan study conducted at the University of Michigan showed that people who believed that they were receiving a pain killer actually produced more pain-killing endorphins in their brains and experienced less pain.

A relatively recent branch of medicine known as mind-body medicine addresses this fascinating and important topic of how the mind influences the body. In this collection, I speak with Bernie Siegel, Andrew Weil, and Larry Dossey about how we might be able to use this understanding to improve our health. I also speak with psychopharmacology researchers Raphael Mechoulam and Rick Strassman about the therapeutic potential of cannabis and psychedelic drugs. Many hallucinogenic plants—such as peyote and ayahausca brews—have a long history of shamanic and medicinal use in healing practices around the world, and may enhance the strength of the placebo effect (i.e., the power of the mind) because of their consciousness-changing abilities.

When I interviewed Dr. Weil he told me about how he had become completely cured of a lifelong cat allergy during an LSD session when he was twenty-eight, and that this experience had a profound influence on his medical perspective. He said that he would use psychedelics in his medical practice if they were legal. Dr. Weil said, "I think they've been a very profound influence. I used them a lot when I was younger. I think that they made me very much aware, first of all, of the profound influence of consciousness on health...Psychedelics can show you possibilities... I think they're potentially tremendous teaching tools about mind-body interactions and states of consciousness."

Perhaps even more fascinating than mind-body medicine is a transpersonal phenomenon known as "remote healing." It seems that what we think may not only affect our own health—it may also directly effect the health of others. When I interviewed Dr. Dossey he told me about numerous controlled, double-blind studies demonstrating that "prayer" can have measurable health effects. The effects of directing positive intention have been demonstrated in dozens of controlled laboratory studies—in people, animals, and even bacteria. Dr. Dossey also told me about studies that demonstrated health benefits from engaging in religious practice, and spoke about the integration of medicine with spirituality. Reflecting on the integration of medicine with spirituality brings one to the notion that sometimes healing the essence of who we are, and reducing suffering, may mean letting go of the physical body.

The Right to Die

Just because medical technologies give us the ability to live forever doesn't mean that we have to do so. The late psychologist, Timothy Leary, was one of the first people to start promoting ideas about life extension; he began doing so in the late 1970s. Attaining physical immortality, he believed was one of the "goals" of biological evolution. Dr. Leary's enthusiasm inspired longevity researchers and helped to popularize ideas about how science would soon conquer the aging process and allow us to virtually live forever.

However, when Dr. Leary was diagnosed with terminal prostate cancer at the age of 76, he said that he was "thrilled and ecstatic" to hear that he was going die. As much as Dr. Leary loved life, he not only accepted death—he embraced it. In the end, he even decided to forgo his plans for cryonic suspension. I think there is an important lesson in Dr. Leary's dying process about the importance of facing the mystery of death with the same openness and sense of adventure that one faces life.

In other words, attaining physical immortality in a human body may not be the final stage for evolving consciousness in this universe. Numerous spiritual traditions—such as Hinduism and many forms of shamanism—assert that healing the spirit sometimes involves transcending the body and moving on to whatever is after death. However, regardless of whether or not consciousness survives death, not everyone may wish to hang around until the final collapse of the universe, and certainly people who are in chronic pain, or who are suffering greatly, should be given the option to leave if they wish.

When I asked Dr. Weil about his views on the controversial issue of euthanasia he said, "I don't think it's appropriate for doctors to be involved in that, although I think patients should be able to discuss that issue with doctors. I think that for people with overwhelming diseases, for whom life has become really difficult, they should have that choice, and that there should be mechanisms provided for helping them with that."

Dr. Jack Kevorkian, on the other hand, believes that physicians should be able to perform euthanasia, and he is currently in prison for second degree murder because he assisted with the last wish of a patient who was suffering from ALS. When I interviewed Dr. Kevorkian about voluntary death I learned that, despite the U.S. government and medical establishment's opposition to euthanasia, eighty percent of the public support a patient's right to die and one in five physicians has admitted to practicing euthanasia at some point in their career. Why, then, is euthanasia illegal? "I think that the U.S. government, medical establishment and pharmaceutical companies are opposed to euthanasia for monetary or financial reasons," Dr. Kevorkian said, "To help correct this situation there has to be an organized public response and outcry—which I believe is now occurring."

While the goals of contemporary Western medicine are healing disease and treating injuries, the goals that one aspires to in the pursuit of optimal health are much larger and more encompassing. This may involve developing an immortal, nanotechnologically-proficient, self-repairing super-body of our own design, or it may involve gracefully transcending this world entirely and discarding our body like a pile of used clothing—but, either way, I think that the primary goal that medicine should aim for is the reduction of human suffering. I think that if we make the reduction of human suffering our number one priority, then the future of medicine does indeed appear very bright.

The Future of Medicine

We are living in truly astonishing times. Although our current healthcare system appears to be crumbling around us, we are simultaneously witnessing a rapidly-advancing biotechnology revolution that promises to forever change the course of human history. New possibilities are emerging everywhere we turn, and there is enormous cause for hope. When we look out onto the frontiers of medicine we see an incredible vista blossoming with possibilities that stagger the mind and border on the miraculous. New advances in medicine promise to help humanity end countless generations of suffering and deliver us into a golden age where disease and aging are merely subjects that we learn about in history class and the boundaries of our physical capacities are limited only by our imaginations.

The following interviews shed some light on where modern medicine may be evolving. They provide a treasure-trove of practical suggestions that anyone can use to improve their health today and they offer an exciting vision of what's to come. These mavericks of medicine provide us with bridges to awe-inspiring possibilities, and they offer us the hope that we can all live longer, healthier, and happier lives.

— David Jay Brown
Ben Lomond, California

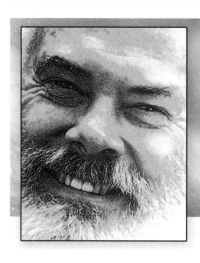

**THE TRANSFORMATIVE POWER
of
INTEGRATIVE MEDICINE**

An Interview with Dr. Andrew Weil

Andrew Weil, M.D., is an internationally recognized expert on Integrative Medicine, which combines the best therapies of conventional and alternative medicine. Dr. Weil's lifelong study of medicinal herbs, mind-body interactions, and alternative medicine have made him one of the world's most trusted authorities on unconventional medical treatments. Dr. Weil's sensible, interdisciplinary medical perspective strikes a strong chord in many people. His recent books are all New York Times *bestsellers and he has appeared on the cover of* Time Magazine *twice, in 1997 and again in 2005.* USA Today *said, "Clearly, Dr. Weil has hit a medical nerve," and* The New York Times Magazine *said, "Dr Weil has arguably become America's best-known doctor."*

Dr. Weil has long had a talent for blending the conventional with the unconventional. He received an undergraduate degree in botany from Harvard in 1964 and his M.D. from Harvard Medical School in 1968. After completing a medical internship at Mt. Zion Hospital in San Francisco, he worked for a year with the National Institute of Mental Health. From 1971 to 1984, he was on the research staff of the Harvard Botanical Museum, where he conducted investigations into medicinal and psychoactive plants. Then from 1971 to 1975, as a Fellow of the Institute of Current World Affairs, Dr. Weil traveled throughout Central and South America, collecting information and specimens for this research. These explorations—where he not only studied plants but indigenous peoples, their medicine and pharmacology—were to have a profound effect on Dr. Weil's medical career.

Dr. Weil has long been interested in altered states of consciousness and how the mind affects health—even before he began studying medicine. He has written extensively about this interest and about how his early psychedelic experiences profoundly influenced his views on medicine. Dr. Weil's first book, The Natural Mind, *was an investigation of drugs and higher consciousness. Because of this interest in altered states of consciousness, Dr. Weil has been honored by having a psychedelic mushroom named after him—Psilocybe weilii, which was discovered in 1995.*

Dr. Weil is the author (or coauthor) of ten popular books, including The Marriage of the Sun and Moon, From Chocolate to Morphine, Health and Healing, Natural Health, Natural Medicine, Spontaneous Healing, Eight Weeks to Optimum Health, *and* Healthy Aging. *He has also appeared in three videos featured on PBS:* Spontaneous Healing, Eight Weeks to Optimum Health, *and* Healthy Aging.

Dr. Weil is currently the Director of the Program in Integrative Medicine at the University of Arizona's College of Medicine. He also holds appointments as Clinical Professor of Medicine, Professor of Public Health, and is the Lovell-Jones Professor of Integrative Rheumatology. A frequent guest on Larry King Live, Oprah, *and* The Today Show, *Dr. Weil is the editorial director of DrWeil.com, and he publishes the popular newsletter* Self Healing. *To find out more about Dr. Weil's work visit: www.drweil.com.*

Dr. Weil lives near Tucson, Arizona. I conducted this interview with Dr. Weil on March 8, 2006. Dr. Weil appeared to be especially interested in the relationship between consciousness and health when we spoke. We talked about some of the most important lessons that physicians aren't being taught in medical school, why it's important for conventional Western medicine to be more open-minded about alternative medical treatments, and how the mind and spirituality effect health.

David: What originally inspired your interest in medicine?

Dr. Weil: My father had wanted to go to medical school but was unable to finish college. It was during the depression. I had a G.P. family doctor who was an influence in that direction. I was interested in science and biology, and I kind of went to medical school by default, because I really didn't know what I wanted to do. I had a sense that a medical degree would be useful to me, and I wanted a medical education, but I really never saw myself being a doctor.

David: How did your early study of botany and the medicinal use of plants in South America affect your views of medicine?

Dr. Weil: That was a huge influence. I think that's one of the luckiest choices I ever made. It really gave me a grounding in natural science. It connected me to the plant world. It got me interested in ethnobotany and uses of plants in other cultures. It exposed me to Native American culture, both in North and South America. It gave me a perspective on drugs that I don't think anyone else in Harvard Medical School had, and it really started me on a career interest in medicinal plants. I think it was one of the major influences in how I think about and practice medicine.

David: What do you think are some of the biggest problems with modern medicine and what do you think needs to be done to help correct the situation?

Dr. Weil: I think it's too reliant on technology. I think it's overly reliant on very powerful pharmaceutical drugs without appreciating their potential for harm. I think it is very effective in many areas, but I think it's very ineffective in large categories of disease that affect people. I think it's doing a very poor job at prevention. I think it neglects, or underplays, the body's potential for healing, which has been a major theme of my work and writing. And I think it's become very divorced from the natural world.

David: What do you think are some of the most important lessons about health that most physicians aren't currently being taught in medical school?

Dr. Weil: I think the major one is that the body has a tremendous potential for self-regulation and for healing, and that's where good medicine should start. You want to figure out how to make that happen or remove obstacles to it. I think that physicians are generally uneducated in the whole realm of lifestyle medicine—that is, how diet, exercise, mental states, and habits all affect health. I think they're very uneducated in mind-body interactions and the spiritual dimension of human health. I think there's almost a complete omission of education about nutrition, about use of dietary supplements, about use of botanicals, about many of these other systems of medicine, like Ayurvedic and Chinese medicine, that are thousands of years old and very effective in many areas. So there are large areas I think of omission in conventional medical education.

David: Why do you think it's important for conventional Western medicine to be more open-minded about alternative medical treatments?

Dr. Weil: First of all, a huge number of patients are using these systems and doctors should know what their patients are doing—if only for the point of view that they might interact or impact the conventional treatments that they're recommending. Secondly, there are a lot of ideas and treatments out there in the world of alternative medicine that are very useful that can compliment these deficiencies in conventional medicine. So that alone is, I think, a reason for doctors to at least be aware that these other systems and methods exist.

David: Can you talk a little about Integrative Medicine and why you think it's important?

Dr. Weil: I think Integrative Medicine is the way of the future. It makes sense. It's increasingly what patients want. It's what doctors want to practice. And I think the real potential of it—which is going to make it a mainstream phenomenon—is that it has the potential to lower healthcare costs by bringing lower cost treatments into the mainstream, while preserving outcomes or even improving them.

David: Can you explain what you mean by the body's "healing system"?

Dr. Weil: I think this is obvious if you watch the way wounds heal on the surface of the body. The body has a capacity to diagnose problems, to repair them, and to regenerate. This exists at every level of the organism, and it seems to me that good medicine should start with that principle, that the body has the ability to heal itself, and wants to get back to a state of health. And that your job as an outside practitioner is to help that process. So you're not putting a cure into somebody. You are impacting, removing obstacles to, and allowing that natural healing power to work.

David: What are some of the basic suggestions that you would make about diet?

Dr. Weil: First of all, the basic theory of my work is in the book *Health and Healing*. I think that appeared in 1983. In a lot of my practical books I've included information about diet. I have a whole book on that subject called *Eating Well for Optimum Health*, and in a cookbook I did with Rosie Daley, *The Healthy Kitchen*, there's a lot of very concise information that people easily can get about basic dietary theory. In my recent book, *Healthy Aging*, I think this is organized most tightly. I talk about an anti-inflammatory diet, but this is really a diet for optimum health. It is modeled on the Mediterranean diet, which I think is the best template to use for designing a healthy diet.

David: What do you think are some of the most important nutritional supplements that one should be taking?

Dr. Weil: I think that everyone should take a good multivitamin, multimineral supplement. I've been arguing that the government should provide one free to all school kids. I think that would do a lot to help correct micronutrient deficiencies, which are especially common in the poor population. I think it would improve school performance, and provide a lot of benefit. I think that people need to know how to read the label of a multivitamin bottle, so that they can tell whether it's worth their money or not. I've given those rules in my book *Healthy Aging*, and they're also available on my Web site. There are some fairly simple things that you look at on the label that tell whether or not this is a good product. The quality of vitamin supplements varies enormously and there isn't necessarily a correlation with price. And there are a lot of not well-designed products out there.

David: What sort of recommendations would you make to someone looking to improve their memory and their cognitive performance?

Dr. Weil: I think, first of all, to use antioxidants, to avoid smoking, and to look at some of the natural products out there which may be useful for that. There's a dietary supplement called phosphatidylserine (PS), which looks useful for memory. There's a product on the market called Juvenon, developed by Bruce Ames at Berkeley, which has two dietary supplements in it that looks useful. Ginkgo biloba may be helpful. But I think a major piece of advice that I would give people is that education seems very protective. The more education you have, I think, the better your memory is and the better it stays as you get older. I think there are some kinds of education that are particularly useful, like learning another language, so I urge people to make an effort to learn another language. You don't have to master it; it's just the act of trying to learn it that seems very useful. And there's one other thing—it looks as if a lot of the neurodegenerative diseases begin as inflammatory processes. So again, following an anti-inflammatory diet, and using natural products that have anti-inflammatory effect. Turmeric looks especially powerful as a memory protectant.

David: What sort of recommendations would you make to someone looking to improve their sexual performance?

Dr. Weil: I think, first of all, one needs to analyze what the problems are, and access whether there is a physical problem that's interfering, or whether there is a psychological problem. So I would say to get help from an expert in the field. I think that Viagra and its relatives for men certainly are better than anything else that has been available throughout history. I think there are a number of natural products, like Asian ginseng, an Indian plant called ashwagandha, a plant from Mongolia called rhodiola, and arctic root. All of these have reputations as being sexual enhancers, especially for men. For women, I think the best thing we have is low-dose testosterone, and that needs to be given on prescription with some careful diagnosis, but it can be very useful.

David: What do you think are some of the virtues of aging and why do you think that it's important that we accept the aging process?

Dr. Weil: I think it's important because it's inevitable, and there's nothing we can do about it—despite what the anti-aging people have to say. It's an inevitable universal process. So I think it's important to get with it, and accept it. I also think that, while aging brings difficulties and problems, there are some things that get better as you get older. I think that you accumulate wisdom. You develop more authority. I think that certain aspects of mental function get better, such as pattern recognition. I think that in cultures where aging is valued, and not devalued as it is here, old people look different. They're valued as major cultural resources, and sources of information, experience, and wisdom. And people look up to them for that reason.

David: What do you think are the primary causes of aging?

Dr. Weil: Ultimately, I think it's the Second Law of Thermodynamics—that disorder increases in systems, and that's just the law of the universe. I think that on the cellular level that means the accumulation of errors in the DNA code. I think that one way you can look at living life is that it's a perpetual struggle between oxidative stress and antioxidant defenses. The main source of oxidative stress is normal metabolism, and eventually oxidative stress wins, because of the fact that disorder increases. So I think that you can look on various levels as to why aging occurs. You can look at damage to DNA, damage to cell membranes, and oxidative damage, but I think the root cause is that this is a law of the universe.

David: What do you think are currently some of the best ways to slow down the aging process and age more gracefully with greater health?

Dr. Weil: My goal is not to slow down the aging process; it's to reduce the risk, and delay the onset of age-related diseases. I don't think it is necessary to get sick as you get older. One of the things that I worry about with the anti-aging movement is that if you're obsessed with slowing down or reversing the aging process it distracts you from that other goal, which is, I think, the really important one. And to do that, I think, it means attending to all aspects of lifestyle. It means learning the principles of good eating, good physical activity, ways of neutralizing stress, using natural products to enhance health, and knowing what you can do on the mental level to protect your memory and other mental functions. So I think it's working in all aspects of lifestyle, and I think we have a lot of that information out there about how to reduce the risk of age-related disease.

David: What role do you see the mind and consciousness playing in the health of the body?

Dr. Weil: I think it's huge. This is an area that I've been interested in, I think, since I was a teenager—long before I went to medical school—and a lot of my early work was with altered states of consciousness and psychoactive drugs. I reported a lot of things that I saw about how physiology changed drastically with changes in consciousness. I just reviewed a paper from Japan; one of the authors is a doctor I know. This is a group of people looking at how emotional states affect the genome. They have shown, for example, that laughter can actually effect gene expression in patients with Type 2 diabetes. Now that's really interesting stuff, and I think that this is the type of research that is generally not looked at here. I think that our mental states—our states of consciousness—have a profound influence on our bodies, and even our genes. And I think they have a lot to do with how we age.

David: What role do you think that spirituality plays in health?

Dr. Weil: Again, I think, large, but it's hard to define spirituality. For me, I make a very sharp distinction between spirituality and religion. Religion is really about institutions, and for me spirituality is about the nonphysical, and how to access that and incorporate it into life. In *Eight Weeks to Optimum Health*, I gave a lot of suggestions in each week about things that people can do to improve or raise spiritual energy, and they are things that at first many people might not associate with spirituality. But they were recommendations like having fresh flowers in your living space and listening to pieces of music that elevate your mood. Some of the other suggestions included spending more time with people in whose company you feel more optimistic and better, and spending time in nature. I think that I would put all of these in the realm of spiritual health.

*David: When I interviewed Larry Dossey he told me about research
that showed evidence for the health benefits of remote healing. What
do you think of the studies done with remote healing that show health
benefits from prayer?*

Dr. Weil: I don't know what to make of them. I think that's really frontier
stuff, fringy stuff, and I'm certainly open to those possibilities. I'm willing
to believe anything, but then I really want to see evidence for it. And I
think that the evidence that has been collected so far for these effects, at
least in the experiments where people don't know that these interventions
are being done, that that's such a challenge to the conventional model,
that there really has to be very solid evidence for it. I'm open-minded,
but unconvinced at the moment.

*David: How have psychedelics affected your perspective on medicine,
and what sort of therapeutic potential do you think they have?*

Dr. Weil: I think they've been a very profound influence. I used them
a lot when I was younger. I think that they made me very much aware,
first of all, of the profound influence of consciousness on health. I have
published and described one of the experiences that I had that was very
dramatic, and this was seized upon by some networks that put it all out
there. This was that I had become cured of a lifelong cat allergy. If a cat
touched me, I would get hives. If a cat licked me, I would get hives and
my eyes would swell. So I always avoided them.

Then, one day when I was twenty-eight, I took LSD with some friends.
It was a perfect day. I was in a wonderful state of mind, feeling totally
relaxed and at one with everything, and a cat jumped into my lap. My
immediate reaction was to be defensive, and then I instantly thought,
well, here I'm in this state, why don't I try to pet the cat. So I petted the
cat and I had no allergic reaction. I spent a lot of time with it, and I've
never had an allergic reaction to a cat since.

So, to me, that's an example of a potential of those drugs, and if they were
legally available I think that I would use them as teaching tools to show
people that you can change chronic patterns of illness, because even if you
aren't cured of an illness the psychedelic may show you that it's possible.
Another experience that I've written about with psychedelics is when I

was learning yoga, and had a lot of difficulty with some positions. The one I had the most trouble with was "the plow," where you lie on your back and try to touch your toes behind your head. I could get to about a foot of the floor and I had horrible pain in my neck. I had worked at this for weeks and made no progress. I was on the point of giving up; just thinking I was too old. I was twenty-eight then. I thought I was too old, that my body was too stiff.

Again, an experience with a psychedelic, where I felt completely happy and elastic, showed me otherwise. I noticed that my body felt very free. So I tried that posture, and I thought I had around a foot left to go when my feet touched the floor and there was no pain. I kept raising and lowering them, and it was just delightful. The next day when I tried to do it I could get to a foot within the floor and I had horrible pain in my neck—but there was a difference. I now knew that it was possible, and I think that's a model for how these drugs can work.

Psychedelics can show you possibilities. They don't give you information about how to maintain the experiences, and if you try to rely on the drug for the experience, the drug stops working after a time. But, in this case, just having seen that it was possible, I was motivated to keep working at it, and in a few weeks I was able to do it. I don't think I would have pursued that if I hadn't seen the possibility. So I think they're potentially tremendous teaching tools about mind-body interactions and states of consciousness.

David: What are some of the new medical treatments that you foresee coming along in the near future?

Dr. Weil: First of all, there are all the high-tech ones, which are great. I think these are fabulous possibilities. Now, whether they will become practical realities or not, I don't know. I would say that a huge area is genomic medicine—the possibility of being able to individualize treatment to patients, including pharmaceutical drug treatment. Just as an example, there's a lot controversy now about soy and its ability to protect from breast cancer. Some of this seems to have to do with how women metabolize soy. Some of them are able to metabolize one of the phytoestrogens of soy to a protective compound and other women are not. If you could identify those women who could do it, then those are the ones you would want to get to eat soy regularly. The other ones, maybe not.

With cigarettes there are a lot of people, especially Asians, who are able to smoke like chimneys all their life and have no increased risk of lung cancer. They have different enzyme systems. It would be nice to identify that group, and then there are some people to whom you could say, you must never smoke because you're at high risk. And to other people we could say, if you want to do it, maybe do it, although you might still be at risk for other problems from it. And the same way with how people respond to pharmaceutical drugs and surgical treatments. So I think that there is this promise out there on the horizon of customized medicine, based on people's genetic makeup. At the moment it's promise; we don't have the practical techniques to do it. The other question is that some of these new techniques may be too expensive to deliver to everybody, so it'll be medicine for the affluent. Anyway, I think there's a lot of stuff like that out there on the horizon that looks great.

David: What are your views on euthanasia?

Dr. Weil: I think it's great that this issue, at least, has been raised to the level of public discussion. I don't think it's appropriate for doctors to be involved in it, although I think patients should be able to discuss the issue with doctors. I think that for people with overwhelming diseases, for whom life has become really difficult, that they should have that choice, and that there should be mechanisms provided for helping them with that. I think the experience in the Netherlands is very positive, and I don't see abuses of it there. So I would like a society where that was possible.

David: What are you currently working on?

Dr. Weil: I'm not interested in taking on another book for awhile. My main focus is developing curriculum for the program in Integrative Medicine, which, eventually, I hope will be in all medical schools, and really increasing the numbers of doctors out there that we've graduated. We now have over three hundred. My focus is really on having that be a new generation of physicians and nurse practitioners who get it, and have this kind of knowledge that's been omitted from medical education. I think that's my main focus. I'm interested in doing more work in radio and television. I may want to write something for kids. I'm very interested in trying to effect public health policy, especially on nutrition, and I'm also looking at ways of reforming the healthcare system. So, all that stuff. And having more leisure time for myself is also high on my agenda.

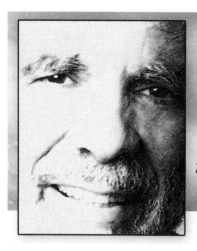

**THE FRONTIERS
of
NATURAL MEDICINE**

An Interview with Dr. Jonathan Wright

Jonathan Wright, M.D., is one of the world's leading experts on natural medicine, nutritional supplements, and bioidentical hormone replacement therapy. He is the medical director of the Tahoma Clinic in Kent, Washington, and he has treated over 2,000 patients with natural hormone replacement since 1982.

Dr. Wright graduated from Harvard University, and he received his medical education at the University of Michigan Medical School. He later specialized in family practice and nutritional medicine. Dr. Wright was a monthly medical columnist for Prevention *magazine from 1976 to 1986 and for* Let's Live *magazine from 1986 to 1996. Since 1994, he's written* Nutrition & Healing *newsletter (1-800-851-7100, www.wrightnewsletter.com)*

He is also the bestselling author or coauthor of numerous health books, including Natural Hormone Replacement For Women Over 45, Dr. Wright's Guide to Healing With Nutrition, Maximize Your Vitality & Potency for Men Over 40, *and* Dr. Wright's Book of Nutritional Therapy.

Since 1982, Dr. Wright and his colleague, Dr. Alan Gaby, have been teaching an annual seminar called "Nutritional Therapy in Medical Practice," based on their experience in medical practice and personal research libraries, which contains over 45,000 medical journal articles dating from 1920 to the present. He also publishes an informative monthly newsletter. To find out more about Dr. Wright's work visit: www.tahoma-clinic.com.

I spoke with Dr. Wright on July 14, 2005. He is a very enthusiastic and entertaining speaker. We spoke about preventing heart disease and osteoporosis, the basics of vitamin therapy, how people can improve their sexual performance, and the importance of treating hormonal decline with hormones that are identical to those found naturally in the human body.

David: What inspired your interest in medicine?

Dr. Wright: I'm not sure. I decided to go into medicine when I was eight years old. I recall a conversation with my parents about the whole thing, and the choices got narrowed down to law or medicine. For whatever reason, I decided that there are too damn many attorneys, and that they spend their time fighting, so I thought I'd go into medicine.

David: Can you talk a little about why you think that hormone replacement therapy is so important for both men and women as they age, and why do you think that taking natural hormones is better than taking synthetic hormones?

Dr. Wright: Hormone replacement therapy is especially important for men and women as they grow older at this particular time in the history of the planet and of the human race. Hormone replacement therapy is something that, in many areas of the world, simply wasn't even possible until about the 12th Century in China. But even though that was many centuries ago, as far as we know, there have been people on the planet for hundreds of thousands of years, perhaps millions of years, and no one could do hormone replacement for most of that time.

Some people have pointed out that the average person's life span was shorter in previous centuries, and perhaps people didn't need hormone replacement because they didn't live to the point where they needed it, and that may be true in some areas of the world. But we have not only Western Biblical references, but we have other writings that refer to some quite ancient people, in the past, who seem to have gotten by without hormone replacement, and lived to a good long age. The name Methuselah, of course, always comes to mind. Then there are some names that—not being a being a Chinese speaker—I can't pronounce. But in Chinese writing, folks are said to have lived for two or three hundred years, and it doesn't appear that they took hormone replacement.

But the differences that may necessitate more hormone replacement in our time than in prior times include what has happened to the food supply, the water supply, and the 50,000 new chemicals that are introduced into the environment every year—without knowing whether they're safe or not. There has been terrific demineralization of the soil, chemical additives to the water, such as chlorine and fluoride, and then there's all the electromagnetic radiations that folks are exposed to that just simply didn't exist two hundred years ago. The list could go on and on, and we don't want do a treatise here on all the enormous environmental changes that have happened. But while we were living in this vastly changing environment, human biochemical systems remained the same.

Therefore, we're seeing a tremendous rise in such things as Alzheimer's disease and senile dementia, which was, of course, so rare in the past. A paper on Alzheimer's disease from a century and a half ago said that people had less than a one percent chance of coming down with the disease, whereas today we're now told that our chances of ending up with Alzheimer's disease or senile dementia is fifteen percent. We also have seen the peak of a very large increase in cardiovascular disease, and thank goodness it's gone down. I believe it was Paul Dudley White who was the first person to actually identify himself as a cardiologist and a specialist in heart matters in the early part of the twentieth century. Before him, we didn't have cardiologists. We didn't need them in the prior century, or the century before. And it's not because people didn't have heart disease back then, it's because it was very unusual. Thank goodness—with no credit, I'm sorry to say, to American medicine, but a lot credit to just public awareness—that the large increase in cardiovascular disease seems to have reached its peak in the late 80s, maybe early 90s, and has subsided a bit again.

The other major thing that people look to hormone replacement for turns out to be osteoporosis prevention, which again, was fairly uncommon until the last century—except for the Inuit of northern Canada. Osteoporosis was fairly rare in this country until, again, the early Twentieth Century when the incidence started to rise, and went up and up and up.

So we have those three major problems—osteoporosis, cardiovascular disease, and senility and Alzheimer's disease are (more or less) one problem. Cardiovascular disease has gone up enormously, and if one tracks it back, a lot of it has to do with the current mismatch between human biochemical systems and the enormously changed dietary and other environmental factors. What has been observed is that hormone replacement therapy is not only perhaps a longevity issue, but it can do a lot to reduce the probability of those three major problems. I think that is fairly definite and very defendable, but only if we use the same hormones that have been found in human biochemical systems for as long there have been human biochemical systems.

I suspect that I'm beating a dead horse, to make a deliberate pun, when I say that putting horse hormones into humans—when those horse hormones are roughly seventy percent different from human hormones, and have never been in human bodies before—was one of medicine's many grievous errors in the last century. If we had been using bioidentical hormones we very likely would have never ever run into the disaster that the Women's Health Initiative turned out to be. But we can significantly lower the risk of those three major risk problems that arose in the Twentieth Century, and continue into the Twenty-first Century, with bioidentical molecules.

We need to be extremely careful about not only the types of molecules, and duplicating exactly what goes on in the human body, but we also need to be concerned about quantities, the route of administration, and timing. It's not very complicated. Actually, the whole thing can be summed up in two words—"copy nature." If we're going to replace the body's hormones, let's use the same molecules, the same quantities, the same timing, and the same route of administration that nature uses. That is the least likely to get use all into trouble.

David: What are some of the symptoms of low testosterone in men?

Dr. Wright: It's debatable, but, for example, when testosterone starts to drop, ordinarily if an aging man is exercising regularly, and trying to keep up a certain muscle mass, he'll notice that it's more difficult to maintain that muscle mass. And we've all heard of 'grumpy grampa.' Well, for some men, particularly in their seventies and eighties, some of the just general grumpy mood can actually be attributed to testosterone being lower than it should be. I've talked with a number of families who say, oh yeah, Grampa's a lot more cheerful, and he's cracking more jokes, ever since he got his testosterone level back up. So that's one of the mental symptoms, and there are physical ones, such as muscle mass problems. Certainly all men, or at least nearly all men, are concerned about their declining libido and sexual performance as they age, and they have problems that could have to do with low testosterone levels. That's not always due to low testosterone, but if we combine several things—such as mental decline, a loss in muscle mass, and a loss in sexual desire and performance—and the more of those things we put together, the more likely it is that it's going have to do with lower than desirable testosterone levels.

David: What recommendations would you make for an aging male to raise his declining testosterone levels?

Dr. Wright: That's somewhat age-dependent, although one can run into that, certainly, as young as one's forties. If one is in one's forties with that, sometimes the problem can be solved by making a reformation in the diet, getting some exercise going, using nutritional supplements in addition to an excellent diet, and bringing in some botanicals. Sometimes a man can bring his own testosterone—internally produced—back up, and it's always preferable to get our own bodies to do that. But let's say we've tried that, or let's say we are at an age where that's not going to work, and then we would use testosterone as a supplement, and bring the testosterone levels back up. I call the supplement a replacement, only because we always have a little testosterone in us. But if it's below the critical amount, we'll bring the testosterone levels back up to—well, you've heard of the Jack Benny theory of medicine, have you not?

David: The Jack Benny Theory? No.

Dr. Wright: When Jack Benny was in his sixties and seventies, he used to get on TV, and he'd do a little sketch where he'd go in to see the doctor. He'd tell the doctor about his problems, and then leaning over to pat him on the back, the doctor would say, "Oh Mr. Benny, all these problems, it's your age." Jack would stop the doctor and say, "Doctor, that's the problem, I'm only thirty-nine." And the doctor would look at him and say, "Oh Mr. Benny, you don't look thirty-nine." And he'd say, "That's the problem, doctor, I don't even look thirty-nine, and I want to be treated as if I was thirty-nine." (*Laughter*)

So one may not want to use supplements to bring his level of testosterone back up to what one might call the raging hormones that one had between the ages of eighteen to twenty-five. But shooting for Jack Benny's area of around thirty-nine or forty is something that a human body of either sex can tolerate quite nicely, and do better with than the levels that are happening as a matter of normal decline by age seventy or eighty.

David: What recommendations would you make for a post-menopausal woman to raise her estrogen and progesterone levels?

Dr. Wright: If she's gone through menopause, and there are no menstrual cycles, one needs to look at all the factors and reach a decision. Now, there are those who say that menopause is natural. So what is a natural medicine physician doing interfering with a natural process such as menopause? The answer to that is, perhaps sometimes we should and sometimes we shouldn't.

But again, to go back to the business of all the environmental changes that have put us all at a lot more risk, one of the first things we should do if we're considering replacing hormones is to ask if there are genetic risks in the family. Have there been heart attacks, strokes, cardiovascular disease? Did someone end up with dementia or Alzheimer's disease? Did they need care the last ten years of their lives when they couldn't recognize all their relatives? That sort of thing.

If one does have those risk factors, then the consideration of supplementing the hormones might be a stronger one. Again, we're not totally replacing the hormones, because women who have gone through menopause do have some hormones. If she has none of those kinds of risk factors, and her mom lived to a robust eighty, ninety, maybe even a hundred, then perhaps she doesn't have to think about it—if, of course, her diet is optimal, her exercise pattern is good, and some dietary supplements are taken.

But there's one other reason why both men and women will sometimes choose to use bioidentical hormones and that is appearance. There's just very little question anymore that the use of bioidentical hormones, past the age when they decline, has a beneficial effect on appearance. With bioidentical hormones over the years—not over the days and months— women maintain a slower decline in the appearance of the skin, the appearance of the muscles, and just the appearance of the entire body. Look, we're all going to get slowly older and die someday anyway, and no one is saying that the bioidentical hormones can even come close to preventing that, but they certainly can slow the rate of decline. If we have a group of women aged seventy to eighty who've taken bioidentical hormones since menopause, and a group of women who've not, one can almost, not quite, but almost always tell the difference.

So one then needs to balance the risks and benefits, and if there's a strong family history of any of the risk factors I mentioned, we can reduce that risk and, perhaps, give "appearance points" too. If there's no family history of that at all, then do we really want to go into it just for the appearance and the antiaging properties? Now that's every woman's—and, while we're at it, every man's—own decision, because we need to look at risk factors regarding whether bioidentical hormones could somehow be involved in some cancers. We have to admit that even women twenty-five years old get cancer, and women in their thirties get cancer, so one can not say at all that bioidentical hormones are totally without risk.

Now there's a lot of debate back and forth in the medical literature (and, after reading Shakespeare, one may wonder why medical writings are called literature, but that's a parenthetical remark) about whether, for example, estrogen in itself triggers the cancer, or whether something else triggers the cancer and then estrogen makes it grow faster. The same thing goes for testosterone, although the case is a little stronger there. It appears that testosterone likely doesn't cause cancer, but if something else triggers it, it sure as hell can make it grow. So that's why properly done replacement by bioidentical hormones is so important. We need to as closely as we can mimic the patterns of a young healthy woman with young healthy hormones.

If I could, for a moment, mention that there are certain estrogens and estrogen metabolites that are known to be slightly pro-carcinogenic, and there are certain others that are known to be anti-carcinogenic, or at least neutral. And in a young healthy woman's body there will be a good balance of those. There will be more of the 2-hydroxyestrogen and the 16-hydroxyestrogen, and more estriol—by far—than the combination of estrone and estradiol. And if we mimic that young healthy pattern as closely we can with the estrogens, and bring in—just as a young healthy woman's body does—some progesterone, DHEA, testosterone, thyroid, and melatonin, we're least likely to run into complications with hormone therapies. It's never ever the supplementation of just one hormone; it's always a concert of hormones working together.

This requires working with a doctor who is really skilled and knowledgeable in how to do all of them. After they've started on hormone therapy, the physician will help the individual carefully measure what's happening, readjust the levels if they need readjustment, and monitor from time-to-time. It's not something where a person can start in on supplementation willy-nilly at a random dose, and hope everything comes out all right. It won't, if we go into it that way.

David: What do you think are the primary causes of aging?

Dr. Wright: I don't think anyone has yet proven that aging isn't something that's supposed to happen. I know that's a weasely sort of answer, but I think that aging is basically something that's going to happen anyway with everyone. There are those of us who think that we can make this lifetime last forever. In addition to doing a disservice to past-life therapists—I mean, what would they do if we all lived forever? (*Laughter*)—I just don't think it is part of the natural universe that anyone is going to last forever. So part of it, I think, is just programmed right into our cells and genes, but it certainly can be accelerated. Now, if we reframed the question to ask, what do I think is the primary cause of the acceleration of aging? Oh, there are many of those.

Even mainstream medicine has started in small corners to beat the drums about one of them—the consumption of refined sugar and refined carbohydrates. *Scientific American* and other publications have published articles written about what they call "advanced glycosylation end-products"—abbreviated cleverly as AGEs. Refined sugar and refined carbohydrates are things that have never ever been part of the human diet before. Perhaps Henry the VIII, who had his little bit of sugar which actually was more costly than gold at the time, or the ancient Egyptians, who also used refined sugar, were among the first. But we don't find it anywhere else for several hundred thousand years. That's just one change, which looks like it's always been with us.

AGEs really stiffen tissues. They stiffen arteries and lead to a constellation of end products that are mostly stiffening. They just make everything go down hill faster. So we can improve that right away, but that's just one island in a whole sea of things that can accelerate one's aging. There are all the chemicals in the environment—for gosh sakes—some of which interfere with mitochondrial function. We all know that mitochondria are the so-called energy engines in cells, and if we interfere with its production of energy then cells are going to age more rapidly. It's very fortunate that research scientists are putting their fingers on more and more of these chemicals that mess up, not only mitochondrial function, but other cell functions.

So, again, it looks like what accelerates the aging process is a lot of the environmental changes that have come on with food refining, industrialization, lack of exercise—all the same things that I think I've been pointing to in a long-winded fashion since the beginning of this interview.

David: Hormone replacement therapy aside, what do you think are the most important nutritional supplements that one should be taking for optimum health?

Dr. Wright: We always have to start with Irwin Stone, Linus Pauling, and vitamin C. It might seem very mundane to be talking about vitamin C as one of the most important nutritional supplements, but if we go to any standard textbooks on genetics or pediatrics they'll tell us that scurvy is a genetic disease. Okay, so what are the implications of that? Having a genetic disease means that there's something missing in the DNA that codes for a certain enzyme that would actually get our own bodies to produce vitamin C—just as dogs, cats, elephants, goldfish, and most other species do naturally. The only species that don't produce their own vitamin C are some primates, guinea pigs, and a few other species. There aren't very many.

Other species produce the vitamin C that's in their bodies. Now, what's been shown—incontrovertibly, by lots and lots of research—is that species tend to produce more of their own vitamin C when they're under any kind of stress. For example, when dogs are given carcinogens their livers produce anywhere from ten to twenty times the vitamin C that they normally produce, until that carcinogen is detoxified with the aid of vitamin C. If you put rats in cages, and force them to run round and round and round, their internal vitamin C production goes up. If you cold water shock experimental animals their vitamin C production goes up. Just about anything that puts stress on the body of an animal—whether it's chemical or emotional—causes the production of vitamin C to go way up. One can actually prove by chemical analysis that when humans are faced with those kinds of stresses their livers attempt to make more vitamin C, but they can't because of the genetic disease.

vitamin C is a universal aid to detoxification. That's why it applies to so many things. Linus Pauling said that we should be at the bowel tolerance intake of vitamin C, but this varies. Is it two grams a day or ten grams a day? Sometimes we need to take more for a few weeks when we're under greater than normal levels of stress. Whatever that bowel tolerance normally is, we should use that much vitamin C at minimum of two intervals during the day. The way vitamin C kinetics is, it should really be three times a day if we can. This way we're going to be maintaining our maximum detoxification vigilance.

I recall a moderately obscure study done at one of the universities in Southern California that claimed that women who used as little as one gram of vitamin C per day could expect added longevity of five years. No kidding. And men who used one gram a day—and that's no where near bowel tolerance—could expect the added longevity of one year. I guess that just allows us guys to catch up with the women. So vitamin C is right at the basis, because it's actually there to correct a genetic disease problem that all human beings suffer from. We just need to take more of it to stay healthy. So I would ask people to start with that particular supplement.

So far as the other supplements go, probably a very well balanced vitamin E comes next. There's been a lot of recent bad press on vitamin E—as we all know—and it was bad press in all senses of the term. The studies addressed something that needed to be criticized, but the press was usually bad criticism. The studies looked at the effects of dl-alpha-tocopherol, which is halfway synthetic, or other incomplete forms of vitamin E. Students of vitamin E point out that there are eight isomers known to be useful and effective as vitamin E—the alpha, beta, delta, and gamma tocopherols and tocotrienols. So, one does need to balance all eight of those isomers if one is going to do a natural vitamin E.

vitamin E, in its fat soluble phase, is as important to the body as an antioxidant as vitamin C is in its water soluble phase. Even though there are certainly antioxidants that are "more potent," there are none that are as important to be widespread around the body as appropriate amounts of vitamins C and E. Now, we've heard that for years. Take your multiple vitamin, and vitamins C and E. But it happens to be true, even for longevity reasons, to get that bowel tolerance vitamin C in there, and the eight isomers of vitamin E in a sufficient quantity. Then, perhaps, one can go on from there to some of the more trendy things in anti-aging.

One of the real important ones is adequate amounts of vitamin D. This has come roaring to the forefront in just the last five to ten years. The university research scientists who have been studying vitamin D—such as Dr. Michael Holick at Boston University and Dr. William Grant in Southern California—have been pointing out that we all would be healthier if we had blood levels of vitamin D that would be achieved if we lived in the tropics. That is, if we got out in the sunshine and didn't burn ourselves to death, but at least got a good tan if we're Caucasian. Those levels of vitamin D can keep us a lot healthier and cut the risk of a whole bunch of cancers, as well as autoimmune disease. That evidence seems to be incontrovertible, and yet mainstream medicine is still telling us to slather ourselves with sun block to the point where our bodies make so little vitamin D from sunshine that we actually put ourselves at risk for more cancers.

So I recommend some real basic adequate vitamin D. I happen to live in the Seattle area, and reaching optimal blood levels of vitamin D from sunshine can be difficult from time to time. Sometimes people do well, and sometimes their levels are low, but they're never in the optimal area without supplements. It's been pointed out that the amount of vitamin D that's optimal for adults appears to be three to four thousand units a day. This not only appears to be so, but I think it's a well established way to prevent a significant portion of prostate and breast cancers for men and for women.

I know I'm really covering basics, but let me do one more, enough to make it through the fatty acids. I'm just amazed at how many folks who think they're on good diets actually don't have enough omega-3 fatty acids in there to act as an overall anti-inflammatory agent. We all know that the omega-3s, combined with vitamin E, are going to quench inflammations all over the body. And I'm not just talking about eating fish, and perhaps taking one's tablespoon of cod liver oil, although that's really a good idea. I'm also talking about the whole free-range cattle movement—free-range chickens, free-range beef, free-range whatever—if we eat animal protein. There are at least a few preliminary studies that have shown that free-range animals have a much better ratio of omega-3 fatty acids to omega-6 fatty acids then do grain-fed animals. Those who do eat meat, if they can, should start switching over to eating the free-range animals. The same thing goes for such things as eggs; when the hens are free-range there are more omega-3 fatty acids in the egg.

All right, so we have the omega-3 fatty acids, vitamins C, D, and E—the basic alphabet, but also some very basic longevity-promoting nutrients. Then after that we could go on to such things as acetyl-L-carnitine and alpha-lipoic acid. Acetyl-L-carnitine and lipoic acid are both endogenous (naturally present in the body) antioxidants that have been shown to restore mitochondrial function and reduce free radical damage. Dr. Bruce Ames has shown that when alpha-lipoic acid extends mitochondrial life, it also helps to revive rats that are getting senile—

and chances are it does that for humans too.

David: What recommendations would you suggest for people who want to improve their sex drive and sexual performance?

Dr. Wright: Believe it or not, humans have not been eating most of the agricultural products that we eat today for the last hundred or two hundred thousand years. I'd refer people to a couple of books on this. One of them is called *The Paleo Diet* by Dr. Cordain from the University of Colorado, and the other one, written almost twenty years earlier, is called The *Paleolithic Prescription* by S. Boyd Eaton and others at Emory University. Those two books make it fairly abundantly clear that most of our biochemical systems—I wouldn't say everyone—but most of our biochemical systems are still adapted to the type of diet that we had as hunter-gatherers.

Now, when I say adapted, I don't want to leave out the Creationists—maybe we were created this way. But most of our biochemical systems are still adapted and/or created to the type of diet that humans have been accustomed to on this particular planet for at least two hundred thousand years as a species that is exactly the same as ours, and millions of years for other species that are very similar to us. Now, this would be diets that do not happen to have any milk and dairy in them—yeah, I'm really talking about sex life folks (*laughter*)—and they have more in the way of animal protein. There are a lot of studies out there that show that vegetarian men and women have lower levels of sex hormones. And that's not at all to disrespect an ethical vegetarian choice—it's just being realistic about it. Animal protein diets are always associated with higher sex hormones and vegetarians with lower ones. These are just the facts. One can make up one's mind about it.

But getting back to that more or less caveman diet approach—that actually does help raise sex hormones if you're older. All right, then we can bring in our basic vitamin supplements and some of herbals that have been used around the world. Different continents seem to favor different ones that help with sex drive. There is a tradition of using ginseng from China. There's yohimbe from Africa, ashwagandha from India, and maca from South America. So, one can either use one of those supplements, or others that our ancestors found useful for that, for literally thousands of years. Or one can use some of the combinations on the market. Some of the marketers have combined many of those things into one supplement, which does make it easier to use. But other marketers have pointed out that you don't get as much of each herb in one supplement. They say that in China people use more ginseng than is ever in these supplements. In India, they use more ashwagandha, and in Peru they use more maca, and so forth. But those traditional things, when studied scientifically, do turn out to have anywhere from small to intermediate effects.

Just for example, a British researcher actually paid some research volunteers who had inordinate vaginal dryness to have biopsies done. He looked under the microscope, and sure enough the cells had atrophied. But in the study he did not have the volunteers take hormones—he had them all take ginseng. And a few months later—I guess they were well-paid volunteers—they all had biopsies done again. He looked under the microscope, and, well, look at that—the cells were not atrophied anymore. In fact, it looked like someone had fed them estrogen, but nobody fed them estrogen, and they could not find that they'd taken any. But it had that effect. So what I'm saying is that these traditional things from the various continents of the planet are indeed very useful. One can bring those in to improve performance before we even think about replacing, or rather, supplementing hormones. It's not really a replacement because they're not totally missing.

David: What do you think are some of the biggest problems with the way that medicine is practiced today, and what do you think can be done to help improve the situation?

Dr. Wright: With your permission, I'll take that in two parts. First, I'm going to be a little bit hard on myself and my natural and alternative medicine colleagues in the area of hormone replacement. Hormone replacement is being done very erratically, and by all kinds of different means that are going to get us into trouble, give the whole field a very bad name, and just possibly bring on some of the unconstitutional governmental retributions that happen when things go wrong. Even though the retributions are unconstitutional, they happen anyway.

Let's take the book out there called *The Sexy Years* by Suzanne Summers.

The tremendous service this book has done us all is to bring bioidentical hormones to the attention of millions of people. The disservice that Ms. Summers does in her book is she says that she's taking two milligrams of estradiol every single day. Now, the laboratory that I work with has done studies of some thirty-five women doing doses of estradiol, ranging all the way from .025 up through .25, .50, 1.0, and up to 2.0 milligrams of estradiol each day. But the dosages in this study were not deliberate. All thirty-five women had different doses because they came in from doctors who were giving them different dosages, so we know it's very disparate out there. And what we found is that women who take more than .25 milligrams of estradiol have excessively high levels of estrone, because estradiol metabolizes into estrone. They have levels of estrone that are equal to the levels that one would find in the third or forth month of pregnancy, which are well above the levels of estrone that a nineteen year old women would be putting out, never mind a thirty-nine year old women.

The rhetorical question in here is: Can it be healthy for Ms. Summers or anyone else taking a larger than "natural" dose of estradiol? She's writing about it in her book, and perhaps some misguided natural medicine doctors will be following that lead. Can it be healthy to be going around with a level of a procarcinogenic estrogen that is higher than any young woman would have in her body during the normal course of her menstrual cycle, and is only achieved for a brief period of time during pregnancy? That's a rhetorical question because obviously that's an unhealthy thing to do, and yet we haven't gotten to any kind of consensus on even doses of these things in the identical hormone replacement field, and many women are being way overdosed.

The same thing goes for DHEA. We see some horrendously high levels of DHEA, and it's metabolized in men who either self-dosed, or were advised by their doctors to be on very high doses because the doctors are only following their blood levels, and one can't find the metabolites in the blood. So this bit of venting criticism here is an introduction to say that we have organized something that's called the Bioidentical Hormone Society. We've had one meeting, and we're going to be holding future meetings. The goal of the organization is to get information out about bioidentical hormones and how people working with them can use them safely. The Website address is: www.bioidenticalhormonesociety.com.

The Web site has the graphics showing the different doses of estradiol and what it does in so far as producing levels of other hormones. You can measure all of this, and make sure it's within safe levels for all of the presently "replaced" hormones. What we hope to achieve through these Bioidentical Hormone Society meetings is to have people pick up on the information, get organized and copy nature. We're getting back to those two fundamental words: copy nature.

Here's another very simple principle that applies to folks with falling estrogen or falling testosterone. Excuse me, but no one has their ovaries or testicles stitched to the inside of their intestines, do they? And yet if we swallow those hormones, what we're doing is we're assuming somehow that those hormones enter the body through the gut. Now, that's an entirely different route of administration than what they really do. When we swallow them they go for the gut, they zing right to the liver, and the liver gets whacked with them. It's been shown, for example, that even when one of the safer estrogens, called estriol, is swallowed, metabolized, and then endometrial biopsies are done, sometimes there are abnormalities that show up. But when it's used in a cream or an ointment that's rubbed into the vaginal area, which is close to where estrogen is delivered in the body by the ovaries, and then endometrial biopsies are done, no abnormalities show up.

When it's taken in the cream that way it's close to where estrogen is delivered in the body by the ovaries. From the ovaries it goes into the pelvic plexus of veins, then all over the body, and, finally, to the liver, where it's taken in. So it's not just dose. It's not just timing. It's also the route of administration. Everything we need to do can be summed up in these two words: copy nature. And only when someone does several double-blind, placebo-controlled, crossover studies that demonstrate that nature is wrong—and you can tell I'm doubtful that will ever happen—should we deviate from what nature does. That's more or less the message that the Bioidentical Hormone Society is to trying to get out.

Now, so far as medicine in general goes, our very biggest mistake has been a century-long mistake. It started in the early part of the twentieth century, and it continues to this day—and that is, relying on patent medicines to heal the body. This has been an enormous mistake, because the condition necessary to patent anything says that it can not occur in nature. But our bodies are made of materials that are entirely natural—a big bunch of water, protein, vitamins, minerals, hormones, essential fatty acids, amino acids, and other things. And then we have adapted to the botanical world. So plant material can certainly cause harm, but not near as much as patent medicines. Patent medicines—by definition— have to be not natural, and if they're not natural then, in a manner of speaking, they're space aliens! (*Laughter*) They're molecules that have never been found on the planet before. Now, what do we think we're doing trying to heal a body that was created or evolved on this planet with space alien molecules?

It's not going to work. The best it's going to do is suppress symptoms, and yet the medical profession has gone along with this for over a century. We do ninety percent of our studies on space alien molecules, the little bit of benefit that they have, and the enormous harm they can cause. And one after another we have to shut them down because they're doing too much harm. Then we go on to the next space alien molecule. One of these days the medical profession is going to wake up and notice that even though we have made enormous progress in diagnostics, diagnostic imaging, in surgeries, and so forth, when it comes to things that we swallow or apply to the body, we're using molecules that have nothing to do with the body that we're treating, and this has caused so many problems. When medicine gets away from that, when it stops putting space alien molecules in the body, and starts using materials that are natural to the body, then there is really going to be a revolution in medicine at that point.

Now, the people who do that are called alternative doctors, but in the early part of the Twentieth Century conventional physicians were using natural material for natural bodies, and we've only been on this detour into space alien molecules for a century. None of our ancestors did that. They applied natural stuff to natural bodies. And with all the science that we have, if we turned our sights to the study of how natural molecules interact with natural molecular structures that are made by our own bodies, we would make some enormous advances, in a hell of a hurry, but we haven't got there yet.

David: What are you currently working on?

Dr. Wright: As you can tell, I'm working on getting the Bioidentical Hormone Society up and running. I'm teaching courses. Dr. Leonard and I are working on an update of our 1997 *Natural Hormone Replacement for Women Over 45*, and that update should be out by the end of the year, or the very beginning of next year. That actually was the first book in the field of bioidentical hormone replacement, and it certainly deserves an update, as there's been enough new information published. So that's one of the main things that I'm working on. I also do a newsletter every month, and that occupies a lot of my time.

David: Is there anything we haven't spoken about that you would like to add?

Dr. Wright: You probably have any number of examples to demonstrate where we can use something natural and replace a whole category of medications, and we're not doing it, but let me just give you one. Something that I worked on for a number of years was the use of D-Mannose for treating urinary tract infections. There are literally millions of folks who end up with bladder infections every year. Most of them are women, but a few are men. Ninety percent of those infections are due to E. coli, and ten percent are due to miscellaneous other factors.

So what does modern medicine—or rather mainstream medicine—do? They use antibiotics and it kills the germ, but, as we all know, it also interferes with gut flora. It kills that normal flora in the gut too. Now we know that the continual interaction between bowel flora and the immune system is one of the things that keeps it strong, and we're giving people literally billions of dollars worth of antibiotics to clear up urinary tract infections that just keep coming back. Well, there is a simple natural substance that will do the job on urinary tract infections ninety percent of the time with absolutely zero effects—and it's a hell of a lot cheaper too.

The stuff is a simple sugar called D-Mannose. D-Mannose is, in fact, produced in the human body in small quantities. There's D-Mannose here and there, and importantly there are D-Mannose residues in the cells that line the bladder. The residues are in the cell walls of those cells that line the inside of the bladder, and that's how E. coli actually is able to do so much infecting. E. coli has the capability to hook inside of the bladder, onto these Mannose molecules, and that's the reason that it isn't rinsed out every time you urinate. It has all these little finger-like projections that attach on to the D-Mannose residues like Spiderman. This allows the E. coli to climb up the walls of the bladder like Spiderman does, where they then set up a happy home and make an infection.

Well, somebody got the bright idea that if E. coli like D-Mannose so much, let's see what happens if we give it to them. So back in the '80s I started working with patients with bladder infections, having them take D-Mannose. For adults the dose was a teaspoon of the powder, and for children less, every three to four hours. Now, what happens is this. Here's the E. coli inhabiting the bladder, hanging on to those D-Mannose residues in the bladder wall. Then instead, here come these great clouds of D-Mannose through the uritors because D-Mannose is not well absorbed. Our bodies don't metabolize much of a dose like that because our bodies don't use very much, so the kidneys just throw it out. Then out it goes, through the kidneys, into the ureters, and then the bladder. So here's the E. coli inhabiting the bladder, hanging on to those D-Mannose residues in the bladder wall. Then here come these great clouds of D-Mannose, and for the E. coli, basically, it's party time because they love D-Mannose. So they literally detach themselves from this D-Mannose residue in the bladder wall, and they surround themselves with clouds of D-Mannose.

So they're happy, and we're happy. Now that they have detached themselves from the walls of the bladder, and they're just swimming in all that fun D-Mannose that they love so much, the next few times we urinate, there goes all the E. coli, and there goes the infection. It works like a charm ninety percent of the time. And all we have to do is take D-Mannose regularly for a couple of days, while we're awake. We don't even have to wake up and take it because of course no urine is leaving the bladder, so it stays full of D-Mannose.

The first case I worked with was a four or five year old child who had a long series of urinary tract infections. She had become resistant or allergic to all kinds of antibiotics, and her parents were being told that she was going to need a kidney transplant by the time she was seven or eight because her kidneys were starting to go. Then they came in to see me. I wasn't so smart; I just knew about D-Mannose dynamics. So I asked Mom if she knew what kind of bladder infections her child had had, and she says, well yes, I have this record book. And, my God, she had two scrap books of every single test her child had ever had, and they were all E. coli infections.

So I told Mom that there's a good chance that we could get rid of this whole problem within a few days. Well, Dad just about walked out of the office. He thought I was some kind of quack, but he asked me, "Can it hurt anything?" and I said "No it can't." So they put her on the D-Mannose, and her bladder infections cleared up. She didn't have another one for four years, when the family was on vacation and they forgot their D-Mannose. She kept taking it until she was a teenager. Then her estrogen came on, which protected her bladder, and she didn't need it anymore. So there are now two or three companies that sell D-Mannose in jars that you can find in any natural food store, and as long as you keep that handy then you have a ninety percent chance of not having to take an antibiotic for your bladder infection. I tell all the people that I treat with bladder infections to give it a day or two, and if your bladder infection isn't gone then you're going to need an antibiotic.

D-Mannose is inexpensive. It doesn't do bad things to the body when it's used that way. It cures the problem. The mechanism of action is known. That's the kind of treatment that we need to be replacing the patent medicines with—things that can be researched out, and they have an effect that's beneficial for us. But also, one might call it an ecological effect if one is into deep ecology, because we make the bacteria happy. Now, if we make the bacteria happy then they just go off and share all their D-Mannose with the other bacteria, and they talk about how nicely they were treated. And if we treat bacteria nicely they don't develop antibiotic or drug resistance do they? Because any life form, if we try to kill it, is going to resist, and that's what happens with bacterial resistance to antibiotics. So that's really the kind of therapeutics we should be looking forward to.

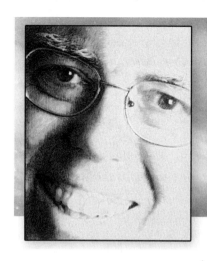

DINING IN THE ZONE

An Interview with Dr. Barry Sears

Barry Sears, Ph.D., is one of the world's leading medical researchers on the hormonal effects of food. He is best known as the author of the number one New York Times *bestseller* The Zone, *which outlines his strategy for controlling insulin levels in the body through diet.*

Dr. Sears developed the Zone diet as a way to keep the body from producing excess insulin. The Zone diet does this by providing a proper balance of protein, carbohydrates, and fats at each meal, and also with supplements of high-dose pharmaceutical grade fish oil. The consumption of carbohydrates such as pasta and bread can cause a sharp spike in insulin production, and if this happens chronically we start to gain weight. This leads to insulin resistance and eventually results in a dangerous condition known as "silent inflammation." Researchers are discovering that silent inflammation is at the root of many major illnesses, such as heart disease, cancer, and Alzheimer's disease. This is why Dr. Sears believes that we should treat our food like drugs.

In addition to The Zone, *Dr. Sears has written nine other books on the Zone diet, including* Mastering the Zone, The Age-Free Zone, The Soy Zone, The Omega Rx Zone, Zone Meals in Seconds, *and* What to Eat in the Zone. *His books have sold more than five million copies and have been*

*translated into twenty-two languages in forty countries. He
continues his research on the inflammatory process as the
president of the nonprofit Inflammation Research Foundation
in Marblehead, Massachusetts.*

*I interviewed Dr. Sears on March 7, 2005. Dr. Sears has a
talent for making complex explanations seem simple and he
speaks with great clarity and precision. We spoke about the
dangers of silent inflammation, the role that eicosanoids play
in our body, the benefits of high-dose pharmaceutical grade
fish oil, and how the Zone diet can lower insulin levels and
dramatically improve one's health.*

David: What originally inspired your interest in diet and nutrition?

Dr. Sears: My interest stems from wanting to avoid an early cardiovascular
death, because everyone on the male side of my family—starting with
my grandfather, my father and his brothers—all died in their early fifties
of heart disease. So I realized about thirty years ago that I had the same
genes, but I had the opportunity to change the expression of those genes.
So this started me on a search to answer the question: What would be the
most appropriate format for reducing the likelihood of premature heart
disease? My background at the time was in drug delivery systems. I
was doing work on intravenous drug delivery systems for cancer drugs,
and then I realized that one could apply the same principals of drug
delivery to food, in order to keep the hormones generated by food within
therapeutic zones—not too high and not too low. So I really shifted my
interest from looking at drug delivery systems to looking at food as a
drug and as a modulator of hormones.

*David: What are some of the dangers of silent inflammation, and how
can people tell if they have a problem with silent inflammation?*

Dr. Sears: One of the problems with silent inflammation is that it's silent.
That's why no one knew much about it for so long. People can't feel it
and we had no clinical test for detecting it. Now that we can look for
silent inflammation in the blood, we find it's everywhere, and it seems
to be the underlying cause of a great number of chronic disease states—

whether it be heart disease, cancer, or Alzheimer's disease. So until we had a way of testing, it we had no way of looking at how to combat it. Now that we can test it, we find the most effective way of reducing silent inflammation is—and this has all been clinically demonstrated—by paying attention to the food that you eat. With the right diet—which is really an anti-inflammatory diet—you could reduce silent inflammation in your body within thirty days.

David: Why is reducing insulin levels so important for reversing silent inflammation, and why do you think that we should think of the food we eat as powerful drugs?

Dr. Sears: Insulin affects a great number of things in the body. Obviously it compounds the storage of sugar, but also the storage of fat. That's why it's excess insulin that makes you fat and keeps you fat. But what people don't realize is insulin can also stimulate the enzymes that make the building blocks of inflammatory eicosanoids. That really became the smoking gun that links obesity to so many chronic disease states—because the more obese you are, the more insulin you're making. And the more insulin you're making, the more inflammation you're generating. So with that linkage we can now say, okay, let's find a way to reduce the levels of insulin, and reduce the levels of the inflammatory eicosanoids that insulin can help generate, to keep one managed in a therapeutic zone. That's why food becomes so powerful, because food effects hormones and hormones are hundreds of times more powerful than any drug. This means that food is probably the most powerful drug you'll ever encounter, but the door could swing both ways. Food can be your greatest ally, or your worst hormonal enemy.

David: Can you talk a little about how the Zone diet can help people reduce insulin levels and control inflammation?

Dr. Sears: The Zone diet is really composed of two parts. One part is for controlling insulin, simply by getting a better balance of protein to carbohydrate on one's plate. And actually this is quite simple—because all you need is one hand and one eye. Here are all the rules you need to know in order to control insulin on a lifetime basis. At each meal divide your plate into three equal sections. On one third of the plate you put some low-fat protein that is no bigger or thicker than the palm of your hand. The other two thirds of the plate you fill until it's overflowing with fruits and vegetables. Then you add a dash of monounsaturated fat, which could be olive oil, sliver almonds, or guacamole. Now what you've done is constructed a very tasty drug that will control insulin for the next four to six hours. The other part of the Zone diet is taking adequate levels of ultra-refined EPA/DHA concentrates [pharmaceutical grade fish oil], because it is fish oil that contains the long-chain omega-3 fatty acids, which at high enough levels have profound anti-inflammatory effects. Combine the two, and you have a powerful one-two punch to control silent inflammation on a lifetime basis.

David: How is the Zone diet similar to a Paleolithic diet?

Dr. Sears: It's similar in that 10,000 years ago there were no grains on the face of the Earth. So let's go back to our example plate. There's plenty of low-fat protein, therefore you'd never use excessive amounts, and the only carbohydrates man was exposed to (and that we are genetically designed to eat) were really fruits and non-starchy vegetables, because they have a low glycemic load. So in many ways the Zone diet is basically going back and making a diet for the Twenty-first Century that is compatible with our genes that still live in the Stone Age.

David: Could you clarify what you mean when you say that "10,000 years ago there were no grains on the face of the Earth"?

Dr. Sears: There was no agricultural development 10,000 years ago so that there was no easy access to grains as a major dietary component.

David: You say that the Zone diet is similar to the Paleolithic diet, and that "our genes still live in the Stone Age." Does that mean that our ancestors always ate meals that had the precise portions of protein, carbohydrates, and fats that you recommend for each meal?

Dr. Sears: The genetic propensity that we have for fat storage was a valuable survival mechanism in the past. Now it has become a genetic liability. To overcome the genetic component we have to control the balance of protein, carbohydrate, and fat the best we can at every meal.

David: How have the studies done on caloric restriction influenced your development of the Zone diet?

Dr. Sears: The only proven technology "to slow down the aging process" has been reducing calories. So people say, well yeah, but who wants to be hungry and deprived the rest of their life? I know I don't. So what you're looking at in terms of the Zone diet is a calorie restricted diet—but yet one without hunger, and one without deprivation. One of the little known, or little appreciated facts of the Zone diet is that it's not about how many calories you eat, it's how much energy you produce, that is ATP [adenosine triphosphate, the body's primary energy molecule]. So this is why you can basically reduce the number of calories in the Zone diet and still have high levels of physical and mental energy, because you're now making larger amounts of ATP with a lesser number of calories. So now you have anti-aging the easy way—basically eating great meals, but you're restricting calories without hunger and without deprivation.

David: You mentioned eicosanoids earlier. Can you talk a little about the role that eicosanoids play in our body and how our diet and insulin levels effect them?

Dr. Sears: Eicosanoids are really your master hormones. They control inflammation, but they also control so much more. They virtually control the release and synthesis of all other hormones. So, in many ways, they're kind of the "Intel computer chip" that runs our body, and yet because of these eicosanoids, every aspect of our physiology is under very profound dietary control. With our diet we control the balance of pro-inflammatory and anti-inflammatory eicosanoids, and the better we maintain that balance the more well we become. Conversely, the more we let that balance get out of whack, making more pro-inflammatory eicosanoids, the more rapidly we move toward chronic disease.

David: You say that "Eicosanoids are really your master hormones." While it's clear that eicosanoids are very important, it's not clear why they are "your master hormones." What makes them more important than, say, pregnenolone or DHEA?

Dr. Sears: Eicosanoids were the first hormones developed by living organisms. They control all other hormones because of their impact on cyclic AMP levels in individual cells that ultimately control the release or synthesis of other hormones.

David: I have a master's degree in psychobiology, and I never learned anything about eicosanoids in my endocrinology classes.

Dr. Sears: When I first wrote the book there were probably five people in the country who could pronounce the word. (*Laughter*) There are many more now, but still it's a very arcane part of endocrinology.

David: You mentioned earlier that taking high-dose ultra-refined EPA/ DHA concentrates [pharmaceutical grade fish oil] is part of the Zone diet. Can you talk a little about the specific benefits of taking fish oil?

Dr. Sears: The primary benefits are the long-chain fatty acids—such as EPA and DHA—which, at high enough levels, have these profound anti-inflammatory effects. By taking these fatty acids we can attack the problem by doing what's referred to in pharmacology as "going upstream." See, most drug companies develop drugs that go "downstream." That is, they try to inhibit the enzymes that make the pro-inflammatory eicosanoids, yet all those pro-inflammatory eicosanoids are derived from arachidonic acid. So the opposite way is to go "upstream," and simply decrease the production of arachidonic acid. It's a much more elegant, much more sophisticated approach, and that's what the Zone diet does. It uses diet and the fish oil to reduce the levels of arachidonic acid, and by doing, so you choke off the substrates to making excessive amounts of pro-inflammatory eicosanoids.

David: How does one know if the fish oil that they are taking is pharmaceutical grade or not?

Dr. Sears: It's hard unless you have a half million dollars of instrumentation in your kitchen, which most people don't. But here's an easy first test. Take your fish oil home, and if it's in capsules, break open the capsules and pour the contents into a small shot glass. Now put that in the freezer and come back five hours later with a toothpick. If the fish oil is rock solid, you can probably believe that the fish oil is the sewer of the sea. On the other hand, if you can put the toothpick through it, and it's either mushy or liquid, then it's probably the good stuff.

David: Why do you recommend that people take fish oil and not hemp seed oil—which contains omega-3 and omega-6 fatty acids in a 4:1 ratio?

Dr. Sears: Hemp seed oil contains short-chain omega-3 fatty acids, and alpha-linolenic acid. Alpha-linolenic acid is very inefficiently converted to the long-chain omega-3 fatty acids that do all the work in controlling inflammation. So if you're willing to basically take fifty to a hundred times the volume of hemp seed oil, you might get the same effect as a much smaller volume of fish oil.

David: Why is it dangerous to have chronically elevated cortisol levels and what can people do to prevent their bodies from producing too much cortisol?

Dr. Sears: The trouble with excess cortisol is that three things can happen. It makes you fatter, because it increases insulin resistance. It makes you dumber because it destroys the nerve cells in the hippocampus, where all your memories are stored. And three, it makes you sicker because it turns off the immune system. So these are three pretty good reasons why you want to control excess levels of cortisol.

Now, how do you go about doing that? The easiest way is to take adequate levels of fish oil, because by reducing inflammation in the body you're reducing the need for the body to secrete more cortisol to keep it under control. The second way to keep cortisol under control is to control blood-sugar levels. If blood-sugar levels drop too low, the brain will send out signals to make more cortisol to break down muscle mass and convert it into glucose. And the third way is an old time-tested way. It's called meditation. You take some time to stop and smell the roses.

So, again, like with insulin and the pro-inflammatory eicosanoids, it's better if you're not increasing those hormones. It's better to actually be decreasing those hormones, and bringing them back into an appropriate zone that's consistent with long term wellness.

David: You say that one can reduce cortisol levels with fish oil. Are there any studies which demonstrate this?

Dr. Sears: In patients with cachexia it is known that fish oil reduces cortisol levels (*Nutrition and Cancer* 40: 118 (2001) and in normal subjects undergoing mental stress (*Diabetes Metabolism* 29: 289 (2003).

David: How does exercise help to lower inflammation in the body?

Dr. Sears: Exercise helps lower inflammation by actually lowering insulin. As I said earlier, it's excess insulin that stimulates that enzyme to make arachidonic acid, the building block of these inflammatory eicosanoids. So by lowering insulin through exercise you're taking another step toward reducing the overall inflammatory load on the body.

David: Why do you think that taking mega-doses of antioxidants may suppress the immune system?

Dr Sears: Because we have to have some bad eicosanoids, otherwise we'd die, and to make eicosanoids—both good and bad—you need a certain amount of free radicals. When you take very high levels of antioxidants the free radicals necessary to form eicosanoids get inhibited, and this puts the body at great risk in terms of its ability to fight off bacterial infections, or to inhibit the process needed to repair injuries.

David: What do you think are the primary causes of aging?

Dr. Sears: I think the primary cause of aging is basically the increased inflammatory burden, and therefore if we really want to talk about anti-aging medicine, we should talk about anti-inflammatory medicine. But if I use the words "anti-aging medicine" I'd be laughed at if I went to Harvard Medical School. However, if I use the term "anti-inflammatory medicine" they welcome me with open arms. I'm talking about exactly the same thing, but again, this demonstrates the power of words to convey certain messages.

David: So do you think that the Zone diet actually reverses or slows down the aging process?

Dr. Sears: Definitely, because we know the Zone diet is a calorie-restricted diet, which we know does slow down the aging process. We know the Zone diet is an anti-inflammatory diet, which also slows down the aging process.

David: You say that aging is caused by an "increased inflammatory burden," that can be alleviated by the Zone diet. Does this mean that our Paleolithic ancestors, who ate the type of diet that you recommend, didn't age?

Dr. Sears: Aging can be defined as the cause of mortality. Today, the cause of mortality is primary chronic disease conditions accelerated by inflammation (i.e. CHD), whereas 10,000 years ago the primary cause of mortality was famine or injury.

David: How long do you think it's possible for human life span to be extended?

Dr. Sears: I think realistically, probably to age 90. For right now, we're at about age 78. But it's not the length of life span that's important, it's really our health-span; that is, longevity minus years of disability. And here our track record is not quite as good. So I think that when we ask what we really want, the answer is basically to live a full life—a life with as little pain as possible, with maximum wellness, and to die when our time comes. The fact is we're all going to die. I'm just saying that we want to die on our terms, and basically in a state of relative wellness. So I think that the great goal is to have the population live a life that is full of vitality and follows what is called a rectangular curve—great vitality and then you die the next day. That's really what we're looking for. To extend life span to over a hundred may not be what we want. If you've ever been to a nursing home, you say, yeah they're living to 100 and 102, but that's not the quality of life I want to go out with.

David: What are some of the new anti-aging treatments that you foresee coming along in the near future?

Dr. Sears: I only really see one: diet. But actually there are three things:

diet, exercise, and stress reduction. None of those can be put into a capsule or pill. Those three things are the verities of human wisdom, and they have to be done on a consistent daily basis to keep your hormones in the zone. That is the key to aging well.

David: A lab in Spain recently found that cannabinoids can help prevent Alzheimer's disease in mice due to their anti-inflammatory properties. What role do you think our body's own endocannabinoid system plays in maintaining health?

Dr. Sears: The endocannabinoid system is interesting because right now the hottest ticket in terms of obesity research is anti-cannabinoids— agents that block the cannabinoid receptor. The cannabinoids tend to give people the munchies. So, researchers found out that if you block that receptor you simply don't get hungry. I think that a lot of the data about what's going into the brain is very interesting. That's why if you see anti-aging reports talking about the cannabinoids being useful, remember that there's corresponding data that says anti-cannabinoids are also useful because they help basically reduce the hunger, and therefore reduce the amount of calories you consume.

David: What are you currently working on?

Dr. Sears: My focus is primarily on inflammation. Right now I'm looking into doing the clinical studies which will demonstrate that you can intervene with diet in a wide number of different disease states, and show statistically significant changes and reversals in a number of them. I've done most of the work to lay the foundation for that. Now it's time to put the money on the table and learn conclusively to what extent we can use food as a drug. This isn't to say that food will replace drugs, but rather that it can help make drugs work better—that is, at lower concentrations, and with less side effects.

David: Is there anything that we haven't spoken about that you would like to add?

Dr: Sears: One last thing is that in America we face a great day of reckoning, which is coming very quickly. That year of reckoning will be the year 2011. That is the year that the first of the Baby Boomers will be able to access Medicare, which is virtually unlimited health care. And as rich as our country is, we do not have the money to pay for the medical liabilities facing us. So we have to either hide our head in the sand like an ostrich, or face the fact that we're going to have significant restrictions and a rationing of healthcare.

But we have a way to circumvent that by treating our food like a drug. By doing this we relieve the great coming burden on our healthcare system, because now people can take responsibility for their future. Rather than waiting for some scientist in the basement of Merck, Sharp, and Dohme to make some pill to save them from themselves, the answer lies in their kitchen. So the question is: As a country, do we have the will to use the kitchen as a food pharmacy, an anti-inflammatory pharmacy, or do we want to sit back and wait for the inevitable, which is basically a complete collapse of our healthcare system? I really hope it's the former and not the later.

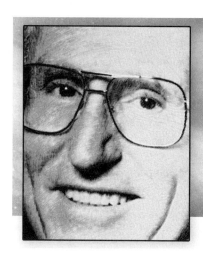

ELATION OVER CHELATION

An Interview with Dr. Garry Gordon

Garry Gordon, M.D., D.O., is one of the world's experts in chelation therapy, nutrition, and mineral metabolism. He is the founder and current president of the International College of Advanced Longevity Medicine (ICALM), and is one of the cofounders of the American College for Advancement in Medicine (ACAM). Dr. Gordon wrote the original protocol for the safe and effective use of EDTA oral chelation therapy, and is the author of numerous scientific papers on the subject. He is also the coauthor of the bestselling book The Chelation Answer.

Chelation is a chemical process in which a metal or mineral—such as lead, mercury, or calcium—is bonded to another substance. This is a natural process that goes on continually in our bodies. Chelation therapy—which employs the weak acid EDTA—has been shown to safely improve blood flow and relieve symptoms associated with atherosclerotic vascular disease in more than eighty percent of the patients treated. Chelation therapy also helps to prevent arteriosclerosis, improve circulation, and remove lead and toxic heavy metals from the body. This results in a myriad of beneficial effects, including improved vision and hearing, as well as better skin texture and tone. It also helps to improve cognitive function by increasing circulation to the brain.

Dr. Gordon received his Doctor of Osteopathy in 1958 from the Chicago College of Osteopathy. In 1962, he received an honorary medical degree from the University of California, Irvine, and in 1964, he completed his Radiology Residency at Mt. Zion in San Francisco. For many years Dr. Gordon was the Medical Director of the Mineral Lab in Hayward, California, a prominent laboratory for trace mineral analysis.

Dr. Gordon is on the Board of Homeopathic Medical Examiners for Arizona, and is a Board Member of International Oxidative Medicine Association (IOMA). He is advisor to the American Board of Chelation Therapy, and was the past instructor and examiner for all chelation physicians. Dr. Gordon is responsible for Peer Review for Chelation Therapy in the State of Arizona.

Dr. Gordon is currently attempting to establish standards for the proper use of oral and intravenous chelation therapy as an adjunct for treating all major diseases. To find out more about Dr. Gordon's work visit his Web site www.gordonresearch. com

I interviewed Dr. Gordon on March 16, 2006. Dr. Gordon speaks enthusiastically about alternative medicine and his excitement is contagious. We spoke about the dangers of environmental toxins and the benefits of chelation therapy, the differences between oral and I.V. chelation therapies, and about how chelation therapy effects bone growth.

David: What do you think are some of the biggest problems with modern medicine and what do you think needs to be done to help correct the situation?

Dr. Gordon: The biggest problem is greed. We have so many people in medicine today who are known to be receiving compensation from a drug company, or from some other company. It's actually gotten to the point that the editor of the *New England Journal of Medicine* actually wrote a book about it. I believe she resigned saying that it's gotten to the point that it's almost impossible to have any honesty in medicine. So, because we have money driving the system, and it is such a huge system, we've lost our anchor. People are no longer functioning primarily to help their fellow man. It's—how can I get ahead? Or can I get a million dollars worth of stock out of this? So the picture that we have today is so drug-oriented, and we've walked away from the medicine that the rest of the world practices.

Western medicine is not the dominant theory in the world. There are billions of people in the world. Many of these people know what plants grow in their area and what these plants can do medicinally. If you're an African Bushman, for example, and you get bit by a snake or you step on something, you know what leaf to use as a remedy. But this knowledge has been lost to those of us here in the Western United States. We pretend that something that is FDA-approved, or that is used by mainstream medicine, has some science to it—whereas, in fact, if you look at it, a lot of it is nonsense.

Everything has to be looked at in view of what we would call the benefit and the risk. What people don't understand is that a drug can get approved in this country on the flimsiest of research—in the following sense. All any drug has to do is be one percent better than a placebo and it can get approved—even if it's killing people! So, here's what's really sad—if I ever killed somebody with vitamin C, they would absolutely drum vitamin C out the door. They'd put it on prescription so that nobody could get it.

But drugs like Celebrex and Vioxx kill people left and right, and they go forward doing this, because they are "approved." But what people don't understand is that the drug companies are allowed to throw away a study that shows that the drug was worse than placebo. They can keep going until they get one out of three studies that says it's slightly better than placebo, and now they've got an approved drug. Then they can turn around and—according to headlines in the *Wall Street Journal* lately—bill people as much as six hundred thousand dollars a year for something that doesn't cost them six thousand dollars.

In other words, the drug companies are giving the drugs a thousand-fold markup, and they feel it's legitimate, because they've got this incredible story behind it. Most people don't realize that if they had simply taken vitamin C they would have clearly outlived however long this so-called new miracle drug makes them live with their cancer. These so-called miracle drugs that are getting approved often only extend life span one or two months. Yet they can legitimately charge an arm and a leg, and they can have side-effects that include death. Whereas I cannot have any such side-effects in alternative medicine. So the system is really just upside down. It's out of control, and it is totally driven by money. It's lost its anchor, which was to do good, and we have a crisis in health today.

The Earth has become so totally polluted that everybody today is walking around with high-levels of styrene, PCBs, and dioxins. They're in every human being we test today, as well as are lead, mercury, and cadmium. These are taking their toll—and not just on humans. It's getting to be more and more extreme. We're seeing problems like birds at a 10,000 foot elevation that are loaded with mercury. For example, at Mount Washington the birds are loaded with mercury that's coming from the burning of coal in China. There is simply no escape from the particulate matter. We have poisoned our nest. We have got to do natural things, which means somehow learn how to use simple things—whether it's garlic, vitamin C, or a high-fiber diet. We have to do something that's natural, but that's not the focus of conventional Western medicine today.

The focus is on giving the patient a drug because their knee is bothering them, and if they have a little bit less pain, then it's an approved treatment. It's okay if you kill patients with the side-effects of the Vioxx and that Celebrex®. So the system today is out of control. We have to go back to our roots and realize that there was a time that we raised the food in our backyard, and we were personally responsible for it. It wasn't loaded with these pesticides that keep the food from spoiling. You buy something at the store, and it lays in your refrigerator for weeks and doesn't turn bad, but you put that in your intestine and the chemicals that are in that food are killing your normal bacteria.

So we have huge problems, but I also see us as being able to extend life span. I believe in anti-aging medicine, stem cell research, and what we're doing today with genetic testing. We're now able to modulate genes with food. From the results of gene tests we can selectively tell people that they need to emphasize this food and avoid that food. We can make foods that will actually lower your risk of ever getting Alzheimer's— even if both your mother and father's side had the disease. You don't have to get Alzheimer's, but you have to have knowledge. Knowledge is the gene testing, and we can modulate genes by getting appropriate natural products—like RNA foods.

So this is a New Age that we're in. We can fight back. But the system at the current time is such that poor folks are being so deluded that they think that if something is an approved drug then it's the right choice. So they go ahead and let themselves be harmed by the Coumadin, when all they had to do was find out about something as simple as nattokinase and buy a natural thing with their own money. It's not going to be covered by these wonderful insurance plans that the government comes up with, which subsidizes the most powerful industry in the world—the pharmaceutical industry. Nobody has the profits that these people have.

Nobody has the power that they have to influence legislation. They actually buy our Congress. So the net result is that it's going to take a period of time for the people to wake up, and this book could do a wonderful job of helping people know that the system they're living under is absolutely not in their best interest. I have people taking chelation therapy, even though it's not covered by insurance, and they say, well, at least if I have bypass surgery that will be covered—not realizing that they've walked into a blind trap, and they have a risk of dying on the table. They have a risk of huge complications, and no real proven long term benefit. But they say, at least it's proven medicine.

Well, it's not proven by any standards because people don't know how to read the research reports. If we took any new drug that gets approved today, and we really went through the data, many people would be shocked at what they saw. For example, when a research report says that a new drug is fifty percent more effective than the last drug, you'll see that many times what they did is they simply administered a higher dose. They had more side-effects, and they increased the price times three. You have to read the damn report and see this. They are absolutely just robbing the American public, and the people who study this are well aware of it.

David: Why do you think it's important for conventional Western medicine to be more open-minded about alternative medical treatments?

Dr. Gordon: The reason it is important is because their patients are beginning to wake up, and their patients are saying, Doctor, isn't there anything else? So that is the beginning of the revolution. When we put on conferences in homeopathy, nutrition, chelation, acupuncture, and body-mind medicine, many conventional doctors appear. When you ask them why they're there, they say that their patients keep asking them, isn't there something else? So it is the patients who are getting the doctors to want to actually learn what alternative and integrative medicine is all about. This is a consumer-driven revolution that we're going to have.

David: Can you tell me why you think that chelation therapy is important, and what the primary differences between oral EDTA chelation and intravenous chelation are?

Dr. Gordon: The reason that chelation therapy is so important is because—from the moment we're born—every man, woman, and child today has an average of a thousand times more lead in their bones than their ancestors. This is because the lead downloads from the mother. In fact, according to the top research in the United States, the best way for a woman to get rid of lead in her body is to have a baby, because the lead goes into the baby. So, from the moment you're born, you have too much lead, mercury, and cadmium in your body. According to Archives of Internal Medicine, these metals are now proven to have adverse effects on your morbidity and mortality. It's documented how the lower you keep your lead level throughout your life, the longer you live, and the less likely you are to get cancer, diabetes, hypertension, etc.

So everybody today needs chelation. This is because we have polluted our Earth. Today the planet has so much lead that even if you're raising grapes to make vinegar in Italy, the vinegar will have lead in it, because the soil has lead. There's no place to escape. Every leaf, every blade of grass, is now probably coated with particulate matter, which comes from the burning of things like coal and is carried on the air. So, the oceans are loaded with mercury. There's nothing you can eat that doesn't have these things. So chelation is the only way you're going to have optimal health—because these metals are poisons to the enzymes in your body that allow you to make the some ten billion new cells you have to make every day, and the ability of our body to repair itself continuously is impeded when enzyme function is defeated.

So, to keep it really simple, the difference between I.V. and oral chelation is that oral is a little bit like washing your car. It's a good idea and it looks pretty good. I.V. is a little bit like doing a Simoniz. It does a deeper cleansing, but not everybody can afford to Simoniz their car. So everybody needs to be doing the oral every day of their life. That way they'll be keeping their body as clean as they can. What we've done is we've taken the oral EDTA and mixed it with other natural products that happen to look and function in the body the same as heparin.

I have replaced Coumadin and my patients don't die of blood clots. 1.4 million people in the United States die each year from what they call a heart attack or stroke, but it's really a blood clot. So, to me, oral chelation is absolutely my only way of assuring that my patients don't show up in an emergency room with fatal hearts or fatal strokes. It's been twenty years now, and we have yet to hear of the first person having a fatal heart or a fatal stroke while taking the oral program that I devised. But the intravenous chelation is a deeper cleansing, so one doesn't replace the other.

The sad thing is that I was overly enthusiastic thirty years ago, and I thought the intravenous chelation was actually reversing obstructive plaque on our arteries, taking away arteriosclerosis. It turns out that in some people it can reverse plaque, but many people still had an eighty or ninety percent blockage in their vessels. However, many of these people still find that their memory or vision improves, their sex life gets better, their feet get warmer, their blood pressure grows more normal, and they can suddenly run upstairs.

The reasons that we've restored health to them are much more tied to the concept of nitric oxide acting as an endothelial relaxing factor, which enhances blood flow through capillaries. This actually turns out to be more important than taking the plaque out of your artery, because now you're infusing the tissue efficiently, and the lead inhibits nitric oxide synthesis. Removing the lead improves the efficiency of nitric oxide, which helps to enhance blood flow and improve circulation. So pollution is one of the reasons that people have poor circulation.

Oral chelation does two things. It takes the lead out, and when it's in the proper formulas that are available today, it replaces Coumadin, aspirin, or Plavix, which has recently been shown to be dangerous. Natural products are safer, but, unfortunately, people have to pay for natural products. They are not going to be "covered" by the insurance. But we have the advantage that we don't do what Coumadin does. Coumadin is proven to help turn your blood vessel to bone. It actually is proven to do that. This means that you really have hard blood vessels, and the harder your blood vessels, the higher your blood pressure goes, and the sooner you're going to die of a complication of vascular disease.

So the need for chelation is universal. We have to make it affordable, and nothing is as convenient as oral chelation. The oral can be as simple as EDTA, which is my favorite molecule. It's four molecules of vinegar, and it has never been shown to cause any damage when taken, as long as there is a reasonable intake of good minerals with it. This is because EDTA is not so clever that it binds only to lead, mercury, and cadmium. It will also take out zinc. So you could have the embarrassing thing of somebody taking a chelating agent, and not taking a good multiple that has zinc, and aggravating the zinc deficiency that much of the American population has. That would not be in their best interest.

So with chelation we do have to do a constant good mineral input, but that's important anyhow if you're going to be healthy. Everybody needs to know that most people are not getting enough selenium. They're not getting enough magnesium. Hardly anyone is getting enough vitamin D, enough vitamin B-6, enough vitamin C, etc. All these nutrients are not adequately present in our diets, so we have to supplement. After we have the supplements going in then people need to be on oral chelation daily from as early as possible. This way, we'll have fewer infections in childhood. We'll have less death and longer life spans.

The intravenous chelation is really wonderful, because it's a deep cleansing. People who put off doing something about their health for years sometimes walk in my office, and it looks like we're going to have to amputate their right foot, or they're going to have to be placed in an old folk's home, because they don't remember their last name anymore. Then the deep cleansing of intravenous chelation can do things that you simply couldn't rapidly enough do with oral chelation to get the patient out of their problem.

David: If EDTA is removing calcium, then how does it effect bone growth?

Dr. Gordon: The interesting thing is that when you take the disodium EDTA it actually stimulates bone growth. Disodium EDTA is the intravenous compound that I initially championed. What happens to people as they age is that their blood vessels inevitably turn to stone. Let's give it a number. At age ten, you have a certain amount of calcium in your aorta. At age eighty, there will be one hundred forty times more calcium in every person's aorta.

So with disodium EDTA, you actually tie up the calcium that's in the blood, so that the body thinks there's a shortage of calcium, and it turns on the parathyroid hormone. The parathyroid hormone then mobilizes that calcium that has been building up in your artery. Provably, we can lower that content of calcium in your vascular tissue, and, amazingly enough, that same parathyroid hormone switch will make you turn on bone growth again. It's a very exciting process. After all, we're the only medical society with two practicing ninety-four year old members. They've had over two thousand intravenous treatments. They have perfectly healthy bones, nice soft arteries, and they are still practicing. They are still able to show up and enjoy working. Anti-aging is part of the chelation treatment. So there's a big difference.

So, because nobody could understand everything I just said, we have largely now switched to the calcium EDTA. Calcium EDTA gives you calcium when we give you the EDTA, and it makes it a painless treatment, taking three to five minutes. This cuts down the cost of the treatment from $120 to around $60, making it available to everybody, because it doesn't interfere with their day's productivity. People can swing by the doctor's office, be there in five minutes, and have the treatment. The treatment is given rapidly, because it's painless, and it will take out as much as ten or twenty times more lead per treatment than we get out of the old treatment.

But it doesn't do that interesting thing that I've talked about of lowering the level of calcium in your arteries, and enhancing the uptake of calcium in your bone, which is done under the parathyroid hormone influence. In fact, if you are a world expert on parathyroid hormone, you'll know that disodium EDTA infusions are called parathyroid tropic hormones.

The old treatment that we've treated ten million people with safely— without a known death—is the treatment used in the Trial to Access Chelation Therapy (TACT) study done by the National Institute of Health. The TACT study, funded for twenty-nine million dollars, is studying the old treatment that I brought to the world. Ten million people have had the benefits of that therapy, and about eighty-five percent of them said they saw enough improvement in their circulation that it allowed them to avoid a proposed amputation of an extremity, a placement in a nursing home because of loss of vision or memory, or the proposed bypass that some hospital was telling them they needed.

We do not do bypass surgeries. I've done no bypasses on any patient in twenty years. I don't do stents. I cancel all of that surgery based on a simple rule. I ask patients the following question: What are the benefits of the proposed surgery that the hospital or the doctor wants to do, and what are the risks? Once people understand that the benefit is extremely weak, and the risks are extremely large, then they can choose to bet their life on what I'm telling them. There has not yet been a single known fatality in twenty years among people who are simply taking EDTA, and I canceled surgery on people who have eighty to ninety percent blocked vessels.

David: Why isn't oral EDTA chelation recommended by more physicians?

Dr. Gordon: I think this is because the standard policy of doctors is to be down on what they're not up on. You see, the scientific literature in this country is entirely controlled. The net result is that if you have a real breakthrough, something that's really going to cure cancer or heart disease, it's not going to be in the *New England Journal of Medicine* or *Lancet* because of the game that is played in this world. We've known from the beginning that this was too big a revolution. If every doctor did what I'm promoting, there would be no huge hospitals, with huge mills. Every year about four to five hundred thousand people have bypass surgery. That's a huge part of our budget. There are a lot of people dependent on that income, so it's hard to make a big change suddenly, because of the economic ramifications. These changes don't happen suddenly. They happen when people start asking questions. But we've treated ten million people. Those people know, and they've told their families that this actually made them able to go back and run their business, or that this got them out of the nursing home. We have documented so many success stories that it's incredible.

David: What do you think are the primary causes of aging?

Dr. Gordon: We have so many different aspects that we talk about today. One of my interests has been the whole problem of the calcium accumulation, because death occurs when the calcium really builds up rapidly. Here's a simple example. In a normal cell you have ten thousand times more calcium outside of the cell than inside of the cell. It takes energy—in the form of ATP molecules—to be able to have that calcium pump pushing that calcium out all of the time. When a cell dies, and it loses ATP, that gradient is suddenly lost.

So instead of there being a huge amount of calcium outside and very little calcium inside the cell, it now becomes the same on both sides. When death occurs that calcium pours across that membrane and the energy pump stops because that energy pump is created when the mitochondria are producing ATP. But in the moment that those high-energy phosphate bonds get saturated with this huge intake of calcium, they turn to stone essentially.

So this is one of about fifteen phases of anti-aging. There's the hormonal implication. There's the problem of pituitary failure, and there's all the problems from what we call the Free Radical Theory. There's the Cross-Linkage Theory. There are so many different theories. I have had the privilege of being part of a medical group called the American College

of Advancement for Medicine (ACAM), and I've been able to observe
that those doctors who practiced what they preached were the ones that
still look remarkably young. I became convinced over thirty years ago,
when I formed the American College of Advancement for Medicine,
along with a few other doctors that we had a basic anti-aging therapy.
But at that time, thirty years ago, I had no idea that lead would turn out
to be so important.

Thirty years ago no one was explaining to me that everybody walking
around had approximately a thousand times more lead in their bones
than we had four hundred years ago, and that that lead gets released
when a woman starts to go through change of life, and starts to lose her
bone strength. That's why women at change of life often start to develop
hypertension, because the lead has been "safely" in storage in the bones,
and now it starts to kill them.

But what I'm finding that's really exciting is the cover of *Scientific
American* that's on the streets today. The cover story talks about the
DNA and the known genes that can influence longevity. In research for
stopping aging, we can take a simple worm called C. elegans and make
it live six times longer than it's ever lived before by playing around with
its genes. There are about seven more of them that we have now, and
they're identified in the *Scientific American* cover story. We now live
in a day and age where we can actually modulate those genes at will.
We can do this with nutrients—called Ribonucleic Acid NutriSwitch
formulas—that allow us to up regulate the SIR, or down regulate the
TOR or the DAF. By doing this, we get these dramatic benefits that
result from the body doing what it does when it thinks there's a drought
or a major change coming, and it switches over to a more economical
form of metabolism.

We've been able to play with these gene-modulating foods and see, for
example, that patients no longer needed Lipitor, they were no longer
borderline diabetic, or they no longer had elevated levels of triglyceride.
We also use this same product on animals, like a dog that's on its last
legs and has got complete renal failure. The doctor said that the dog will
die in days, and we'd simply give the dog one of these Ribonucleic Acid
NutriSwitch formulas, and in two days the dog goes back to functioning.

In human beings the kidney function goes back to normal, and they don't need dialysis.

So the most exciting thing for me today is what I would call gene therapy, which, for me, would be to modulate genes using foods. And you can't really successfully do that without measuring genes on people who are doing that today. What's really exciting then is once you get people optimized, then to look into the stem cell revolution, which is here. We're doing stem cells successfully on patients. We've restored vision. We've restored functioning in people time after time, and we can turn on stem cells in your own body using magnetic field therapy, using a converted MRI, or we can inject stem cells. But my position is related in the following story.

Several years ago somebody called me and they said this eighteen month old child is blue, his heart is filling the lung area, and we're going to have to do an emergency heart transplant. I said, "Why would the new heart last any longer than the old one unless we find out what was wrong with the child?" Did that heart fail because there was a carnitine deficiency? What was the underlining cause? But, if I treat the underlying cause first, then putting a new heart in might be more appropriate because it would have a chance to survive. And I've successfully done this. But what's interesting is that when we corrected all those defects that one can measure, then the child was no longer blue and the heart went back to normal size. So I didn't need to do a heart transplant.

But with stem cells, I will need to do stem cell therapy on seventy and eighty year old people who are not functioning well. However, the stem cell therapy would be a lot more successful if I first optimized all the defects. One of the most important areas of defect today is called methylation—which includes glucuronidation, acetylation, and all the different methods by which we do our detoxification. Methylation is also the key factor in the body for the production of things like carnitine and coenzyme Q-10, but even more importantly methylation is the way that we keep all of our infections under control and successfully repair the ten billion cells we have to make each day. When we do these gene tests, and we look at the methylation genes—there are forty different ones— we find that there are what we call single nucleotide polymorphisms, or SNPs, that are abnormal. The more of these that someone has, the sooner the person will have serious aging and or other illnesses.

But we can modulate those genes by telling the person that he or she has this defect. For example, let's say that you have a defect with a particular gene that means that you can not excrete heavy metals. So we have to do this to you, and we're going to put you on these kinds of products. And you have a defect in methylation, so we're going to give you some RNA products that will help to handle that, and you may need lots of methyl donors, such as trimethylglycine, methylsulfonmethane, and the lists go on. But we live in a New Age today. I'm certainly planning on practicing when I'm age one hundred, and I'm really very confident that we can all live to a hundred and twenty years of age. I believe that we're all entitled to it, if we merely take care of this incredible machine—our body—have some respect for it, and begin to understand something about how it works.

David: What are some of the new anti-aging treatments that you foresee coming along in the near future?

Dr. Gordon: The number one anti-aging treatment that I see is that everyone is going to have to maintain cleanliness, because if we all have dioxin PCBs, lead, mercury, etc., we have to detox everybody. That's simple. Number two, everybody today is infected. If you become an expert on infections you realize that it's not just the avian flu that we should be worried about, and it's not the Ebola virus. It's the infections we all carry around in our bodies today, and that includes everything from the Epstein Barr virus to Herpes to mycoplasma to Chlamydia. Everybody alive today is filled with infections.

So my anti-aging programs involve, essentially, one, that I adequately nutrify the body, because no one that I test today has adequate levels of selenium to offset the huge levels of heavy metals that are in our bodies. No one has adequate levels of magnesium. No one is getting adequate levels of vitamin D. The levels of vitamin C are far too low. So we have to do the nutrification. Then we have to do the detoxification, which would be dealing with the heavy metals, as well as lowering the level of dioxin PCBs, etc., getting people into organic foods, getting them to eat right for their blood type, and all these simple things.

Then we have to look at lowering the total body burden of pathogens. It's in mainstream literature (*Circulation*, the journal of the American Heart Association) that the higher the level of pathogens that you have—like Chlamydia, CMV, or any of these other things—the sooner you will die. So, obviously, we don't have drugs that handle all of those kinds of stealth infections that are in everybody today, so I use oxidative therapies. This includes everything from high-dose vitamin C, to things like ozone ultraviolet blood irradiation, immune modulation, and other therapies that we can use so that you can help lower the total body burden of these infections.

Then, the last thing, which I am very excited about, is genetic testing. I'm now having all of my patients do gene tests which show the number of SNPs they will have out of forty. I had one person come back with thirty-one abnormalities out of forty. That person obviously was not functioning well. That was an autistic child. But when we see what the problem is, then we can get the child back to full functioning, going back to normal school, etc. So once you know what's wrong, you can correct for it.

Then, once you've optimized the body, stem cells are going to be extremely important. We have people using magnetic field therapies, sleeping on magnetic pads that allow their body to much more efficiently carry out the heavy metals, as well as turn on the switch to make our own stem cells—because we're loaded with stem cells. If you fall down and tear all the skin off your arm, you'll cry about it, but you know the skin is going to come back. So we have stem cells in our brain. We have stem cells everywhere. One safe switch to turn it on seems to be putting people into a strong magnetic field, which, of course, would be like a converted MRI. I can have people go back to full functioning, even though they've been told they need a heart transplant. We do that all the time. We cancel heart transplants routinely.

We're very close to being able to do that with people who might have needed a brain transplant, because their brain is not working properly, but we can let our body do that with our stem cells, and increasingly stem cells will become available. The University of Oregon is doing some studies right now working with very handicapped children, and the day is coming rapidly that we will all have access to affordable stem cell infusions that will work dramatically. But they're going to work much more dramatically in people who have chosen to optimize their body by dealing with all aspects of it, taking care of nutrition, lowering the total body burden of toxins, lowering the total body burden of pathogens, and then optimizing the body for its dietary intake and dealing with stress, all of these other aspects. Obviously, today, we know enough to have everybody on a really good dietary program to deal with antioxidants, but chelating agents happen to be the most powerful antioxidant there is.

In other words, once you tie up the trace metals in the body that are excessively present with a chelating agent, you've dramatically lowered the level of free radical pathology. So I'm extremely optimistic about the therapies that we have. And, obviously, the facts are that at a certain age all of us start losing our hormonal levels, and so I do hormone replacement. I have people taking melatonin and DHEA, as well as applications of progesterone and testosterone. We have a natural hormone replacement for women today that's extremely safe, that replaces all of the work that these people have done working with so-called herbal therapies that really never worked. For women with hot flashes, we now have found something in Northern Thailand that really works in the body like natural estrogen called *Pueraria mirifica*.

So we have to support the hormone levels in the body. But let's look at how all this ties together. If you go to a lot of conferences on aging, you'll see many people talking about human growth hormone injections. Well, that's interesting, but what was wrong with my pituitary gland that it stopped producing enough growth hormone? Why did it stop working? If we look at an autopsy study, in addition to seeing that the aorta has turned to stone, we'll find that the pituitary gland—the master gland in the body—is an organ that has high content of cystine. Because cystine is a chelator, it has sucked in the mercury that's been in your body. In other words, you don't have the same level of mercury, lead, cadmium in each tissue of your body; certain tissues get uniquely poisoned.

Some of them are poisoned because the tissue is infected, and that infection, very cleverly, helps hold on to toxic metals so that the body's immune system doesn't attack the infection. But in the case of the pituitary gland, we have shown that it is extremely high in mercury, and when I do the chelation long enough, to lower the level of mercury, amazingly enough that patient's human growth hormone levels start to go back to what they were at a much earlier age. So it all ties together, but I have to do a lot of hormone replacement therapy anyway.

David: Is there anything we haven't spoken about that you would like to add?

Dr. Gordon: I just want to really make it very clear that we live in a day and age of genetic testing. Just yesterday, after nine years of study, the Welcome Trust in England is finally going to start doing intensive gene tests on three thousand people—between ages forty-five and sixty-five—and follow them for the next twenty years. But we are already doing things. If you look at the literature, some of the reports will tell you that gene testing is five to ten years off. At this moment, we have over eleven hundred people using our autism-answer Web site, and they're all patting each other on the back saying, Aren't we lucky we found Dr. Gordon and Dr. Yasko? We're doing the gene test on our kid after no one could help. We spent a hundred, two hundred thousand dollars and no one could get our child back to school. Our child couldn't speak. She never said a word. We can take a fourteen year old child, who has never said a word, and in six months have the child stand up and read a poem that she's written. So it's an exciting time that we live in. The answers are here. We don't have to wait forever.

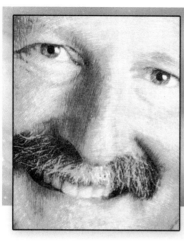

UNDERSTANDING AND TREATING CHRONIC FATIGUE SYNDROME

An Interview with Dr. Jacob Teitelbaum

Jacob Teitelbaum, M.D. is a board-certified internist and a leading researcher in the field of Chronic Fatigue Syndrome (CFS) and Fibromyalgia (FM). He has a specialized practice for CFS/FM and pain patients in Annapolis, Maryland, and is director of the Annapolis Research Center for Effective CFS/ FM therapies. Dr. Teitelbaum is also the author of several books, including From Fatigued to Fantastic, Pain Free 1-2-3!: A Proven Program to Get You Pain Free Now!, *and* Three Steps to Happiness: Healing Through Joy.

Dr. Teitelbaum received his medical degree from the Medical School at Ohio State University, and in 1980, he became Board Certified in Internal Medicine. For over two decades he has worked with CFS/FM patients. His motivation to specialize in this area of medicine began with personal experience. In 1975, Dr. Teitelbaum had to drop out of medical school when he himself contracted CFS/FM, and this had a profound influence on the course of his medical career. Although he recovered enough to resume his medical school training a year later, CFS/FM symptoms persisted for many years, and this motivated him to become an avid reader of the scientific medical literature, where he came across many studies that he had not learned about in medical school.

Applying this research, Dr. Teitelbaum began to treat his patients with nutritional and herbal therapies, hormonal supplements, anti-infectious treatments, physical therapy measures, and sleep support. Much to his surprise, these previously untreatable patients started to improve dramatically. Dr. Teitelbaum was amazed as his general internal medicine practice began to fill with patients who were flying in from around the country. He has now effectively treated approximately 2,000 patients with CFS/FM related disorders.

In addition to having written several books, Dr. Teitelbaum has written numerous articles on CFS/FM, including the recent landmark paper "Effective Treatment of Chronic Fatigue Syndrome and Fibromyalgia—A Randomized, Double-Blind Placebo-Controlled, Intent to Treat Study," published in the Journal of Chronic Fatigue Syndrome. *Dr. Teitelbaum has also designed a line of nutritional supplements and support formulas, and all of his royalties from the sale of these products goes to charity. To find out more about Dr. Teitelbaum's work, visit his Web site: www.endfatigue.com*

I interviewed Jacob on October 11, 2004. Jacob is open-minded, curious, and very enthusiastic about alternative medicine. He has a very upbeat perspective on life in general, and he laughs a lot. We spoke about the etiology of Chronic Fatigue Syndrome, the relationship between CFS and FM, how to sleep better and increase mental clarity, and other effective treatments for CFS/FM.

David: What inspired your interest in medicine, and how did your experience with Chronic Fatigue Syndrome in medical school influence your medical career?

Jacob: I've wanted to be a healer since I was a little kid. I tend to be very empathic, and if somebody was hurting I could feel what they were feeling. When I was seven or eight years old, I still remember how I'd want to hide behind a corner, and just wiggle my finger and make people who were hurting feel better. So that's always been my goal. If you look at my high school yearbook, you'll see that it says that's what I'm going to be. I've felt this way for as far back as I can remember. Part of being a Jewish kid is the expectation that you're going to be a Jewish doctor, but that's my nature. Part of being empathic is being a healer.

Because I had Chronic Fatigue Syndrome in medical school, I was forced out of school for the year. It also forced me on the road. I was basically homeless, because my dad had died when I was about seventeen and I had no money. I had a scholarship, loans and work study, but since I was out of school, I had none of that, and I couldn't work because I was too sick. So I was homeless, and I was living on the road. I discovered that on the road you meet fascinating people. I met all these healers and fascinating people along the way—people who were teaching some fascinating areas I had never heard about in medical school.

Also, I grew up in an old Eastern European Hassidic family and Hassidic community, so the healing arts are very natural. Science is natural, and using healing was natural. So these things were all becoming second nature as I met people that were teaching energy medicine, naturopathy, and all different things along the way. So I healed up enough, in part because of that—probably in large part because of that. I think that's why I recovered, as opposed to staying sick, because of the energy work that I was doing and learning. It really kept me open to that as I learned the hard science, instead of just getting closed down. In medical school, they would teach that anybody who does any of this stuff is a quack, but I knew better.

Using the chakra system, I could do an energy scan, feel a tumor, and send the person for a test and find it there. You see people get better. You see it and experience it. Then I would also look at the medical literature aggressively for just about everything, not just prescriptions, but also for natural remedies. In my training this encouraged me to not just look at the three main journals, and a specialty journal, that most doctors read, which are basically paid for by the drug companies. They're basically big advertisements for the medications. They think it's science, but what they ignore is that if the drug company pays for the study, it has a much greater effect on the outcome then whether it's placebo-controlled or not.

The medical journals wouldn't dream of publishing something that wasn't placebo-controlled. But what they publish is almost only articles related to medications that are paid for by the drug company, or by people who are working for the drug company and getting money from them. So it's a big advertisement, and that creates a selectivity and bias that's just very strong against natural remedies. And that's all doctor's hear about. But I would look at studies from literally dozens of different journals. I discovered that the smaller journals don't draw as much drug money, and they do more basic research. They're much more open to just publishing what science shows works, and just giving the straight data. So it got me interested in being open-minded to natural remedies as well as prescriptions.

I learned to recognize that there are many tools in the healing tool kit. In medical school all you come out with is a hammer, and everything looks like a nail. But when you start to do comprehensive medicine, you have a hammer, so if you have appendicitis you can do surgery. But if you have back pain, instead of having to cut the person open, you can give nutritional support or hormonal support. You can use willow bark, for example, which has been shown to be more effective than Motrin®. You almost never have to send anybody for back surgery, so you don't have to whack everybody with a hammer. You could use gentler things that are more effective and more appropriate, because you have an entire tool kit.

Around five years ago, there was a forest fire and my office burned down. It just took it out, and I saw this as a good thing. The universe knew I was about to burn out, because I'd been doing all that research, writing, lecturing, and teaching, in addition to running a practice, raising my five kids and the rest. The universe knew I would either burn out or the office would burn down, and it always takes care of me. So the office burnt down. It gave me a chance to sit back and think, okay, what do I want to rebuild out of the fire? What do I want to let stay in the ashes? So that's all good stuff. But when the office burnt down, I had over 14,000 research study reports in my files that went up in smoke, and that's only a tiny percent of what I read, because most studies aren't worth the bother. Now I still know the stuff, because it's in my head. However, when it first went down, it left me feeling like I got kicked in the stomach.

But this stuff is all accessible anyway, and it actually turned out to be a good thing. So this is what my work is based on, and when people say it's not evidence-based medicine, and that they see no evidence that natural remedies work, that's because they won't look at the thousands of studies that show that it works. (*Laughter*) Then they can honestly say that they haven't seen any evidence. It's like Sgt. Shultz in the old Hogan's Heroes. He would say, "I see nothing!" Well, that's what the priests of high medicine are like in academia and the rest. It's like they see nothing, and they will support no data that shows natural remedies work. If anybody does a study they will peer-review it into the ground, coming up with nonsense reasons to not publish it. If it is published, they question the journal, and they won't look at the data. Then they can honestly say that they don't see anything. But it's a religion. It's scientism, and basically, if they had their way, they would keep people from having access to the vast panoply of safe and effective therapies.

David: Can you talk a little about what you've learned about the etiology of Chronic Fatigue Syndrome?

Jacob: Yes, Chronic Fatigue Syndrome is basically like blowing a fuse. It's like the circuit-breakers you have in your home. If you plug in too many heaters, for example, or blow-dryers—boom!—off go the lights because you've blown a circuit or a fuse. The fuse that you blow in Chronic Fatigue Syndrome is called the hypothalamus, and that's a key control center in the brain. It controls temperature regulation, sleep, hormonal function, and the autonomic nervous system which regulates blood flow, blood pressure, and pulse. Because the hypothalamus is blown, those four systems are off-line in Chronic Fatigue Syndrome.

Now the way that that acts as a circuit breaker is like this. You can view Chronic Fatigue Syndrome, and its painful cousin Fibromyalgia, as an energy crisis, where you're calling on your body to supply more energy than it's able to supply—and you can only overdraw your bank account for so long before things start bouncing, so to speak. So, since the hypothalamus is so energy-dependent, because it's doing so many things in a small area, when you are outstripping your energy supplies, that's the place that goes first, and that's why it acts as a circuit-breaker.

David: How does Chronic Fatigue Syndrome lead to immune system dysfunction?

Jacob: It does this in several ways. Chronic Fatigue Syndrome is integrally tied in with the hormonal functions of the hypothalamus, which control the immune system, and poor sleep also causes immune dysfunction. There's also the problem of not making enough energy in your muscles, so the muscles get stuck in a shortened position, just like with rigor mortis when somebody dies. The muscles don't have enough energy, so they don't go loose. The muscles become rigid as a board, and when they go rigid, they hurt. So there are a number of ways that it causes direct immune dysfunction, as well as ways that are not quite as direct; they're basically one step removed from that. Then, because the immune system is not able to have the energy it needs to fight infections, you get these infections, which put more demand on the immune system, when it's already on its knees. Then it basically just starts firing off wildly, trying to fight all these infections, and then it exhausts itself. That's why the change is biphasic. We have an overactive immune system followed by an exhausted immune system.

David: Can you talk a little bit more about the relationship that you see between Chronic Fatigue Syndrome and Fibromyalgia?

Jacob: They're the same thing in most people. The body doesn't care what name we call things. What's going on is what's going on. You can call it Fibromyalgia, Fibrositis, Chronic Fatigue Syndrome. If the person, in addition to fatigue, insomnia, and brain fog, also has widespread muscle pain—which most of them do—then they have Fibromyalgia.

David: What role do you think vitamin deficiencies and diet play in Chronic Fatigue Syndrome and Fibromyalgia, and how might taking nutritional supplements and improving one's diet help improve symptoms?

Jacob: Oh, it's a major role. Remember we talked about blowing a fuse because you can't make enough energy? So the question then is how do you make enough energy so that you can turn that fuse back on? I use the acronym T.H.I.N.S. to help people understand how to do this. The initial T is for toxins, which you want to eliminate. H is for hormonal support.

I is for infections, which need to be treated. N is for nutritional support. And S is for sleep support. Those are the things that make energy, keep energy, and eliminate the energy drain. So people who have this disease need proper nutritional support. Actually, the American public in general is horribly nutritionally deficient—and it's not that they're deficient in one nutrient. They're deficient across the board, and the reasons are multiple.

One reason is that we get an average of one hundred fifty pounds of sugar per person added to our diet every year. Soda has almost one teaspoon of sugar per ounce. So if somebody goes to the 7-11 and gets one of these 64 oz Big Burps, that's 64 spoons of sugar, and sugar supplies 18% of our calories. Another 18% of our calories come from white flour. So 36% of our diet is nutritionally wiped out before you ever get out of the starting box. Then you have food processing, and you have all the different bowel infections that people get that decrease absorption and increase nutritional needs. So most Americans are nutritionally deficient, and it's not just with a single nutrient. In Chronic Fatigue Syndrome and Fibromyalgia, it gets even much worse because you have both increased needs and decreased absorption. So the question is, what do you do?

We used to give people dozens of vitamin tablets and different supplements to take, because there are about forty or fifty different nutrients that they're low in. But after awhile that started to get insane. It was just too much for people. So there's a vitamin powder that's out now which makes it easy. People take one drink and one capsule, and it replaces thirty-five tablets of supplements. You have to make it easier for people, or they're not going to be able to do it. Because of my teaching role, I have a policy that 100% of the royalties for any products that I make go to charity.

For example, we just gave a hundred thousand dollar grant to do a study on autism using NAET, which we have found to very effective. NAET is an acupressure-applied kinesiology technique, and we've seen it make autism go away a lot of times. It's just amazing. So the money gets used for charity or research, and I just don't get any of it. I think this allows for more objectivity, and it's also more fun for me to have the money go that way. So I don't take money from any company for any products that I recommend, because when people start selling me stuff I tune out, and

I didn't want that to happen. The teaching is too important, and I didn't want that to get in the way of it.

David: You said that the cause of Chronic Fatigue Syndrome and Fibromyalgia is the hypothalamus being blown out. Would you recommend any type of hormonal treatment then to help correct the situation?

Jacob: Absolutely. Remember the acronym T.H.I.N.S. H is for hormonal support.

Nutritional support is easy. Avoid sugar and increase water because the hormone that holds on to water is low. Take the Energy Revitalization System vitamin powder, which simply maintains good solid nutritional support in general. Most people find a high-protein diet feels better than a high-carb diet, but everybody is different with that. Except for sugar, it's most important that people eat what makes them feel good, because there's no one diet that's right for everybody.

Then with hormonal support, it's important to be clear that blood tests are hopelessly unreliable, and they miss the majority of people who benefit from and need hormonal support. So thyroid is usually low if people are tired and achy, cold-intolerant, and suffer from weight gain. If they have two or three of those, they deserve a trial of thyroid hormone, period, regardless of what the blood tests show. Tens of thousands of adults are dying a year, in addition to tens of thousands more neonatal deaths and miscarriages, because people are not being treated for their low thyroid. Generally, it's better to use the natural hormones than the synthetic ones, because they're the same thing that the body makes. So Armour thyroid is excellent and very helpful.

Then there's adrenal support. The adrenal is our stress handler, whereas the thyroid is like our gas pedal—it's like the thermostat that says how much energy you're making. The adrenal gland is what helps you handle stress, and in our modern society we put so much stress on our bodies, because of the environment, because the fast pace of things, things like that. We exhaust the adrenal glands, and you can tell that that's going on because you get these hypoglycemic symptoms. This is basically when you get very irritable, when you're hungry, when your blood sugar drops, people around you recognize that if they don't feed you NOW, you get so irritable that they feel like you're going to kill them. Fortunately, natural adrenal hormones and glandulars (e.g. Adrenal Stress End) can be given in low dose very safely and can be dramatically beneficial.

You can use natural hormones safely. Testosterone deficiency needs to be treated in women as well as men. Treating a low testosterone in men using natural hormones decreases the risk of angina, improves diabetic control, and decreases cholesterol. Now you don't want to go to super-high levels like the body builders, that's dangerous. But you don't need to do that with hormones generally. So the hormonal support is critical and the blood tests are horribly unreliable.

David: You spoke about the role that sleep deprivation plays in Chronic Fatigue Syndrome and Fibromyalgia. What suggestions would you make to help improve someone's sleep patterns?

Jacob: The hypothalamus is the sleep center, so it's not a matter of poor sleep hygiene. It's a matter of the sleep center is not working. So, first of all, I like to start with natural remedies, and there are herbals. I think the best herbals for sleep are wild lettuce, Jamaican Dogwood, theanine, and hops. Passion flower and valerian are also okay. All six of those are in a product called Revitalizing Sleep Formula by Enzymatic Therapy, so they can get them all in one capsule.

5-HTP is good, but is expensive and takes six weeks to work. It also causes weight loss, and because the average weight gain in this disease is 32 pounds, that's helpful for people. It also decreases pain. Taking calcium and magnesium at bedtime also helps.

Melatonin helps too, but only one half milligram. A half milligram is all it takes to totally bring a low melatonin level up to normal, and the studies show that for most people that low dose is every bit as effective as a higher dose for sleep. I have concerns when someone starts taking a massive dosage of hormones. Even if they're natural, I don't think one should take a dose that brings us above what the body normally would have.

David: Are there any other herbal remedies that you would recommend for treating chronic fatigue syndrome in general?

Jacob: Oh, there's a whole host of things. Go to my web site at vitality101.com, and click on "treatment protocol". It's the bottom link on the left. And if you go through it section-by-section—for sleep, for treating yeast, for treating pain—you'll see dozens of different herbals that are recommended, and how to use them.

David: Are you familiar with Jay Goldstein's work and his book Tuning the Brain? *What are you thoughts regarding his ideas about neurosomatic medicine, and his approach to treating chronic fatigue syndrome by reconfiguring neural networks through pharmacologic modulation?*

Jacob: Oh yeah, Jay is brilliant. Jay and I used to tease each other—you know the story of the five blind men and the elephant? They go feel around, and one feels the back leg and says, "It's a tree trunk." The other felt the trunk of the elephant and said, "No, it's a snake." And one felt nothing at all and said, "You're all crazy." That's what it's like in Chronic Fatigue Syndrome. I tease that I have the left thigh and leg of the elephant and Jay's got the trunk. He's working specifically on the brain chemistry to alter things downstream, and the good thing about that is you'll sometimes see dramatic effects with a single medication.

The downside is that since you're goosing one part of the system, but not bringing up the rest of the system, the benefits often tend to wear off over time. With my approach it takes more treatments, but you're actually fixing the problem. But Jay is brilliant, and his work is wonderful. He just got burnt out because he just ran into so much opposition from the medical system, the National Institute of Health (NIH) groups, those kinds of things. They are so resistant to any change that does not come from within the NIH or academia, and certainly if it comes from natural remedies.

Their resistance is like a religious faith, and I applaud their religious faith, but what they're doing is religion, it's not science. Their blind faith against anything natural takes on the fervor of heavy-duty fundamentalism, and I honor and I appreciate their faith. I just think that the people who want to use natural remedies have the right to their religious beliefs too. The science supports the use of the natural remedies. So Jay got the same kind of slamming from them, and he finally just gave up.

David: What advice would you give to someone to help them find a physician who understands conditions such as chronic fatigue syndrome and fibromyalgia?

Jacob: Go on my Web site. I see people from all over the world, but it's two to four hours for a new patient visit, and I only see people five or six days a month, because the rest of the time I'm teaching. But the Web site has the tools that everybody needs. I actually hold the patent on a computerized physician. If you go to the patent office, I'm the one that has it for computerized doctor, because we needed that to reach six million people. So people can go on the web site, put in a detailed history, put in their lab tests (and get a prescription for the lab tests to take to their local lab if their doctor won't give them one), and it will analyze all of that, make a complete medical record of their case, and tell them exactly what they need to do to get well, because treatment is different for everyone. If you have a hundred people you could have a hundred different treatment protocols, so it tailors the treatment to each individual case.

Then there's also two referral lists on the Web site. One list is of doctors who want to see people with chronic fatigue syndrome. We don't charge people to be put on the list, so one list is anybody who just wants to see people. Many of these people are clueless, but at least they want to see people with CFS, as opposed to the physicians who start crossing themselves and running out of the room if they hear you've got chronic fatigue syndrome. Then the second list gives the people that I've trained, who have done two or four day workshops, and that group has at least gotten the basic foundation and training. So people can go online from anywhere around the world, and see who's in their area.

David: What are your thoughts about human longevity, and what do you think are the best ways to slow down the human aging process?

Jacob: We often talk about humans causing more mass extinctions than any other life form in history, but that's not correct. The life form that

caused the most mass extinctions in the history of the planet, that we
know of at least, is algae—because algae made this incredibly toxic
substance that they put into the environment called oxygen. Now oxygen
is very oxidative. If you put oxygen with iron it rusts and becomes iron
oxide. So oxygen is very toxic and it causes wear and tear. Now, the
species that survived were adaptive enough to actually not just learn
how to live in an oxygen-rich environment, but how to use it to make
energy. It's a little bit like in Judo, where you turn your opponent's force
to your own advantage.

So, a couple of things if you want to stay young and live a very long
life—or as I put it, die very young very late in life. Number one is sleep,
because studies show that things that raise growth hormone can slow
aging. For example, if you have sex three times a week you look ten
years younger. This is from a study out of Scotland, and it was postulated
that that's because of the growth hormone release. So if you want to
increase your growth hormone, get deep sleep, get exercise, and have
sex. That's how you raise growth hormone naturally. I don't like growth
hormone shots because I'm not convinced of the safety. They're also
expensive, and they're a pain. So raise it naturally by following the
"rough" prescription that I just gave you.

Two, get good nutritional support. The antioxidants are critical. The
vitamin powder—the Energy Revitalization System—is a real easy
way to do that, so you get solid overall nutritional support. You're not
going to get it out of a single tablet. Too much has been pulled out of
our diet for that, and there's too much stress on the body. So get solid
nutrition. Then the T in T.H.I.N.S. is toxins, so detox. It doesn't mean
that you need to avoid every toxin. You can't do that in the American
environment—it's pretty much impossible. But don't spray a can of bug
spray in your house for God's sake. That's poison. That's why it kills
bugs. There are safer ways to control pests, such as using boric acid.

We had this big line of ants coming into my house recently because
they found the cat food bowl. So we could have sprayed the hell out of
them, which would have kept them away for about two days, and then
killed us more than them. But we just put the cat bowl in a bigger dish
that had water in it, so the ants couldn't get to it because there's a little
moat around it. So you can poison yourself, or you can just use common

sense.

I often gave lectures in the schools to the third graders on nutrition. When I was first starting this practice, I would say that there's a very simple rule of thumb—if you can't read what's in the ingredients because the words are so complicated, don't eat it. If the ingredient list says that it contains chemicals with names that start with something like tiulated, futalated, hydroxy, or whatever it is, then avoid it. Also avoid sugar. But words like flour and milk—you can read that. But these big long chemical names, that's probably not very good for you. So just use common sense with it, but don't make yourself nuts.

So avoid heavy toxins, get the hormonal support that really prolongs life, add nutritional support and sleep, and those are the key things basically. There's a concept that I call Vitality 101, which says, feed your body—get proper nutrition, avoid sugar, and get plenty of water. Use your body—get exercise and have sex, things like that. And rest your body—get eight to nine hours of sleep a night. And if you do that, you can die very young very late in life. These things are not hard to do. There's a policy that I have—you never take away something that's giving a person pleasure without substituting something equally pleasurable. So, for example, I'm going to say avoid sugar, but I'm going to add the three magic words—except for chocolate. I think chocolate is a healthy food, and so are other things that give you joy. I'll tell you the fourth thing for Vitality 101, which is the most important for staying young and alive late in life—follow your bliss. This means do what feels good.

David: What advice would you give to someone who is looking to improve their mental performance?

Jacob: Again, nutritional support and sleep are critical. Then, if they have low thyroid the brain is not going to work very well. If they're tired, achy, gaining weight, and cold-intolerant, they probably have low thyroid. So start with the vitamin powder. It'll have a dramatic effect on giving your brain what it needs to function properly. Get eight to nine hours sleep a night. A hundred years ago the average American got nine hours of sleep a night—as many people got ten hours as got eight. We're sleep-deprived, and because of this our brains are not going to work too well.

So first of all, make the time for sleep. Then second, take what you need to get solid sleep. There are many natural remedies like we discussed. You do those two simple things and you're going to improve function markedly. Then make sure your hormonal levels are okay. Make sure your testosterone and your thyroid levels are not too low. But let me give you a quick primer on blood testing. For most blood tests the normal range is based on what's called two standard deviations. This is just a statistical norm. What that means is that they take a hundred people, and measure the blood test. The highest and lowest two and a half out of a hundred are considered abnormal, and the other ninety-five percent in the middle are defined as normal. That's all the normal range means for most tests.

So say you wanted to define a normal shoe size. We take a hundred people at the mall, look at their shoe size, and you get a normal range of maybe four to thirteen. That would get ninety-five percent of people. So say you had a shoe problem, and I measured your shoe size, and you were wearing a size five. I'd say, "No it's normal. There's no problem. It's in the normal range." I see you lost your shoes, so I'll just take one out of the pile, and as long as it's in that range, it's ok. You would put it on and say, "I can't get into this thing." Then I'd measure it again, and I'd say, "No the test says it's normal. It's just fine."

The analogy I just gave you is almost exact. You have to look at the symptoms. Are you tired? Are you achy? Are you cold intolerant? Do you have weight gain? Then you have low thyroid, and you deserve a trial of natural thyroid hormone. So consider thyroid, testosterone, and adrenal support. If any of those three are low your brain is not going to work very well. Taking the treatments to bring these up to normal, if they're low, could make a big difference. So start with getting nutritional support, get your eight to nine hours sleep, treat your hormonal system, and treat any infections or toxin exposures. But that's kind of Vitality 102 at that point. I'd start with 101 for most people.

David: What do you think are the key steps to happiness, and how do you think happiness promotes healing?

Jacob: My book *Three Steps to Happiness: Healing Through Joy* talks about that. These are the keys steps. Number one would be to be authentic with our feelings. A lot of us are taught we're not supposed to be angry, hurt, pissed off, or whatever, and the thing is you're going to feel how you feel. So simply be authentic with your feelings and feel your feelings, but you also need to know how to let go of them when you're done feeling them, and start feeling good. So the book talks about how to get in touch with your feelings, and how to let go of them when you're done.

Number two is that you want go ahead and stop being a victim, because as long as you have a sense of victimization you're giving up the power to control your life—in which case, you're dead meat. I'm going to broaden that out. If you're caught up in blame, fault, guilt, judgment, comparisons, expectations, you are putting other people in charge of your happiness, and that's a real bad idea. So part of not being a victim is no blame, no fault, no guilt, no judgment, no comparisons, and no expectations, on anybody else or on your self. Now, you can be really pissed off at somebody, and that's fine. But that's different than blaming them. You create your own reality. If something happens, it's what you created, and don't blame yourself either—because no guilt and no blame apply to you as well. Just recognize, oh okay, that's what it is. Is that how I want it to be? And if not, then how do you want it to be? And change it.

Then that brings us to step three, the most important step, which is follow your bliss. This means do what feels good. That's why we have feelings. Our brain tells us what we're programmed to do to get approval. Our church, synagogue, parents, school, T.V. sets, and society said we needed to be good boys and good girls and get approval. That's what our brain tells us, or to get attention in some cases, in which case then we can be the bad boys. But either way, it's to get attention and approval. But that's not authentic to who we are; that's just what people are telling us.

Our feelings tell us what's authentic for us. When you're authentic, and you're at one with your spirit—which is what authentic means—it feels good, because spirit always feels good. That's what spirit it is—a place of bliss. So if you're feeling good, then you're connected with spirit. You're tapped in. When you feel bad it's cause you've cut yourself off. You're in a place of thinking or believing that's not authentic, and that's why we have feelings. So we can get past this computer program we have and get into who we are. So if something feels good I recommend you keep your attention on it. Joseph Campbell, who had studied religions throughout history, and all over the planet, when asked to summarize in one sentence what he had learned from all of these, put it very brilliantly. He said, "Follow your bliss".

David: What is your perspective on the concept of God, and how has spirituality played a role in your view of medicine?

Jacob: Oh, to me the concept of God is that it's all one. In other words, if everything is God, Goddess, Spirit—whatever you want to call it—it's all one. It's all connected, and that means that all that's going on is God looking at God's self. So it's all simply different perspectives, and that's a fascinating thing. That means nobody is cut off from God, whether they're atheists or whatever. You don't have to believe in God for Spirit to love you and be present, so it means that nobody is right and nobody is wrong. It's all simply different perspectives, which is very freeing, because now you don't have to battle anybody. You just have to do your own thing.

This also allows us to recognize our own connection to spirit, which is very healing, because it allows that energy to flow into us, and allows us to stay whole and connected. So that's a very powerful thing. I mean, my whole life is about Spirit and about God, or Goddess. To think of God as only a man sounds like an insult to God. It's pretty limiting, because God is everything. It also means that nothing and no one is better or worse than anybody else. And there's this critical thing that happens, because that's been the touchstone through much of my life— to recognize I am the equal of all beings, and no one is lesser than me. That means there's nobody that I meet that's better than I am, or that I'm better than them. We're all different perspectives of God. We're all equal, and we're all divine, everybody.

David: What are you currently working on?

Jacob: My next book, *Pain Free 1-2-3!*. I'm interested in addressing those areas that are poorly dealt with in modern society, and this is why I spent twenty-five years teaching people about fatigue, vitality, and

Chronic Fatigue Syndrome. The next area that I'm addressing is pain management, which is horribly dealt with by doctors, and this is what the new book is about. *Pain Free 1-2-3!* will teach people how to get pain free using natural and prescription therapies. They can use either or both. It's comprehensive, and it guides people step-by-step. If this is what you have, then here's how you handle it, and this is what you have to do to get pain free. So that's an awesome book.

So that's where I'm moving into right now. Then I want to take on the biggest crime and most devastating thing in our society. You know how we look at suicide bombers in the Middle East, and we say, God, these people must be insane—sending their children out to kill other children and die. But then if we look at ourselves, we realize we're teaching our children that if you suffer you're going to Heaven, and if you feel good and have a joyful life you're going to go to Hell. I think that's more psychotic. So that's where the three steps to happiness are so important. It's like I tell the docs, if you help people to get healthy so they can go back to a life they hate, you've done nothing for them. I think that's a really important concept. You want to get healthy so you can get a life you love. And the flip-side of that is having a life you love helps you to be healthy. It goes both ways. So it's those areas that I'm interested in. It's a mix of teaching people what they can do to get healthy, but also teaching them how to get a life they love—so that it's worth it.

David: Is there anything that we haven't discussed that you would like to add?

Jacob: If I could just say one thing, if there's one message I could get out for people, it's follow your bliss. It's do what feels good, because that's authentic to you. There's no one thing that's good for everybody to do—to eat this or do that. I can only give you general principles. It's by following what feels good to you that you check in with your own intuition, your own inner wisdom, and that's how you know what's good for you. So that's what it boils down to.

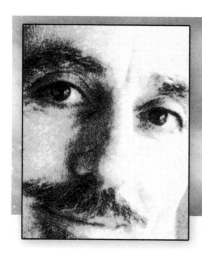

EXPLORING THE FRONTIERS of ANTI-AGING MEDICINE

An Interview with Dr. Marios Kyriazis

Marios Kyriazis, M.D., is both a clinician and a researcher in the field of anti-aging medicine. He has made significant contributions in the science and application of anti-aging medicine, and he is considered one of Britain's leading longevity specialists. Dr. Kyriazis is one of the world's experts on the subject of how carnosine effects the aging process, and his research into the effects of this mighty amino acid dipeptide have revealed how it can offer a number of unique and substantial health benefits.

Dr. Kyriazis has a postgraduate degree in Gerontology from the King's College, University of London, and another in Geriatric Medicine, granted by the Royal College of Physicians. He is also a Chartered Biologist and a Member of the Institute of Biology for his work in the biology of aging. Dr. Kyriazis is the founder and medical advisor to the British Longevity Society, and he is a certified member of the American Academy of Anti-Aging Medicine. He is also an adviser to several other age-related organizations.

Dr. Kyriazis has extensive experience with nutritional supplements and anti-aging drugs. He is the author of several books on these subjects, including The Anti-Aging Plan, Stay Young Longer—Naturally, The Anti-Aging Cookbook, The Look Young Bible, *and* Carnosine and Other Elixirs Of Youth.

*Dr. Kyriazis lives in Hertfordshire, England. I interviewed
him on November 6, 2004. Dr. Kyriazis has a warm and
thoughtful manner about him. We spoke about the best ways
to slow down the aging process, his research and clinical
experience with carnosine, and how just the right amount of
stress can actually benefit our health.*

David: What do you think are the primary causes of aging?

Dr. Kyriazis: When I think about the primary causes of aging, I divide them
into two groups—fifty percent genetic and fifty percent environmental.
From the environment we get free radicals, glycosylation, and hormonal
changes. At the moment I don't think there is anything that we can do
about the genetic part, but we can of course influence the environmental
part of aging. So I am working in clinical medicine to offer ways of
counteracting the environmental causes, or the environmental basis of
aging.

*David: How do you differentiate between the biological symptoms of
aging and those bodily changes that are actually caused by one's belief
about aging?*

Dr. Kyriazis: It depends at what level one looks. I am more interested
in the clinical level, although I have done biological research as well.
I think there are different ways of looking at it. Biology will start with
the molecules and the cells, and say this is an age-related phenomenon,
a disease-related phenomenon. From my point of view, I see individual
patients. People usually come to see me because they have an age-related
illness. So they come with, say, heart disease, or a prostate problem,
which are age-related. Then when we expand on the actual causes of
their problem, they want to know more and find out about other age-
related processes which may affect them. So it is a combined thing. I
don't necessarily make a distinction myself in my work.

*David: What do you think are currently the best ways to slow down, or
reverse the aging process and extend the human life span?*

Dr. Kyriazis: I offer a combination of different therapies affecting the
entire body. For example, I recommend antioxidants and anti-glycator

drugs or supplements. Apart from the ordinary vitamins and nutrients, I recommend carnosine, DHEA, and other hormones, depending upon whether the individual is deficient in those hormones or not. I also recommend a nutritional lifestyle and exercise—but not ordinary exercise. It's a combination of different unusual exercises (which I discuss in my book, *The Anti-Aging Plan*), plus mental and sense exercises as well.

I try to make it easy for the individual to follow this, because many times people think that it's much easier to just take a tablet or a capsule, rather than change their lifestyle. But I think it is very important to find a way to motivate the individual to change their lifestyle. So, in other words, it's a combination approach of different things all working together. Some people say, oh take four different supplements, or four different hormones, and you are covered. I don't agree with that. I think that there are so many different aspects of aging, and that we need to use different treatments, a multi-pronged approach. So that's what I say to my patients.

David: Can you talk a little about some of the beneficial effects your patients have had with carnosine supplements?

Dr. Kyriazis: Yes. I think I was the first person to use carnosine for anti-aging purposes. Carnosine has been around for quite some time, and athletes used to use it to enhance muscle and performance. But I began using it specifically for anti-aging back in 1999. And the first person who took carnosine under my guidance still takes it today, five years later, and everyone says how young she looks generally. Her head hasn't got a single grey hair—not one—although she's now 48 or 49. This corresponds with experiences we have had with other patients. In other words, they generally look younger. Their hair grows better, and it stays black, or whatever color it is, but not grey. Many people experience increased energy. Mental performance, memory, and other brain functions improve as well.

But I always say to people that carnosine is not something that you can notice yourself. It's something that works inside the body over the long-term, over ten or twenty years to prevent all the different age-related processes and damages that happen. I see carnosine mainly as a preventative treatment, not so much as an immediate treatment for some specific disorder, or to be noticeable. It doesn't immediately produce noticeable effects, although there are ways of doing different biochemical tests, blood tests, and so on that show an overall improvement over the years.

I use carnosine on patients who are normally healthy, who don't have a disease. For example, I don't use it on people who have muscular dystrophy or other muscular diseases. I think some people take it for that, but I don't know whether it works or not. So it is difficult to differentiate and see a noticeable improvement on a healthy person. It's much easier to notice if somebody is ill and he or she gets better after taking it. But this supplement is mainly used by healthy people in the long-term.

David: Can you talk a little about carnosine's anti-glycosylation effect, and how it protects the body from dangerous cross-linked, oxidized proteins?

Dr. Kyriazis: Everybody thinks that free radicals and oxidation are the main causes of aging, but there's another important one, which is glycosylation, and this happens all the time. It is due to glucose or other molecules attaching to proteins. This causes cross-linking and "advanced glycosylation end-products" or AGEs. I would say that this causes more damage to the body than free radicals, and carnosine prevents this damage in different ways.

First of all, it prevents free radical attacks because it's an antioxidant. But it is also an anti-glycosylator. In other words, it prevents the proteins from being cross-linked. If two proteins that are not supposed to attach to each other become attached and combine together, then they become useless. That's what happens in cross-linking, and carnosine prevents that. Carnosine is like a shield that protects proteins. So when two proteins come together, they don't attach to each other. They remain free to function normally.

So the first stage is that carnosine prevents glycosylation in the first place. The second stage is that if glycosylation has already happened, if the two proteins have become cross-linked, carnosine will facilitate the removal of these useless proteins. Actually, our body is trying to eliminate abnormal proteins all the time, but with aging this rate of elimination slows down. Therefore, we have an accumulation of abnormal proteins. But carnosine speeds up the rate of elimination, so all the junk material we have in our body gets eliminated quicker.

There is also some evidence that carnosine can actually break the existing bonds between the two cross-linked proteins. So if the proteins have become attached to each other, and they are cross-linked, in some circumstances carnosine can break the bond and allow them to be free again, and to function normally. So carnosine has three different benefits in addition to being an antioxidant.

David: What kind of dosage do you recommend a healthy person take?

Dr. Kyriazis: I started with fifty milligrams a day, but now I recommend a higher dose—perhaps about two hundred milligrams a day. I know that some people use a thousand or more milligrams a day, but I don't see the reason for that. I think about two hundred milligrams a day, in association with other supplements, should be enough for a healthy person.

David: What are your thoughts about using N-Acetylcarnosine eye drops—which breakdown into carnosine in the eye—as a way to protect the health of one's eyes?

Dr. Kyriazis: This is also a very promising development. I was involved with advising the different researchers at the companies that are now marketing acetylcarnosine. The things that carnosine does as a tablet don't work as well as when it is used as an eye drop. But acetylcarnosine as an eye drop is quite resistant to the enzymatic processes that break down carnosine. Carnosine is broken down by the enzyme carnosinase, and if we give carnosine eye drops it would soon break down before it can have a chance to work properly in the eye. But acetylcarnosine is resistant to carnosinase, therefore it is not easily broken down in the eye, and it remains around to produce its effects. But acetylcarnosine as a capsule or a tablet in the body is not as effective as simple carnosine in tablet form. So we have this difference between the two. One is effective as a tablet but not as an eye drop. The other one is effective as an eye drop but not as a tablet. This is due to the enzyme carnosinase in the eye, which breaks carnosine down easily.

David: What sort of benefit does acetylcarnosine have on the eyes?

Dr. Kyriazis: It helps the eye in different ways. Most importantly, acetylcarnosine helps patients who have cataracts. There's quite a lot of research showing that carnosine not only prevents the formation of cataracts, but most importantly it reverses existing cataracts as well. So it can be used as a treatment for existing cataracts, and one can actually avoid the need for an operation. This is something that not many people know. But I think it's a very good development, and now it's being promoted all over the world. I was in Russia a few days ago, where we had a seminar examining the beneficial effects of acetylcarnosine on cataracts. There are also benefits with other eye diseases. For example, it helps people who suffer from glaucoma or macular degeneration. It also helps people who wear contact lenses, or people who work in front of the computer and get tired eyes or itchy sore eyes. It has been shown that acetylcarnosine eye drops work very well to prevent all these eye conditions.

David: In general, what sort of relationship do you see between stress and health, and how can a certain degree of physical or mental stress— such as through caloric restriction—actually benefit our health?

Dr. Kyriazis: This is based on the concept of hormesis. Hormesis means that after mild stimulation different biochemical processes are activated that try to repair the mild damage that happens to the body, and in trying to repair this damage they also repair any coexisting age-related damage. So we are able to activate this process by different means so that our body will then repair the damage on its own. And research shows that we can activate it with different things—like putting an experimental animal in high-gravity conditions, high temperature, or increasing radiation. But these concepts don't apply to human beings.

Concepts that do apply to human beings are stress and stimulation by, say, calorie restriction, or by certain physical exercises, mental exercises, or by keeping the body active in different ways—by keeping it alert, by not following certain routines, by constantly changing one's lifestyle and keeping the body constantly stimulated. This activates hormesis which repairs damage in different parts of the body. So although people say stress is bad for you, I think what they mean is that excessive stress is bad for you. Mild stress isn't bad for you, and, in fact, mild stress is beneficial. I don't think that people who try to avoid stress altogether are doing themselves any favors.

I think that we should keep ourselves mildly stimulated all the time. And looking forward to the future, we are working with some of the scientists who developed the concept of hormesis to develop a type of mechanical stimulation. For example, putting human beings into something that is equivalent to a fairground ride, where they go into increased acceleration, which simulates hyper-gravity, or mildly increased radiation through a sauna. This would be like a small booth, and when people go in, it is very hot. But instead of having only heat, in addition you have mildly increased radiation. So people go and have their sauna, their steam bath or whatever, but there is also background radiation to stimulate their hormetic mechanism. And that would be commercially available, but at the moment it's not. It is still under investigation. But apart from ordinary stress and stimulation there could be mechanical ways of stimulating hormesis.

David: What advice would you give to someone who is looking to improve their mental performance?

Dr. Kyriazis: I would recommend a combination of constant mental stimulation, mental exercises, with supplements or drugs that have been shown to improve mental performance—like hydergine, ginkgo biloba, vinpocetine, and bacopa. Bacopa is a Ayurvedic medicine Indian plant product. I recommend you use this with acetylcarnosine and Alpha Lipoic Acid. I think it's important to try to alternate the treatment, to not have the same treatment all the time. For example, for one month, have a combination of ginkgo biloba with Alpha Lipoic Acid. The next month have vinpocetine with vitamin E. Then the next month change it again, and keep rotating the treatment. Don't have the same treatment all the time. And have that in association with brain exercises, like I mentioned in my book. There are different exercises that stimulate different parts of the brain. Some stimulate the left side of the brain, and others the right side. Other exercises stimulate memory, coordination, learning, and observation.

David: What sort of relationship do you see between one's mental state and their physical health?

Dr. Kyriazis: I think one's mental state is very important. It has been shown that there is quite a distinct relationship between the way we feel and the way our body behaves. People who have a positive outlook on life, who engage in positive thinking, and are always cheerful have higher degrees of different immunoglobulins. In other words, their immune system is working at peak form, and that prevents not only infection, but also cancer and different age-related processes as well. If our immune system is working at full power, then we don't age quickly.

There has been research on people who engage in positive thinking about their cancer, particularly breast cancer, and the studies have shown that the more positive these people are the more likely they are that they'll be cured, and the less likely that the cancer will come back. That has to do with the immune system. Positive thinking and having a positive attitude stimulate the immune system. For example, I had a patient who was always thinking positively, and seeing the positive side of life. She developed breast cancer, and she was always saying that the cancer is not going to win, she will win. And she managed to survive against all odds by only the power of her mind. All the doctors were saying that she won't survive further than three months, or six months, and she survived five years. I believe that was because of her positive attitude.

David: You discuss a number of alternative health therapies in your book, The Anti-Aging Plan*, such as acupuncture, aromatherapy, biofeedback, homeopathy, and herbalism. What sort of advice would you give to someone who is interested in exploring some of these alternative or complementary therapies?*

Dr. Kyriazis: It is quite difficult to give scientific advice, because I don't think there is quite a lot of research supporting each of those therapies in relation to aging. There may be research supporting therapies in relation to age-related diseases. For example, hydrotherapy is very good for people who have arthritis, sore joints or sore muscles. If they went into a course of hydrotherapy, aqua-aerobics, or something like that, they would benefit exceedingly. But there isn't any research examining the effects of these therapies on the actual aging process itself, so it is more clinically-oriented than biologically-oriented.

I also say to people that if something doesn't work for them then they should try something else. Don't give up. There's always an answer to something. There is always a treatment to our illness. Something that works for somebody else may not work for you, or the other way around. Sometimes one's friends may experience a benefit from using a particular therapy, but that doesn't mean that it'll work for you too. Up to a point, I tend not to base my advice on published research—because I think that sometimes the individual may experience benefits even if there is no scientific research behind the therapy at all. In other words, science has not caught up yet with the benefits that these therapies have to offer.

So, basically, I recommend that—in association with your health practitioner—you find a therapy that is suitable for you and try it for, I would say, around two months, more or less. Something like that. If it works, continue it. If it doesn't work, leave it and try something else. The very fact that you are exploring different therapies is a form of mental stimulation, which contributes to mental health and brain health. So keep looking. Keep searching.

David: What are some of the new anti-aging treatments that you foresee coming along in the near future?

Dr. Kyriazis: I think one of the most promising is a crosslink breaker. It's a drug called Alagebrium, and it's manufactured by Alteon Corporation in the States. This has been shown to actually revert age-related damage—not only prevent it, but revert it, because it breaks existing bonds between the crosslinked proteins. This has been used now in reverting blood pressure, because glycosylation causes thickening of the arteries, and thickened arteries result in high blood pressure. Because this drug reverses glycosylation, that means it also reverses blood pressure, heart disease, and stroke—before the damage happens. But it is mainly used for reversing and curing blood pressure—not just masking symptoms, but actually curing blood pressure. So that's one drug.

We have other therapies with stem cells, which are also commercially available. They cost quite a lot of money, but they are becoming available, both in the States and in other parts of the world. They are actual stem cells by injection, like the new treatment for wrinkles called Isolagen. This is based on stem cell research, on taking blood from your own body, or cells from inside your mouth, growing them, and then injecting them back into the body to reverse wrinkles.

So basically there are quite a few things on the horizon which would become not only available but also accessible to many people, because they won't be as expensive as they are now.

David: What are you currently working on?

Dr. Kyriazis: I have several projects, but the main one that I'm working on now is to try to devise more exercises, and look into the scientific basis of stimulation and aging, like we discussed before with hormesis. I'm trying to see what else we can find to stimulate the body, to work against aging. There is quite a lot of research showing that different forms of stimulation from mental exercises, mental stimulation, or living in an enriched environment has a positive beneficial effect on several biochemical and anatomical changes, both in the brain and in the immune system. So I'm trying to get a clear understanding of these mechanisms, and come up with clinical ways, patient-oriented ways, for making use of these benefits.

David: Is there anything that we haven't discussed that you would like to add?

Dr. Kyriazis: I always recommend for people to try and explore their own therapies. Try to find new things, new therapies, and new avenues. Keep an open mind, and a positive mind. And accept your age. If somebody is forty or sixty or seventy, it doesn't really matter. What matters is whether they have the characteristics of youth—which is strong muscles, clear memory, a good immune system, and a good sex drive. If you have all these characteristics, and you're happy, then so be it. It doesn't matter how old you actually are. I'm not so much involved with or interested in cosmetics, although I have done quite a lot of research in that area. But I don't think the way one looks is important. I think the way one feels is important. So if you feel happy, active, and full of energy, then that's fine. It doesn't matter how you look.

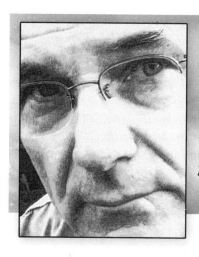

MANUFACTURING
the
AIDS VIRUS

An Interview with Dr. Peter Duesberg

Peter Duesberg, Ph.D. is a professor of molecular and cell biology at the University of California at Berkeley. He is a pioneer in retrovirus research, and he was the first scientist to isolate a cancer gene. More recently, Dr. Duesberg has gained recognition for his theory that abnormal chromosome numbers are the causes of cancer, which challenges the conventional mutation theory. However, he is probably best known for challenging the widely-held theory that HIV is the cause of AIDS.

Dr. Duesberg earned his Ph.D. in chemistry at the University of Frankfurt in Germany in 1963. He isolated the first cancer gene through his work on retroviruses in 1970, and he mapped the genetic structure of these viruses. This, and his subsequent work in the same field, resulted in his election to the National Academy of Sciences in 1986. He was also the recipient of a seven-year Outstanding Investigator Grant from the National Institutes of Health, before he called the HIV-AIDS hypothesis into question.

Dr. Duesberg is the author of Inventing the AIDS Virus, *and his articles challenging the HIV/AIDS hypothesis have appeared in scientific journals worldwide including* The New England Journal of Medicine, Science, Cancer Research, the Proceedings of the National Academy of Sciences, *and*

Nature. *On the basis of his experience with retroviruses, Dr. Duesberg concludes that it is impossible for HIV to be the cause of AIDS, and that AIDS is, in fact, a nonviral disease. He has instead proposed the hypothesis that the various American and European AIDS diseases are brought on by the long-term consumption of amyl nitrites or "poppers" and other recreational drugs, and/or by the use of the extremely toxic drug AZT, which is a chain-terminator of DNA synthesis that was originally developed for chemotherapy of cancer and is now prescribed to prevent or treat AIDS.*

Despite Dr. Duesberg's impressive track record, and the fact that his ideas about AIDS are truly compelling if one studies them carefully, he has found himself at direct odds with the medical establishment since he began talking about his controversial AIDS hypothesis. Many AIDS researchers and drug companies have reacted hostilely to Dr. Duesberg's hypothesis. For example, when I interviewed neuroscientist and AIDS researcher Candace Pert from Georgetown University, and I asked her what she thought about the scientists that don't think that the HIV virus is responsible for causing AIDS, she replied, "These people are nuts."

However, some other scientists think differently and strongly respect Dr. Duesberg's ideas—including Nobel laureates in chemistry Kary Mullis and Walter Gilbert. Duesberg, Mullis, and Gilbert all point out that there is no direct experimental evidence that HIV causes AIDS, and that there are numerous problems with the HIV-AIDS theory. For example, not everyone infected with HIV gets AIDS, and not everyone with AIDS symptoms is infected with HIV. In fact, the symptoms of AIDS vary from continent to continent, and a medical diagnosis of AIDS is often made simply by testing positive for HIV antibodies in the presence of a disease such as tuberculosis or cancer. However, instead of engaging in scientific debate, according to Dr. Duesberg, the only response from the scientific establishment has been to cut off funding to further test his hypothesis.

To find out more about Dr. Duesberg's work, see Harvey Bialy's biography Oncogenes Aneuploidy and AIDS: The Scientific Life & Times of Peter H. Duesberg *(North Atlantic books, Berkeley CA, 2004), or visit Dr. Duesberg's Web site at: www.duesberg.com.*

I interviewed Dr. Duesberg in December of 2005. We spoke about why he thinks that it's a mistake to assume that the HIV virus is the cause of AIDS, why so many researchers are resistant to examining the idea that HIV may not be the cause of AIDS, and what he thinks the real cause of AIDS might be.

David: What originally inspired your interest in molecular biology?

Peter: The idea that there are cancer viruses, and thus ways to understand cancer and perhaps prevent or cure it by vaccines, inspired me forty years ago. I was young enough to ignore, or better, not even know objections.

David: If you could just briefly summarize—what are some of the primary reasons why you think that it's a mistake to assume that the HIV virus is the cause of AIDS?

Peter: Here are four out of many more "primary reasons":

First, AIDS is not infectious. For example, between 1981 and 2004, 930,000 American AIDS patients had been treated by doctors or health care workers. But, despite the absence of an anti-AIDS vaccine, there is not a single case report in the peer-reviewed literature of a doctor or health care worker, who has ever contracted AIDS (rather than just HIV) from any one of these 930,000 patients in now twenty-five years. Likewise, not one of the thousands of HIV-AIDS researchers has ever contracted AIDS from HIV, nor is there an AIDS epidemic among prostitutes anywhere in the world.

Second, like all other viruses, HIV induces anti-viral immunity, which is the basis of the HIV/AIDS test. But, unlike any conventional viral epidemic or individual disease, AIDS is not self-limiting by anti-viral immunity and thus not likely to be caused by a virus.

Third, unlike all other viral epidemics, AIDS in the U.S. and Europe is highly nonrandom: A third of all patients are intravenous drug users and about two-thirds are male homosexuals, who have used nitrite inhalants, amphetamines, cocaine and other aphrodisiac and psychoactive drugs for years before they develop any one or more of the twenty-six different AIDS-defining diseases. In addition, most HIV-antibody-positive people are now prescribed inevitably toxic DNA chain-terminators as anti-HIV drugs. But these terminators are AIDS by prescription, because they were designed to kill cells (for chemotherapy) and are thus also immunotoxic. Thus the AIDS epidemic does not spread randomly like a conventional viral epidemic and coincides with toxic drug use.

Fourth, there is no HIV in AIDS patients. Instead, only antibody against HIV or traces of HIV nucleic acid can be found in typical AIDS patients. But, conventional pathogenic viruses are abundant and not (yet) neutralized by antibodies when they cause diseases.

David: Can you talk a little about why you think that recreational drug use is the primary cause of AIDS among gay men?

Peter: There is both correlative and functional evidence in the AIDS literature that nitrite inhalants coincide with Kaposi sarcoma and other AIDS diseases among homosexual users, and that nitrites are cytotoxic, immunotoxic and Kaposi-sarcomagenic. It is also known for decades that the long-term use of amphetamines and cocaine cause weight loss, immunodeficiency, dementia and other AIDS-defining diseases. It is the long-term use of such recreational drugs alone or in combination with anti-HIV drugs that American and European AIDS patients have in common.

By contrast, millions of HIV-antibody-positive people from without these risk groups are AIDS-free. For example, since 1985 there are one million HIV-positive people living in the U.S., but only about 30,000 of them (three percent) have any one of the twenty-six AIDS-diseases per year—namely exactly the minority of them that uses recreational and anti-HIV drugs.

David: Why do you think that there is such a high correlation between HIV and AIDS?

Peter: The correlation is a hundred percent because AIDS is defined by the U.S. Center for Disease Control, and thus for the world (!), as one or more of twenty-six previously known diseases, if they occur in the presence of antibody against HIV. For example, all tuberculosis patients, who have antibodies against HIV are called AIDS patients. By contrast, HIV-free tuberculosis patients are still tuberculosis patients. Thus, the one hundred percent correlation is an artifact of the AIDS definition, rather than a natural coincidence.

David: When I interviewed neuroscience and AIDS researcher Candace Pert I said to her that, "A few scientists that I've spoken with told me that they don't think that the HIV virus is responsible for causing AIDS."

When I asked her what she thought about this idea she said, "...These people are nuts. The evidence is clear, and it's the most elegant scientific story. There was a movement against HIV research, and the main champion was Peter Duesberg. There were some personal animosities against the power and the money that the early AIDS researchers got, and there are a lot of political aspects to this. But beyond a shadow of a doubt—and I'm speaking as somebody who studies data in the lab— there is just no doubt about the fact that HIV is the cause of AIDS.

There's just so much elegant science behind it. Just let me site one little tidbit that tells you how clean the whole thing is. There are two primary receptors that the AIDS virus uses to enter and infect cells. One of them is called CCR-5. It turns out that a small percentage of Caucasian Europeans don't have that receptor. They have a genetic mutation where the receptor should be, and it's missing a major chunk of it in the middle. Now those people who have that mutation, no matter what risky behavior they indulge in, they do not get HIV disease...Then, of course, you can show clearly in the test tube that you can artificially make cells that have this receptor and they will become readily infected with the viruses that use this receptor. And if the cells don't have the receptor then they don't.

*That's summarizing like hundreds and hundreds of papers that elegantly
address this, so there's no doubt that HIV causes AIDS. Duesberg may
not like some of the HIV virologists, and their style and all, but it's just
so silly. And it's sad, because they've created a movement that's been
very destructive. My understanding is that out in California some of
these people are like Luddites. Some of the activists—not all of them,
but some small percentage—have gotten this into their head, and have
stormed research labs. They've gotten very angry and very crazy, and
it's complete rubbish. I have no doubt in my mind. I'm a hundred percent
sure about this."*

How would you respond to Candace?

Peter: Take for example Candace's "tidbit" of the "elegant science" of
AIDS, that "a small percentage of Caucasian Europeans don't have that
receptor" for HIV and "no matter what risky behavior they indulge in,
they do not get HIV disease"—which means according to the CDC: no
dementia, no diarrhea, no Kaposi sarcoma, no tuberculosis, no yeast
infection, no lymphoma, no cervical cancer, no weight loss, no fevers,
no pneumocystis pneumonia etc. Elegant indeed!

Fortunately in the U.S., God must have distributed Candace Pert's
elegant HIV non-receptors otherwise: Here the majority of the
heterosexual population has no HIV-receptors and therefore does not
get AIDS! Instead, God must have distributed good HIV-receptors
in the U.S. non-randomly to male homosexuals, junkies and a few
hemophiliacs and transfusion recipients, which make up over ninety-
five percent of the American AIDS cases. Lets thank God that our
mainstream heterosexuals—from our president to our leading HIV-
AIDS researchers—are genetically protected against this "deadly" virus
via defective HIV receptors, and are therefore AIDS-free—ever since
this virus is said to have arrived in the U.S. over twenty years ago.

*David: Why do you think that so many researchers are resistant to
examining the idea that HIV may not be the cause of AIDS?*

Peter: Scientists are selected for instincts that help them to get funding,
recognition, invitations to meetings, access to publications and awards.
None of these are available to scientific minorities. On the contrary,

minorities are excommunicated at many levels from the consenting majorities, even from personal contacts with mainstream colleagues. Those are strong incentives for scientists not to "examine" unpopular ideas.

David: What do you think it will take to convince the scientific establishment that HIV is not the cause of AIDS?

Peter: It will take hypothesis-independent funding of research. If funding were available for non-HIV-AIDS hypotheses, AIDS would probably be solved very shortly on the basis of the drug or chemical AIDS hypothesis—as shown in our paper "The chemical bases of the various AIDS epidemics: recreational drugs, chemotherapy and malnutrition," published in the *Journal Biosciences of the Indian Academy of Sciences* in 2003, with support from private sources. According to this hypothesis AIDS is caused by recreational and antiviral drugs.

This hypothesis is already confirmed by exact correlations, and could be easily tested experimentally in animals and epidemiologically in the millions of human volunteers, who are HIV-free recreational drug addicts and develop AIDS-defining diseases under their old names. If confirmed, this hypothesis could readily solve AIDS by banning the inevitably toxic anti-HIV drugs and by warning the recreational drug users against the AIDS consequences of their drugs or lifestyle.

David: Are there any new developments since the publication of your book Inventing the AIDS Virus *that you think are important for people to know?*

Peter: In principle, no. The HIV-AIDS hypothesis has recycled the same unproductive ideas and arguments for invisible or undetectable HIV, for toxic anti-HIV drugs, and excuses for failing vaccines in various formulations, for twenty-one years.

We have pointed this out in two papers since *Inventing the AIDS Virus*, which was first published in 1996. One of these papers, "The AIDS dilemma: drug diseases blamed on a passenger virus" by Duesberg & Rasnick was published in *Genetica* in 1998. The other paper, "The chemical bases of the various AIDS epidemics: recreational drugs, anti-

HIV drugs and malnutrition," by Duesberg, Koehnlein & Rasnick, was published in the *Journal of Biosciences* in 2003.

These papers analyze old and new paradoxes generated by the HIV hypothesis, and address new and old evidence for chemical AIDS, namely AIDS caused by recreational drugs, antiviral drugs and malnutrition.

David: What are some of the ways that you think a prevailing scientific paradigm can limit our medical understanding?

Peter: By becoming a monopoly able to control funding and publication, as is the case now with the HIV-AIDS monopoly and to a slightly lesser degree with the oncogene-cancer monopoly.

David: What do you think should be done to help improve medical research in general?

Peter: Generate a free market for scientific ideas in which funding depends on logic, scientific principles, and useful results, rather than on approval, or better yet the blessings of "peer-review." Since the "peers" represent the established scientific monopolies their self-interest demands "science" that confirms and extends the status quo— rather than innovation, which threatens their considerable scientific and commercial investments.

The only way to achieve innovation is to replace the so-called peer-review system by a system modeled after American courtroom juries, in which only jurors without any investments in the case on trial are judging the merits of a case.

The claim that only established "peers" have the knowledge to decide on AIDS, cancer, Alzheimer's etc. is not consistent with their failures to explain or cure these diseases. And is not consistent even with the spirit of our constitution, where neither the law nor the health of the citizens should be left solely to the powers of the "experts." The claims for exclusive authority of "scientific peers" are no more valid than those of their legal counterparts nor those of their predecessors who wrote prescriptions in Latin, or those of their theological counterparts who determine what's moral or ethical via special connections with God.

David: What do you think are the primary causes of aging?

Peter: I don't know. It's an interesting question. But, if I were to work on it, I would look at the three factors that generate the un-aged prototype: (1) The karyotype or species-specific chromosome combination; (2) The genes; and (3) The differential expression of thousands of genes or "epigenetic" controls that generate differentiated phenotypes. I would plan experiments which compare karyotypes, genes and gene expressions of un-aged prototypes with aged counterparts.

David: What do you think are currently the best ways to slow down, or reverse the aging process and extend the human life span?

Peter: The answer would depend on the experiments proposed in my last answer. But it is already known from the experimental literature that the life-span can be much extended, by about a third, and the cancer-risk reduced by minimizing the metabolism and cell divisions by limiting the diet. So aging could probably be slowed down by minimizing the inevitably fallible processes that replicate chromosomes and genes, and maintain differentiated function by limiting metabolism via the diet.

David: What are some of the new medical breakthroughs that you foresee coming along in the near future?

Peter: I am very skeptical—indeed I am scared—of a "new medical breakthrough" from the very same medical establishment, which prescribes inevitably cytocidal DNA chain-terminators to hundreds of thousands of healthy people solely because they have made antibodies against the non-cytocidal retrovirus HIV!

David: What are you currently working on?

Peter: The currently prevailing cancer theory postulates that cancer is caused by four to seven gene mutations. However, despite over thirty years of efforts, it has not been possible to find one or a combination of mutant genes in cancers that are able to transform a normal cell to a cancer cell, or are able to cause cancer in an animal.

In view of this I am now studying the chromosomal theory of cancer.

This theory is based on the fact that the numbers or structures of chromosomes of all cancers are abnormal.

However, since the currently prevailing cancer orthodoxy holds that gene mutations cause cancer, I am again working on cancer without funding from any non-private, "peer-reviewed" agencies, such as the National Cancer Institute, despite over fourteen grant applications.

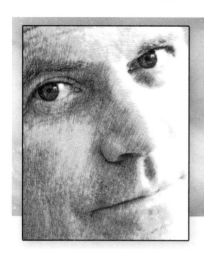

**REDIRECTING
the
IMMUNE SYSTEM**

An Interview with Dr. Kary Mullis

Kary Mullis, Ph.D., won the 1993 Nobel Prize in Chemistry for his invention of the polymerase chain reaction (PCR), which revolutionized the study of genetics. The journal Science *listed Dr. Mullis' invention of PCR as one of the most important scientific breakthroughs in human history.*

PCR is a technique that allows chemists to easily, and inexpensively, replicate as much precise DNA as they need. This solved a core problem in genetics. Before PCR, the existing methods for making copies of those particular strands of DNA that one was interested in were slow, expensive, and imprecise. The brilliance behind this invention, as well as its utter simplicity, lies in PCR's ability to turn the job over to the very biomolecules that nature uses for copying DNA. PCR multiplies a single, microscopic strand of genetic material billions of times within hours. The process has many applications in medicine, genetics, biotechnology, and forensics.

When the Royal Swedish Academy of Sciences awarded Dr. Mullis the Nobel Prize, they said it had "hastened the rapid development of genetic engineering" and "greatly stimulated biochemical research and opened the way for new applications in medicine and biology." Just flipping through any current issue of the journals Science *or* Nature *one will encounter advertisements for PCR systems every few pages. In addition to revolutionizing the study of genetics, it's also influenced popular culture and science fiction. Because PCR has the ability to extract DNA from fossils, it was the theoretical basis for the motion picture* Jurassic Park. *In reality, PCR is the basis of an entirely new scientific discipline, paleobiology.*

Dr. Mullis earned his Ph.D. degree in biochemistry from the University of California at Berkeley in 1972. He has authored several major patents, and has received numerous, highly prestigious awards—including the Japan Prize in 1993, the Thomas A. Edison Award (1993), and the California Scientist of the Year Award (1992). He was inducted into the National Inventors Hall of Fame in 1998.

Dr. Mullis is the author of the book Dancing Naked in the Mind Field, *an autobiographical account of his fascinating, and sometimes mind-bending adventures, which makes a compelling case for the existence of greater mystery in the world around us.*

Dr. Mullis is currently a Distinguished Researcher at Children's Hospital Oakland Research Institute. He also serves on the board of scientific advisors of several companies, provides expert advice in legal matters involving DNA, and is a frequent lecturer at college campuses, corporations, and academic meetings around the world. He is the inventor and founder of Altermune, LLC. To find out more about Dr. Mullis' work, visit his Web site: www.karymullis.com

In the following interview Kary and I discussed his current research, which offers tremendous hope as a medical treatment for dealing with virtually any type of pathogen by engaging the immune system in a novel way.

David: Can you tell me about your latest research project?

Kary: I'm in the process of starting a project which involves a way to redirect the immune system from one target to another, by using a chemical linker that will link an immune response that you have made for one thing to a new target, a target to which you would now like to be immune.

David: How far along are you with this project?

Kary: We already know how to do it, and the experiments that we've tried to do it in with baby rats have worked. In the experiments, we were able to take an immune response in baby rats that was made for this irrelevant organic chemical called phenylarsonic acid, and redirect that to this bacterium that would normally kill rats in a couple of days. By using this method, we made it so that the bacterium wasn't able to grow in them at all. The bacterium that we injected in them, *Haemophilus influenzae*, would have killed them within two days. We gave them the organism first. Then, right after that, we gave them the thing that was going to protect them, and it worked in a really big way. The untreated rats that got the *Haemophilus influenzae* had something like a million microorganisms per milliliter of their blood in 24 hours. It grows really fast in a baby rat. The ones that got our treatment had none that were detectable, which in our protocol is less than 20 per milliliter. So it was a big deal.

That experiment was a contrived experiment. We didn't start with a human that had been accidentally exposed to some pathogen. We started with some rats that had been intentionally exposed, and we knew exactly when and how much. We think that we can take that same system and adapt it, not only to humans, but to just about any human pathogen that we can define beforehand.

For instance, people have defined the pathogen that causes anthrax. We can isolate and grow it in the lab. We can make something that will bind to it. In fact, there are lots of people who have already made things that combine with anthrax. What this invention does is take the thing that combines with anthrax, and use it as one end of a linker, the other end of which binds to the immune response that we already have. The invention is called Altermune, and it defines a class of drugs. In the case of the rats, we injected it in them. Hopefully, we're going to be able to produce Altermune type drugs that you could ingest, so you won't even have to have them injected. But if you've just been infected with smallpox, you won't mind an injection.

David: What are some of the other potential applications that you see for it?

Kary: Most of the possibilities that immediately come to mind have to do with infectious disease. The way we've dealt with modifying our immune system since 1794—when Jenner discovered vaccination—hasn't changed. We vaccinate ourselves for all kinds of things, and we do it in that way—by giving ourselves a damaged or dead copy of what we would like to be immune to. We inject it into your body, and you make an immune response to it over a period of a few weeks or months. Sometimes we have to give it to you on several occasions during that time. You make a whole bunch of antibodies, some of which will bind directly to that thing that we stuck in you or anything like it, and it permanently affects your immune system.

You can make someone immune to anthrax by vaccination, but if it has negative side-effects, they're permanent. The Altermune method takes an immune response that you already have and temporarily redirects it to some target to which you now want to be immune. For the method to work, you have to be prepared for it by having the pathogen in hand, in a fairly purified form. For most of the organisms that we're worried about in terms of bioterrorism, we do.

That's what causes the worry about them—people have been working on them, and they're around. Things like cholera or smallpox, all kinds of terrible things that people have been plagued by, and most of the people in the civilized world are no longer immune to them.

David: The implications sound staggering. What about diseases like cancer and AIDS?

Kary: Everybody asks, what about cancer? Cancer is not at all like an infectious disease, in the sense that every cancer cell is not like every other cancer cell, even in the same tumor. Cancer is a tough one. First, I'm going to deal with diseases that we know the exact nature of, where an organism is responsible for it, and the absence of that organism will cure it. That's most infectious diseases.

AIDS doesn't fall into that category. Nor does it affect many people despite the press that it gets. Plus, the AIDS scientists say you can cure HIV if you want to, but you still can't cure AIDS, because the disease has already done something to you. In terms of an infectious disease, it's kind of an oddball thing. I don't think most of the research is reliable and I am not willing to spend a lot of effort on it. I'm one of the few outspoken people who say that there's no good scientific evidence that the diseases that are called AIDS are really caused by the retrovirus called HIV—in spite of its name. I've had a lot of trouble from people over that issue, because many are convinced that it does. But my assessment is that it is an unsupported and unsubstantiated belief.

There are all kinds of possibilities for the first Altermune targets, but we're going to concentrate on potential bioweapons. There's a list of about twenty different pathogens that people have associated with various biological warfare programs. Most of them came from the Soviet Union, but some of them were developed in the U.S. before 1969, when we stopped making them.

There's fear that some of the pathogens have been produced intentionally and are still out there. How long is it going to be before somebody gives himself smallpox, flies to New York, and walks around for a couple of weeks until he dies? How many people would he infect? How many people would they infect? We have vaccines that may or may not be protective—nobody knows for sure. They might not work fast enough. They're slow in terms of producing their results. With Altermune drugs, you don't have to grow a new immune response; you use a full-strength immune response that you already have in place. You just divert it to the target that you now have in mind—and it's immediate. The chemistry is actually pretty complicated, but chemists are pretty clever these days. I'm glad to be one.

**

In May, 2006, Dr. Mullis added the following addendum about his present activity:

I have several years ago imagined that a particular kind of linker molecules could be employed as drugs against various infectious agents. The molecules would be designed on one end, to correspond, if not exactly, then functionally, to mimic an epitope for a pre-existing immune response, so as to attract antibodies or other immune system effectors. In most cases, the immunogen responsible originally for the immunity in question would be best suited for this function if it were easily synthesizable.

On the other end of the molecule would be a targeting moiety derived from a molecular evolutionary selection, as in the Selex method for aptamers, or the phage display method for peptides. This dual function molecule would serve as a linker between an active immune response and something which the drug user would like to be immune to now. Something like a new strain of influenza or an antibiotic resistant strain of Staphylococcus aureus. I have stewed and brewed over this for some time and am presently being issued a U.S. patent covering the general concept, and am in the unfortunate position for a totally scientific character of having to play business and set up a company to practice the new art and hopefully buy my wife, Nancy, a new house. I've named it Altermune.

On the philosophical side, I am comforted by this new activity. Our brain has created quite a complex, rapidly changing world for our trusty, but blind immune system to function in. The immune system deserves some help from all those brains driving around rapidly spreading diseases.

And I was thinking that my last twenty years would get easier and things would get simpler. The best laid plans of mice and men do often go astray.

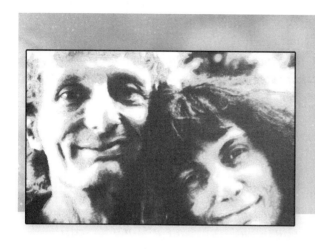

**THE LIFE
EXTENSION
REVOLUTION**

**An Interview with
Durk Pearson
& Sandy Shaw**

Durk Pearson and Sandy Shaw co-authored two of the first and most widely read books on the subject of human longevity— Life Extension: A Practical Scientific Approach *and* The Life Extension Companion—*which triggered a large amount of popular interest in the subject (including my own), and their many television talk show appearances have reached a large number of people over the years.*

Although, perhaps, the ultimate goal of medicine all along, the idea of extending human life in otherwise healthy individuals was a relatively novel concept for most people when Pearson and Shaw published their first book back in 1982. How many people could have predicted back in the early eighties that in just a few years after the publication of Pearson and Shaw's groundbreaking book that there would be such a huge worldwide interest in life extension, anti-aging, and preventative medicine? Pearson and Shaw were not surprised by this new and growing interest and were, in fact, anticipating it.

Pearson and Shaw have been studying life extension since 1968. They are largely self-educated. Pearson graduated from MIT with a triple major in physics, biology, and psychology, and Shaw graduated from UCLA with a double-major in chemistry and zoology. However, most of their knowledge comes from consuming scientific and medical journals with a voracious appetite, talking with colleagues, and experimenting on themselves. In this manner, they have become two of the most well-informed people on the planet regarding the biochemical mechanisms of aging, and they continue to study it full-time. Pearson and Shaw then apply this knowledge in designing nutritional supplement formulations for their own use, some of which are available commercially.

Pearson and Shaw have also been very politically-active over the years with regard to protecting people's rights in America to access nutritional supplements, and to easily obtain available accurate information about the supplements which may benefit their health. To this effect, they wrote the book Freedom of Informed Choice: FDA Versus Nutritional Supplements *(Common Sense Press, 1993), and won a landmark lawsuit against the FDA—Pearson v. Shalala— charging the government agency with unconstitutionally restricting manufacturers from distributing truthful health information (which was viewed as a violation of the constitution's First Amendment guarantee of free speech) that could save many people's lives. This was a landmark achievement for the dietary supplement industry and for the availability of truthful scientific information to consumers.*

This interview occurred on December 16, 2005. Durk and Sandy are responsible for inspiring my own interest in life extension and they have long fascinated me. The couple makes a great team, often completing one another's sentences, and bouncing ideas and facts back and forth off each other as they speak. It's as though their nervous systems are symbiotically intertwined, and the breadth of their knowledge is staggering. It doesn't take much to get them talking passionately about their favorite subjects—life extension and freedom. A few questions can ignite an information explosion. We spoke about how fish oil can improve cardiovascular health, about how the FDA tried to suppress this information, and how they legally forced the FDA into reversing their unconstitutional attempt to suppress the distribution of truthful information.

David: What do you think are the most important nutritional supplements that people should be taking?

Durk: Let me just preface my answer to this question by stating that we're dealing with a system here—a system for handling free radicals and for doing a lot of other things—and just saying, here are the most important three or four nutritional supplements—really does a disservice to people. This is because free radicals are in fact handled by a rather elaborate system that's evolved over the past few billion years that the planet's had oxygen, and just having one of them doesn't really do you anywhere as much good as having a set of them. But if I wanted to mention just one, I would say EPA and DHA, particularly DHA found in oils from cold water fatty fishes. The reason for that is that it can reduce the risk of a sudden-death heart attack by anywhere from about fifty percent to eighty percent, depending on the dose. As little as two meals per week of fatty cold water fish could give you about a forty to fifty percent reduction on your risk of sudden-death heart attacks.

Sandy: Three hundred thousand people die of sudden-death heart attacks every year in the United States, so if all of those people were taking the recommended amounts of fish oil supplements, or the two fatty fish meals a week, then there'd be about fifty percent fewer that would have died. In other words, a hundred and fifty thousand people would not have died.

Durk: They're very inexpensive, very safe, and very effective. You see these sorts of heart attacks on TV all the time. Somebody has a heart attack, the ambulance arrives, and they defibrillate and resuscitate the person and everything is okay. Well, it doesn't work that way outside the hospital, because they have to get that defibrillator to the person within a few minutes.

Sandy: But most of the incidences of fibrillation occur outside of a hospital, usually in a person's home or where they work, and they don't get to the hospital right away. If you lose several minutes, by that time you've either already died or you've suffered irreversible brain damage, so if you do survive you're in a very damaged condition.

Durk: Under the usual conditions, your brain starts dying after about five minutes from a lack of circulation, which occurs when your heart fibrillates—just vibrates and stops pumping blood. Incidentally, that's what happens when you are electrocuted. At about ten minutes, your brain is irreversibly and completely gone. A response time for a really good paramedic operation is about eight minutes. So you can see that there's not much of chance for revival, and in fact, paramedics in the field are actually able to revive about two percent of people whose hearts have gone into fibrillation from a sudden-death heart attack. The DHA is very effective in preventing this from occurring. It doesn't stop the heart attack from happening, but it turns a sudden-death heart attack, which gives you very little chance, into a...

Sandy: ...survivable heart attack, where you do recover, and you don't have irreversible damage to the brain. You can have a full recovery.

Durk: They can get you to the hospital, and then they can do angioplasty, or put in a standard, quadruple bypass or whatever.

One thing that's very important for people to know about this is that the FDA tried to suppress this information...

Sandy: ...about the benefits of fish oil. We actually sued the FDA in 1994 because they would not permit a health claim that fish oils may reduce the risk of cardiovascular disease.

Durk: It's not that they merely would not permit it; they actually issued a regulation that stated that it was a crime to state that the cold water fish oils, with omega-3 fatty acids, could reduce the risk of cardiovascular disease. It was actually illegal. They specifically made it illegal.

Sandy: So we filed suit for violation of the First Amendment, because they were not permitting the communication of truthful information.

Durk: At the time we filed suit against them in 1994, there were one hundred and seventy-four papers on the subject in the scientific literature. A hundred and seventy of them supported our position; four did not. The four that did not were very small preliminary studies that didn't have the statistical power to detect the fifty percent reduction in sudden-death heart attacks. During the seven years that we litigated against the FDA, one million Americans died premature preventable deaths.

Sandy: Half of the three hundred thousand people dying every year from that wouldn't have died if they'd have been taking fish oil. However, dietary supplement companies, and also food companies offering fish, couldn't tell people about the benefits of fish oil. And because of that, people simply didn't have the information.

Durk: Since the legal case was resolved in our favor in 2001, you're now starting to see claims on fish oil supplements, and recently the FDA even caved in and is allowing claims on fish. So I think we're going to see a very dramatic reduction in people dying of heart attacks as a result of this.

Sandy: I wanted to add that one of the ways that we study the effects of the various supplements is to look at metabolic pathway charts. You see, what happens with free radicals is that they're handled by a chain of antioxidants in the body. It's not just one or a couple that take care of the free radicals that are constantly around in the body. They're constantly there because you're producing them naturally through metabolic activity, and your body has got to handle these free radicals.

The metabolic pathways show you that once a free radical scavenger like vitamin C reacts with a free radical, then it becomes a free radical itself. It becomes an ascorbyl radical. That radical then has to be taken care of by another antioxidant. Glutathione usually takes care of the vitamin C radical, and converts vitamin C back to its reduced state.

Durk: And the way vitamin E works is that it becomes a free radical when it either gives up or attracts an electron. When it has an unpaired electron it's called a tocopherol radical, and that's less reactive and less dangerous than what you started out with, which might be, say, a hydroxyl radical, but it's still dangerous. So the vitamin C hands off the unpaired electron to reduce the vitamin E radical back to vitamin E.

Sandy: Exactly, and this is one reason why clinical trials, where people are supplemented with just one antioxidant, like vitamin E or vitamin C, have not shown very good results. Because, what happens when you give people a large excess of vitamin E, is you end up with a bunch of tocopherol radicals after the vitamin E reacts with the free radicals. The vitamin E is just doing what it should do, but then you don't have enough of, let's say vitamin C, in order to take care of the tocopherol radicals and convert them back to vitamin E.

Durk: If you go back ten or fifteen years and look at the medical literature for large-scale, double-blind, placebo-controlled trials, like where researchers gave people things like large doses of vitamin E, the epidemiological data are positive in terms of vitamin E providing cardiovascular protective effects. However, if you look at the more recent trials it seems that vitamin E isn't working any more. What's going on here? Were these huge early trials wrong? No, what's going on is very simple.

Essentially everybody who is a subject in these new trials is at relatively high cardiovascular risk, or they wouldn't be in trial. You can not afford to have most of the people in trial not be at high risk or the statistical noise will overwhelm the signal you're trying to find. However, almost everybody who is at high cardiovascular risk nowadays is taking a statin. Now the statins work by suppressing the synthesis of a compound called mevalonate, which is used to make cholesterol. This is how the statins work; they block cholesterol synthesis. However, mevalonate is also used to make a substance called Coenzyme Q-10, which is part of the single electron transfer chain controlling chemistry in the mitochondria.

Sandy: It's also part of the pathway that converts the tocopherol radical back into vitamin E.

Durk: So if a person is taking a statin, it's very important that they replace the missing coenzyme Q-10, particularly if they're taking vitamin E. We would suggest if someone's taking a statin that they take a couple hundred milligrams a day of coenzyme Q-10. If they're not taking a statin, but are taking vitamin E, we suggest about 120 milligrams a day. Your ability to synthesize the coenzyme Q-10 degrades as your mitochondria get worse and worse with age.

Sandy: There's another example of the FDA suppressing information. The FDA does not provide any information about this in the Physician's

Desk Reference, the PDR, or the drug inserts for the statins. All this information is approved by the FDA, so it's only FDA information, and they do not provide any information concerning the fact that you have lower levels of coenzyme Q-10 because your ability to synthesize it is decreased by statins. Actually, Dr. Julian Whitaker—a colleague and a friend of ours—petitioned the FDA to have a warning put into the statin literature that people should take coenzyme Q-10 because they're less able to make it. The FDA refused to do it, so people still don't know about this.

Durk: In fact, Merck Pharmaceutical has a patent on the combination of any statin plus coenzyme Q-10 that dates back to 1990. What happens though is that nobody—even Merck—is producing a combination of a statin and coenzyme Q-10. One of the reasons for that is that it's far more difficult to get FDA approval of a combination of drugs than of a single entity.

Also, by the time that they found out about the effects of statins on coenzyme Q-10, the approvals for the statins alone were well under way. It would have delayed the introduction of statins by years if they said, okay, we have to start over again with a combination of a statin and coenzyme Q-10.

Sandy: Moreover, there's a legal liability problem. If people all of a sudden find out that they were at risk by taking statins because they didn't have coenzyme Q-10—and that alone could cause heart damage—then there is the possibility of having a huge number of lawsuits.

Durk: It's very much like the cigarette companies. Some of them, the smaller ones have actually done a lot of work on developing safer cigarettes—R.J. Reynolds, for example. However, there's a legal problem with coming out with a safer cigarette. First, the FDA won't let you say that it's less carcinogenic. Secondly, that's also an admission that your prior cigarettes were more carcinogenic and more dangerous.

Sandy: Whether something is true or not is not the standard the FDA uses in deciding what they will allow you say—it's whether or not you meet the agenda that they have for regulating information. For example, the FDA will not allow any information concerning the use of a natural product that is sold as dietary supplement in the treatment of disease, and yet there is a considerable amount of information that supports doing so. For example, fish oils have been used to treat people who have a very high risk of having a cardiac arrest from fibrillation.

Durk: For example, a friend of ours, his mother had very severe cardiac arrhythmias. She would have about half a dozen attacks a day, even though she was taking multiple prescription drugs to help prevent the cardiac arrhythmias. She wasn't expected to live a year.

We said, continue with the prescription drugs, but add the cold water fish oil, a couple grams a day of EPA plus DHA, plus about four grams a day of taurine, which is a natural nutrient that stabilizes electrically-active tissues against excessive stimulation.

Sandy: Like the heart, the brain, and the eyes, for example.

Durk: She's now down to having an arrhythmic episode about once every six months, instead of half a dozen times a day, and is doing just fine.

Sandy: But that's just a case that we know about. This information is in the literature. It's been in peer-reviewed, scientific publications, that people who have a high risk of arrhythmia can be treated with fish oils, and the fish oil is actually safer than the anti-arrhythmic drugs that people are being treated with these days. Believe it or not, if you don't get exactly the right dose, if there's a little bit too much, they can cause arrhythmias.

Durk: We have a lawsuit against the FDA concerning this. There is a dietary supplement called SAM-e, S-adenosyl-methionine. It occurs naturally in every living cell. It takes part in about two hundred different reactions in every cell, primarily methylation reactions.

Sandy: It's extremely important for regulating the turning on and turning off of genes. I mean, you're talking about a very basic function here.

Durk: And there is a government report, a meta-analysis from the Agency for Healthcare Research and Quality that examined the literature on SAM-e for treating three different conditions: depression, osteo-arthritis, and liver disease. And what they found is that the prescription drugs were better for liver disease but that for treating osteo-arthritis and depression the SAM-e was quite effective and quite comparable to the prescription drugs. It works much faster in treating depression than Prozac. It works much slower than Celebrex® in treating osteo-arthritis, but by an entirely different mechanism. It's not a painkiller like Celebrex; that's why Celebrex works within a couple hours after you take it. However, if you stop taking the Celebrex, or other painkillers—whether it be naproxen, aspirin, or whatever—the pain relief goes away and you're right back where you were before. That's because those drugs do nothing to treat the underlying mechanism of damage, whereas the SAM-e actually stimulates repair.

Sandy: Now that's serious, because the government itself published this report. It was published by a government agency and it's available at seven public government Web sites, so there's nothing secret about this information. It's already available, and what we proposed to do was simply distribute the information widely—to people who don't know about these seven Web sites.

Durk: Yeah, we just wanted to print it up, and incidentally, right on the first page of the government report, permission is explicitly given for anybody to reprint it, right on the very first page. Reading two hundred pages off a CRT screen is a real bummer. Reading it nicely printed is a whole lot easier on your eyes.

Sandy: Would you believe that the FDA is spending taxpayers' money to fight us, simply because we want to distribute information that's already been made public? This is information that the government itself has made public in official statements.

Durk: The FDA is not claiming that the report is false, misleading, or erroneous in any way. What they're saying is that SAM-e is a legal dietary supplement—so long as you don't sell the report. If you sell the report, that turns it into an illegal, unapproved new drug.

Sandy: So our counter-argument to that is, if it's legal unless you provide certain information—and therefore the only issue that exists is the communication of the information—then that makes it a pure First Amendment case.

David: What do you think are the primary causes of aging?

Durk: One of the most important mechanisms is free radical damage in the mitochondria. Dr. Denham Harman's Free Radical Theory of Aging and Age-Related Diseases is holding up very well.

Sandy: But one thing that he actually realized quite early on was that most antioxidants do not get into the mitochondria—where the free radicals are generated. That's actually where you have the most serious problem with free radicals—inside the mitochondria themselves.

Durk: Remember, the mitochondria are your little sub-cellular energy factories. They produce the universal energy molecule ATP by burning carbohydrates and fats, and they do this by a free radical mechanism. There are single electron reactions going on there on purpose. That's an essential part of the way it works, so you can't just suck up all the free radicals. For example, cyanide will do a beautiful job of killing you—and the reason it does this is because it sucks up those single electrons in the mitochondria so you can't make ATP and you die.

Sandy: Yeah, so it's a perfect free radical quencher, which just goes to show that you have to be selective about free radical quenchers. Not just anything that prevents free radicals is going to be good for you.

Durk: A recent paper in *Science* reported that it is possible to stimulate biogenesis of new mitochondria in old cells.

Sandy: That means making new mitochondria. This is critically important when you consider that part of the aging process involves the decreasing numbers of mitochondria per cell, whereby you end up with less energy per cell, because the mitochondria are converting all the energy. But that's what happens with aging—you end up with fewer and fewer mitochondria per cell. Also, a lot of the ones that still exist are damaged and not working too well.

Durk: And leaking a lot of free radicals.

Sandy: One way that you can make new mitochondria is through exercise. One of the beneficial effects of exercise is that it stimulates the biogenesis of mitochondria. So that's one good reason to do exercise, but there's other ways of doing it.

Durk: Arginine, particularly in conjunction with choline and vitamin B-5, that is pantothenate, is able to do this. This increased the production of endothelial-derived nitric oxide.

Sandy: Nitric oxide synthase is the enzyme that makes nitric oxide, and there are three forms of it. One of those forms of nitric oxide synthase is in the endothelial cells, which line blood vessels.

Durk: And it's not only there, it's in all other cells and organelles called caveolae, which are little sub-organs inside of the cells.

Sandy: This endothelial nitric oxide synthase is critically important for preventing cardiovascular disease, for example. A major factor in what happens to people when they get cardiovascular disease is that their endothelial nitric oxide synthase is no longer producing the nitric oxide that they need to keep the blood vessels open.

Durk: So the people end up hypertensive. But it's a lot more than that. Without this endothelially-derived nitric oxide, which is made from arginine, what happens is you don't get a bunch of new mitochondria. However, you can stimulate the biogenesis of mitochondria with compounds that either mimic nitric oxide or nitric oxide itself—and I think is a tremendously important finding in terms of life extension.

Sandy: Arginine is used by nitric oxide synthase to make nitric oxide.

Durk: And acetylcholine is what stimulates the endothelial caveolae synthesis of nitric oxide from arginine. You can make the acetylcholine from choline and pantothenate, that is vitamin B-5.

David: What are some of the new anti-aging treatments that you foresee coming along in the near future?

Durk: I think we're going to see a lot more work on stimulating

mitochondrial biogenesis. Just as an example, the erection drug Cialis®
works by inhibiting the enzyme that breaks down cyclic GMP. Now
cyclic GMP is the second messenger for nitric oxide, and it's in the
pathway of mitochondrial biogenesis.

Sandy: In other words, the cyclic GMP actually takes the information
that the nitric oxide release is providing and then transfers that to other
parts of the metabolic pathways, which continue to pass down the
message.

Durk: And long-acting, cyclic GMP-inducers—ones that work in
things like skeletal muscle, and in neuronal tissue, as well as the smooth
muscle in the penis—may increase longevity if they're long-acting
like Cialis, and they're not too selective. I think that this could help
with mitochondrial biogenesis, and they may be life extension drugs,
although this hasn't been tested. A lot of drugs have been developed
for erectile dysfunction and have been thrown out because they weren't
sufficiently selective for the particular enzyme subtype that occurs in
the smooth muscle in the penis. I think they need to go back and look
at a lot of the drugs that have been thrown out, and examine their effect
on lifespan in mice.

Sandy: One of the real problems right now in the development of life-
extending substances is that nothing is going to be approved by the FDA
for life extension—not prescription drugs, and certainly not dietary
supplements. You can't even provide information about how dietary
supplements can be used in the treatment of disease. There are still a large
number of people that are fighting this in the courts, and by appealing
to the political process. We're involved in litigation and are a part of
that. But until it is possible for people to provide truthful information
concerning potential life-extending effects, then people aren't going to
be finding out about this research.

Look at what the NIH is getting now—some $40 billion a year that
they're spending on scientific research. Well, most of the biomedical
research that's done you never find out about. Unless you're reading
the journals like we do, the only way that you're going to get that
information is occasionally the media will cover something. But that's a
very short-term appearance. So you're not going to get that information

into a product that then can be sold to people on the basis that it does a certain thing, because you can't provide that information.

Durk: Incidentally, we won in the U.S. Court of Appeals, for the district of D.C., in a case against the FDA called Pearson v. Shalala in 1999. They ruled three to zero that it was unconstitutional for the FDA to be prohibiting these four claims which we had brought—one of them was the fish oil claim.

Sandy: Yeah, one of them was that fish oil may reduce the risk of cardiovascular disease, and that it was unconstitutional for them to prohibit those claims.

Durk: The FDA asked for a rehearing, and that was turned down eleven to zero. Not only was it turned down eleven to zero, normally when that happens there's just a note, a one-word note: refused. In this case they wrote another page and a half blasting the FDA for not getting it. In fact, the FDA had actually told a federal judge, the FDA lawyer, that they didn't think the First Amendment applied to them. That was at a magistrate settlement hearing before a federal magistrate. Now that's really scary.

Sandy: It just goes to show where the FDA comes from. They didn't think the First Amendment applied to them?

Durk: They didn't appeal it to the Supreme Court, probably because realizing that if they did they'd lose on that, and they'd lose even more.

Sandy: That's undoubtedly the reason they did it.

Durk: So what they did is they actually announced in the federal register that their regulations have been declared unconstitutional, but they also announced—and this takes your breath away—that they were going to continue to enforce them.

Sandy: That is, until they had developed a process and decided what they were going to do. So, in the meantime, until they decided what they were going to do about it, they were going to continue to enforce these unconstitutional regulations.

Durk: Now, our attorney Jonathan Emord said nothing like that had happened since the Civil War, when Lincoln tried to arrest Chief Justice Tawny and put him in prison. The executive branch of the government normally just does not ignore the courts—or I should say defy? They weren't merely ignoring it; they were willfully defying the courts. So what we did is we asked the judge for a declaratory judgment.

Sandy: The judge at the district court level.

Durk: The Court of Appeals returned it to the district court for final action in terms of enforcing their ruling. She ordered the FDA to rescind the regulations, and they published this thing—no, we're not going to be withdrawing them, even though they've been declared unconstitutional. So we asked the judge for a declaratory judgment that the FDA decision makers were willfully and knowingly violating our constitutional rights. The response from the judge was quicker than anything we've ever seen from a federal court. It was just a few weeks, not six months or a year. The declaratory judgment comes back—they're willfully and knowingly violating our constitutional rights. At that point, we warned them that we are going to sue them as individuals.

Sandy: And take their homes, their cars, everything!

Durk: Yeah, to impoverish them, and sue them for all the legal fees that we have paid to date. A couple of weeks later they decided, whoops, no, we're not going to enforce these anymore.

Sandy: But it took two years. Our victory in Pearson v. Shalala occurred in January 1999, but it took until 2001 before they stopped enforcing the unconstitutional regulations. All this additional stuff had to go on, and the final threat to sue them individually was what did it.

Durk: And during those additional two years another 300,000 Americans died from preventable sudden-death heart attacks.

David: Couldn't they be charged with murder?

Durk: Unfortunately, no. They've got sovereign immunity. However, all I can say is the FDA is not at the scale of Chairman Mao or Joe Stalin, who killed maybe 60 or 80 million people, or Hitler, who killed about 20 million. But they're getting pretty close to Pol Pot.

Sandy: With the fish oil claim you're talking about over a million people who died unnecessarily—and that's just one claim.

David: What do you think are some of the strengths and weaknesses of Western medicine?

Durk: I think the greatest strength is the mechanistic viewpoint. That is, a disease is caused by a mechanism or mechanisms. If you understand what those mechanisms are you can rationally design a process for intervening in those mechanisms to prevent the disease from causing damage and to eliminate the disease.

Sandy: For example, one of the things that you can do is this. Suppose that you know about some prescription drugs that are able to provide some effective treatment for a particular disease, but you don't want to take those drugs. There could be a variety of reasons. They might be dangerous. They have nasty side-effects. Or they're extremely expensive. You may not want to take them, but what you can do is study the mechanism whereby the drug works. The way that the drug affects the disease is by affecting a part of a metabolic pathway. You look at that pathway, and that tells you what the target of the drug is. It also tells you if you're able to target that particular part of the pathway with something else, then you may be able to treat a disease that way. So then what you can do is look at a large variety of natural products. There's a lot of research being done now on the mechanisms of things like flavonoids that you find in fruits and vegetables that are very healthful, on how they work.

Durk: And the curcuminoids that you have in the spice turmeric, which appears to be able to reduce the risk of Alzheimer's disease and cardiovascular disease. And the mechanisms are becoming understood, it's not just that you feed the mice this stuff and they have less Alzheimer's.

Sandy: It's that you have more of an idea of why the substance is having the beneficial effect. You know a lot more than just when you take something it gives you a beneficial effect.

Durk: On the other side, that's the great weakness of the traditional medical systems, like Ayurvedic medicine and traditional chinese medicine. The mechanisms that they talked about were like "hot" and "cold." They're not really biochemical mechanisms.

Sandy: Yeah, it's not helpful.

Durk: But they didn't know enough chemistry to have that. However, the good news is that a lot of Ayurvedic universities and traditional chinese medicine universities are now looking at the basic mechanisms, and guess what? Chinese red yeast rice, which has been used for at least two thousand years to strengthen the pulse—that is the distant pulse at your wrist—well, guess what? The reason it works is that it's got lovastatin and some analogs of lovastatin in it.

Sandy: Yes, it's a natural constituent in the red yeast rice.

Durk: So if you understand mechanisms you could go a whole lot farther, a whole lot faster, a whole lot more effectively. The greatest weakness of Western medicine is the FDA. A great many things are never going to get approved because of the high approval costs. For example, most natural substances, you really can't patent them.

Sandy: And it's just as well. I mean, you don't want somebody to be patenting orange juice or something.

Durk: Legally, these natural substances are a discovery rather than an invention, and you can not patent a discovery. And without a patent you can't afford to do the research necessary for FDA approval.

Sandy: And then because of the FDA you can't provide the information about any treatment effect. For example, there's a recent study that showed that people who drank three eight ounce cups of orange juice a day had a significant increase of twenty-one percent in their HDL level. That is a very substantial increase in HDL. This was a small group of people, but it was a significant effect.

Durk: That's the sort of increase you get with the four dollar-a-day statin—if you got one of the best ones.

Sandy: But you can't provide that information. It's just one of the many things that the FDA will not allow you to communicate.

Durk: As we win more and more cases, and establish more and more precedents about being able to say what's truthful and non-misleading, eventually more and more information is going to get out—because of this litigation that we and others, including friends of ours, are involved in. What we're trying to do is to strip the FDA of its unconstitutional power to suppress truthful, non-misleading information about the health effects of dietary supplements.

Sandy: Certainly they'll complain that that's going to be a hassle and a half, because then they're going to have to do all this sorting, and go through all these claims to make sure that there's not going to be any frauds. There are always frauds out there, but that's no excuse. That is simply no excuse for prohibiting truthful information from being communicated. Enforcing the fraud laws is their problem. They've got to work out how they're going to enforce the fraud laws. In fact, if you look at what they're doing with their budget, they're not putting very much money at all into enforcing fraud laws, and they have a lot of money. Most of their budget is being used for salaries and stuff. They're not protecting the public from frauds.

Durk: In fact, when Pearson v. Shalala was finally enforced in 2001 (when we got the ruling that they were willfully denying our constitutional rights) we forced them to cave in by threat of personal suit, stripping them of their sovereign immunity, which you can do under those conditions, and personally suing them. They held a public seminar about the effects of Pearson v. Shalala, and they actually said publicly they were spending more money on fighting our First Amendment law suits than anything else—than any single other item in enforcement. And there are lots and lots of obvious frauds out there, with people selling magical water which will cure cancer and crap like that.

Sandy: One of the problems with having the truthful communication of information is that it would upset the way that they do things at the FDA, because right now the FDA favors drug companies. There's no doubt about it. The drug companies are in bed with the FDA. The FDA is in bed with the drug companies.

Durk: The big drug companies. The reason for that is that the big drug companies want high approval costs so that the small drug companies can't get drugs approved. Then the small drug companies have to sell out to the big drug companies at a nickel on the dollar.

Sandy: That's precisely right. So what the FDA is trying to do is to reserve treatment information for only drugs, in that way there's no competition from dietary supplements. Supposing that you could advertise that fish oil could be used to prevent arrhythmias, then you'd have a competitor for the anti-arrhythmia prescription drugs. The FDA doesn't want that because the drug companies selling these drugs don't want that. And that's the reason that you have this battle going on.

Durk: Then after retirement high FDA officials either end up going to a pharmaceutical company, a paid for chair of medicine of some sort at a university, or they go on to the board of directors and receive six figure salaries for doing nothing, or working for them in their legal department. If you have taken care of your pharmaceutical company buddies, you really get rewarded when you retire from the FDA.

Sandy: Anyway, the two of us would like to live a long time. This is something that we've been thinking about since 1968 and studying the literature to the extent that we can, and that involves a lot of searches. We subscribe to about twenty-five scientific journals and medical journals, and we read them.

Durk: The cost of all this—including the journals, computer searches, scientific texts and so forth—is about $15,000 a year.

Sandy: That's how we keep up with what's going on, and hopefully we will be able to live a lot longer than we otherwise would have. But the thing is that until the market is opened up, so that it's possible to have competition based on truthful information concerning the effects of all

substances—whether they're drugs, foods, or dietary supplements—
we're going to have this slow progress in anti-aging medicine.

David: How long do you think that the human lifespan can be extended?

Durk: If you take a look at a plant like the chaparral bush you'll discover
that it is as genetically-complicated as human beings, it's a multicellular
differentiated type thing with a lot of terminally-differentiated cells, and
yet they live 12,000 years. I see no reason in principle why human beings
couldn't live a lot longer than now—not necessarily 12,000 years, but
nevertheless a lot longer, like the tortoises. Some of the sea tortoises live
well over two hundred years. Even more interesting is parrots, which
have a higher body temperature and a higher metabolic rate. There are
certain species of parrots that live over a hundred and fifty years. That's
not in the wild; I mean in captivity, where they're well taken care of,
protected from predators, and have their food given to them everyday
and so forth.

Sandy: But, nevertheless, people don't live in the wild either. Not really.
(*Laughter*)

Durk: Exactly, and I see no reason, in principle, why people couldn't
outlive the longest lived parrots, because, as I said, they actually have a
higher body temperature than human beings.

Sandy: It really depends on finding out how aging takes place, which is
being studied. There's a huge quantity of information about aging, and
the body of literature is growing at a dramatic pace. Researchers are
studying how aging takes place, the different critical points in the aging
process that control a lot of what's taking place, and ways that you can
alter how the critical points are functioning.

Durk: Now the government funding of research on aging mechanisms
has both an up and a down side. The up side, of course, is that they're
funding a lot of research, and much of this research is really interesting
and good. The down side is something that Milton Freeman pointed
out back in the early 1980s—that it can cause scientists to go astray. If
you're offered a lot of money to do research here, and not offered any

money to do research over there, you're going to do research here rather than there.

Sandy: For example, for years a huge amount of research has been done on calorically-restricted animals, looking at what changes take place in the animals compared to the animals that are normally fed—that is, that eat as much as they want. Of course this is a very interesting thing, but in the long run this is not telling anybody anything other than, maybe if you starve yourself you can extend your lifespan. In fact, it's still not even established that this mechanism would increase the maximum human lifespan.

Durk: I'd love to see some research done on the metabolic differences in parrots versus human beings—old parrots versus old human beings. Particularly, I'd like someone to look at mitochondrial biogenesis, because parrots have to fly and that's a very energetic task. And yet, even a hundred year old parrot can still fly. I mean, how many hundred year old humans can run a hundred yard dash—in 20 seconds, let alone 10?

Sandy: Another thing about birds is that they have very high blood-glucose levels. In humans, when you have high blood-glucose levels it causes all sorts of problems. You can end up with diabetes, but even if you don't get diabetes, high blood-sugar levels causes a variety of chemical changes. For example, glucose attaches to protein molecules. It's something that happens very readily, and as you age you have more and more proteins that have been altered by glucose.

Durk: This could result, for example, in kidney failure. Even though the parrots have much higher levels of glucose, they don't have these problems. They have some sort of anti-glycation mechanism that either prevents the glycation from occurring in the first place, or reverses it after it happens.

Sandy: Exactly, and I'd sure like to know how that works.

Durk: I know. If a way could be found that could prevent or repair glycation, that would be real good news for a whole lot of diabetics.
Sandy: It will also be a way of slowing aging, because as you get older

these glycated proteins are major factors in the increase of free radical activity, and they decrease the ability of proteins to function.

Durk: They cause loss of elasticity in elastic tissues. They can act as antigens that will stimulate autoimmune diseases. I mean, there are all sorts of nasty things they could do, and yet you've got parrots living for well over a century.

Sandy: If we were the ones that were giving out the money, we'd be giving it for different things. But you know what; we'd never take that job, because we don't want to be giving out other people's money. Another problem with this government-funded research is that, in the end, it's just another special-interest group. It makes the scientists into another special-interest group that are all begging for money from the government. If you read the scientific journals now, it's sort of pathetic—disgusting in fact—how researchers are always complaining that they're not getting enough money. But what's enough? How do you define enough? When you're getting the money from the government, there's never enough. So it's become part of the political process which the two of us avoid like the plague.

David: One of the people that I interviewed for this collection is John Guerin, who started the Ageless Animals Project. According to John, there are a number of animals that don't appear to age. For example, a healthy whale was captured at the age of two hundred and eleven years.

Durk: How did they determine that the whale was two hundred and eleven years old?

David: They used a technique called aspartic acid racemization. Recent research by Jerry Shay at the University of Texas in Dallas showed that whales can live over two hundred years in good health.

Durk: I'd really like to see the scientific references to that, because whales operate at a relatively high body temperature too. They're not cold-blooded, like a sea tortoise.

David: Rockfish don't appear to age either. Rockfish caught around

Alaska have been discovered to be hundreds of years old.

Durk: Well, rockfish operate cold, and free radical reactions double for every seven degrees Fahrenheit. So I can see how a fish that's living just above the freezing point could live a real long time, because that's going to suppress the hell out of free radical reactions. However, when you're dealing with a warm-blooded animal like a whale, that's a whole lot more interesting. Whales are hot like parrots and people.

David: What suggestions would you make for someone who is looking to improve his or her memory and cognitive performance?

Durk: The first thing is you take a look at the raw materials that are required for it, and one of them is choline. Acetylcholine plays a very important role in memory in the brain, and it's very easy to increase the amount of choline and acetylcholine in the brain. There was a paper in *JAMA* which showed that by the time you get into your sixties the amount of choline that you are transporting into your brain drops. It gets into your brain by active transport.

Sandy: Yeah, this is either choline that you're taking as a supplement or choline that you've gotten from your diet. It's in the bloodstream, and is able to get across the blood-brain barrier—but that's where the bottleneck takes place.

Durk: It is active transport that moves the choline into the brain, and by the time you're in your sixties you have maybe twenty or thirty percent of the transport capability moving choline into your brain that you had as a young adult.

Sandy: But you can overcome that by taking a choline supplement.

Durk: If you don't have enough choline in your brain, your brain will actually take apart nerves to scavenge the choline from phosphatidylcholine.

Sandy: Nerve membranes, actually. You have phosphatidylcholine in the nerve membranes.

Durk: And the cholinergic nervous system is a "use it or lose it" type system. That is, the activity of cholinergic nerves in the central nervous system causes the release of neurotrophic factors that keep the nerves alive. If you don't have enough cholinergic activity the nerves start dying back.

Sandy: It's just like muscles that aren't used. The same kind of "use it or lose it" type thing.

Durk: So choline works very nicely. You increase the amount of choline turned into acetylcholine with cofactors that are involved in the synthesis. If you look up on the metabolic pathways chart, one of them is vitamin B-5, calcium pantothenate (pantothenic acid). That works through coenzyme A to increase the acetylation of the choline to form acetylcholine. Another thing that you can do is to take betaine, also called trimethylglycine. It's another methyl donor. A considerable amount of choline gets eaten up, not to make acetylcholine, but to provide methyl groups—because methylation is an important reaction for all sorts of things, including gene control.

Sandy: So if you have a lot of betaine your choline doesn't have to be used for the methyl group and it can be used to make acetylcholine.

Durk: Right. Of the choline that you take, a lot of it gets oxidized into betaine, and by providing the betaine you can reduce that loss. Another thing that you can do is provide other ingredients for neurotransmitters. For example, phenylalanine can be used to make the neuromodulator betaphenethylamine. You need vitamin B-6 and you need copper. It's interesting to note that, according to the old FDA standards, before they lowered the amount of vitamin B-6 that they recommended, something like sixty percent of the population was getting less than the RDA of B-6, which is necessary to form noradrenaline, dopamine, and betaphenethylamine. So you can take a formulation containing phenylalanine and vitamin B-6, and a little bit of copper. Forty percent of the population is not getting the RDA of copper.

David: What suggestions would you make for couples who are looking to improve their sex lives?

Durk: One of the things that I would suggest is that about 45 minutes before sex they could take something that will provide them with more nitric oxide, particularly the man—that is an arginine, choline, vitamin B-5 formulation. Another thing is, of course, a drug like Viagra® or Cialis®. I think that Cialis® is more interesting. First, because the timing isn't anywhere near as critical. It's effective for thirty-six hours, and secondly, because I really do think that Cialis® may have life-extending effects mediated by mitochondrial biogenesis.

Sandy: I think it's important to realize that we're saying that may have that effect.

Durk: May. Repeat, may have that effect.

Sandy: This is a hypothesis.

Durk: But, in the meantime, you can have a lot of fun with it!

Sandy: Hahahaha.

David: What are you currently working on?

Durk: Well golly, in addition to our suits against the FDA, we have a ranch with cattle with mitochondrially-elite genomes—and that's really proving to be very important.

Sandy: Yeah, we selected the cattle so that they were very efficient in feed conversion, and an awful lot of the genes that are involved in feed conversion are those that are used by the mitochondria, because the mitochondria are the center of energy conversion.

Durk: The mitochondria are also what are responsible for being able to survive a blizzard, a drought, or a famine, and they have lot to do with the ability to produce calves and feed them to adulthood.

Sandy: Right, because the mitochondria have their own genome. A lot of people probably still don't know this but the nuclear genome—the genome that's found in the cell nucleus—contains most of your DNA, but not all of it. There's a separate genome that is in the mitochondria.

That's their own genome, and the genome of the mitochondria is handed down only from the mother.

Durk: If you look at ranching publications you'll see full page ad after full page ad for prize bulls, bull semen, and so forth, and you do need to have good bulls if you want to have good calves, because fifty percent of the nuclear genome is supplied by the bull. Also, some of the proteins that are produced by the nuclear genome are imported into the mitochondria. But there's a limit as to how far you can go if you don't have the right mitochondrial genome to start with. So we developed a selection process to get a very good and efficient mitochondrial genome. In fact, it's so efficient that our calving efficiency this year is ninety-seven percent.

Sandy: Ninety-seven percent of the cows had calves. And remember, these cattle are living like wild animals. They have to take care of themselves in the winter. There's nobody out there helping them have a calf. They're doing that all on their own.

Durk: Most ranchers consider themselves doing well if it were in the low to mid eighties, and the University of Nevada brags about their experimental cattle herd. They had a ninety-one percent calving efficiency this year, but they admit that they have calving barns. The calves are born in the barns, and they have veterinarians on call 24 hours a day to help the cows. Ours did it all by themselves out in the field. Ninety-seven percent is absolutely unheard of.

Sandy: So what we did was we got the cattle from herds where they had these very widely distributed cattle over thousands and thousands of acres, and where the cattle were basically taking care of themselves. They were also from these areas where there's very little scrub to eat. They're able to manage on very small amounts of food.

Durk: What we did was we found the worst ranges in Nevada, and Nevada's got a lot of desert. It's got a lot of pretty hard scrabble range, and I found the worst I could find. The rancher was going out of business there. I didn't buy the cattle that hung around the ranch house and got supplementary feed during the winter. I waited until they were just catching what they call the "wild cows", where a whole team of cowboys might catch one or two or three of them a day, far, far out in the middle of nowhere. And, incidentally, the winter range for these cattle was--so help me God—a place called Last Chance Gulch (*laughter*), which is a canyon coming off Death Valley. And, man, I have never seen such a barren place. (*Laughter*)

Sandy: So it worked like a charm. Our cattle do extremely well.

Durk: So to make sure that our hypothesis about the cattle was right, for two winters we put them up in a seventy-four hundred foot high valley during the winter—something that you'd never do if you were in your right mind. And they not only survived, they had calves during the winter.

Sandy: Yeah, that's amazing.

Durk: And the calves survived.

Sandy: And we keep the same maternal line, so we're continuing with the maternal genome for the mitochondria that we selected them for.

Durk: Yeah, it doesn't get diluted by the bulls. A hundred generations from now it'll be the same mitochondrial line.

David: When I interviewed British biochemist Aubrey de Grey for this book he suggested that we move the DNA from the mitochondria into the cell nucleus as a step toward extending human life.

Durk: I think that there may be problems with that. It's an interesting hypothesis. Aubrey de Grey thinks that maybe we should move the DNA from the mitochondria into the nucleus because there's far less free radical activity in the nucleus than in mitochondria. Now, the thing is a lot of genes have moved from the mitochondria to the nucleus. It's happened over the past couple of billion years. So it's already happened to some extent. What I think is that it's going to be very difficult to move the remainder because if it weren't it would have already happened. Many of the genes that are involved in specifying proteins for the mitochondria, in fact, are now found in the nucleus.

Sandy: Yeah, and presumably they remain there because it was an advantage to the animals that had that happen.

Durk: I suspect that if you move the remaining genes from the mitochondria to the nucleus you'll end frying the nucleus, just like the mitochondria fry themselves. But you've only got one set of genes in the nucleus, whereas a typical cell has about twenty thousand sets of mitochondrial genomes in twenty thousand mitochondria.

Sandy: Yeah, because remember that there's a tradeoff. It's true that the mitochondria genome does not have anywhere near the kind of DNA repair mechanisms as the nuclear DNA, but there's a lot more of it. There are large numbers of mitochondria in each cell, so you have a large number of sets of the mitochondrial genome in each cell, whereas you only have one set of the nuclear DNA in each cell. So it's a tradeoff. And I think that if we're able to use those mechanisms that we were discussing before, for increasing the number of mitochondria, and regenerating the mitochondrial genome, then, actually, it could be an advantage to leaving the genes in the mitochondria.

David: Is there anything we haven't spoken about that you would like to add?

Durk: I think that one of the things that people really need to look at is the government entitlement systems for people as they age. They are really completely unsustainable, and if something isn't done about it now there's going to be a crackup and perhaps even a war between generations. And that would be very bad for life expectancy.

Sandy: Yeah, when you think about it, the Constitution was a very noble model for a government, but perhaps they didn't realize the problems that it would cause. And maybe you couldn't even write this into a constitution, really. The problem is that once people find out that they can vote for benefits to themselves, and that other people's stuff can be taken and given to them, it just becomes very difficult to control that. I mean, how do you prevent people from taking advantage of a system where you can just vote yourself money out of somebody's else's pocket?

Durk: It's inherently unstable. Now, one of the ways of dealing with that would be to have a system where to increase a tax you might require a three-quarters vote, or to expend money in an appropriations bill you might require three-quarters vote, effectively. If one quarter plus one vote voted against it, then the money couldn't be spent. That would be a very effective limit on spending money. But, of course, you're going to have a very hard time getting that put into the Constitution nowadays, because so many people are getting so much money from the federal government.

Sandy: Actually, you put anything that you want to into the Constitution, but you can't change people's natures. That's a problem that we're going to have to deal with. Whatever the Constitution is that you have, people can decide that they want to misunderstand or modify the meaning of what was originally put into it, so as to get benefits for themselves at someone else's expense. That's a problem.

Durk: One thing we'd like to suggest that you do is interview a gentleman named Don Ernsberger, who we've known from the 1960s.

Sandy: He's an aide to Congressman Rohrabacher.

Durk: Dana Rohrabacher. Don Ernsberger has written a bill, which Rohrabacher has introduced, which would eliminate most of the problems with the high cost of drugs.

Sandy: That bill was introduced last year.

Durk: Yeah, and what this does, effectively, is it eliminates the Kefauver amendments to the Food, Drug, and Cosmetic Act. Before the Kefauver amendments of 1962 the FDA simply ruled on safety. They left efficacy determinations to the marketplace, to doctors and patients. And in fact a good economist by the name of Sam Pelzman examined the record since before and after 1962, to see whether the Kefauver Act resulted in fewer ineffective drugs, and there's no difference in the percentage of drugs that are ineffective. But the proof of efficacy costs an order of magnitude more than proof of safety. So that's a big part of the cost and it's also a big factor in slowing down the availability of drugs. Another factor that really jacks up the cost of even generic drugs is the FDA's

Good Manufacturing Practices (GMPs), which are 747 pages of bad manufacturing practices.

Sandy: Yeah, they have them for drugs, and they're about to introduce them for dietary supplements.

Durk: Effectively, they prevent the use of modern techniques, such as statistical quality control, which is what turned Japanese products from a laughing stock that was synonymous with crappy quality to the best products in the world. You can not use that under Good Manufacturing Practices.

Sandy: With the Good Manufacturing Practices they actually design your plant for you. It's a lot more than telling you how to manufacture. They tell you how your plant needs to be laid out, and where your various machines have to be located. Also, you'll notice—and this has been the case since the 1930s—you have no 4th Amendment rights anymore. The FDA doesn't require a search warrant in order to go in and examine your plant. They send inspectors around. Those people don't need warrants. These are warrant-less searches, and nobody's thinking anything about them, I guess, because they've been around so long.

Durk: Now, the Health Freedom Act would eliminate the requirement for GMPs on off-patent, generic drugs imported from overseas. The FDA would be allowed to test them for purity, and if they meet the same purity specifications as the American drugs that the FDA has approved, then that's it. It doesn't allow importing drugs that are in violation of a valid U.S. patent. But what this would mean is that you would be able to get a suite of antihypertensive and antihypercholesterolemic drugs for fifty cents a day instead of five dollars a day. So this thing about the Medicare drug benefit would be irrelevant. Nobody would be screaming for help to pay for their drugs if everyone could get everything they needed for four bits a day.

Sandy: All of the reputable economists agree that if we're going to have regulations concerning manufacturing, then what you should have is a standard that the final product has to meet. The final product would have to meet the standard, and that would be how they would regulate it. But that's not the way the FDA does it. Rather than that, what they have for the Good Manufacturing Practices is they design the entire process of how you do the manufacturing. It's an incredibly complex list of regulations, and it's probably impossible for anybody to really comply with all of them.

Durk: The thing is, the biggest barrier between life extension and people is the FDA, by far. It's not ignorance. It's the FDA.

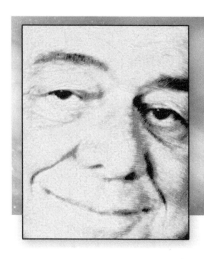

**SHATTERING THE BARRIERS
OF MAXIMUM LIFE SPAN**

An Interview with Dr. Joseph Knoll

Joseph Knoll, M.D., is a Hungarian neurochemist and pharmacologist. He is probably best known for developing the drug deprenyl (also known as Selegiline), the first selective MAO-B inhibitor, and he has researched the properties of deprenyl for over half a century.

Dr. Knoll is also the author of the recently published book The Brain and Its Self: A Neurochemical Concept of Innate and Acquired Drives *(Springer, 2005), which summarizes his life's research and his fascinating speculations about the relationship between brain activity and culture. In this book, Dr. Knoll describes how his experience as a Nazi concentration camp survivor helped to inspire and motivate much of his scientific research. Although his parents were sent to the gas chamber when he was a teenager, Dr. Knoll survived because he spoke fluent German and was chosen to serve as the personal servant to the Chief of the SS guards. After the war, in 1945, Dr. Knoll returned to his native city of Budapest. He earned his M.D. from the University of Budapest in 1951, and later became a professor and the head of the Department of Pharmacology at the Semmelweiss University of Medicine in Budapest.*

In the early 1950s, Dr. Knoll helped to pioneer research into the physiological basis of innate and acquired drives in animals. Trying to make sense of his experience in the Nazi concentration camp, Dr. Knoll became interested in how animals acquire new drives. The research that resulted from Dr. Knoll's interest in this subject centered around studying the brain changes in rats that had been trained to have an acquired drive for an unnatural object—a glass cylinder. This acquired drive—which urged the animals to search for, and jump to, the rim of a thirty centimeter-high glass-cylinder, and then crawl inside—would often override the animals' instinctive drives for food and sex.

Dr. Knoll first synthesized deprenyl in his Budapest laboratory in 1961. He showed that deprenyl improves the availability of dopamine, and slows its age-related decline by acting as a selective MAO-B inhibitor. Even more importantly, according to Dr. Knoll, it has an enhancer effect, and it helps maintain healthy brain cells, particularly in the dopamine-producing area of the brain known as the substantia nigra—the area of the brain that degenerates with Parkinson's disease. For this reason, deprenyl has been used as an effective treatment for Parkinson's disease. It has also been shown to be an effective treatment for Alzheimer's disease and other brain disorders that result in cognitive decline.

Deprenyl has been shown to have many uses as a cognitive enhancer. It is a moderate-level stimulant and antidepressant that has been shown to improve memory, protect the brain against cell damage, alleviate depression, extend the life span of laboratory animals, and heighten sexual desire in both men and women. This impressive substance is available by prescription in the U.S., and although it is primarily prescribed to help people with Parkinson's disease, memory disorder problems, and sometimes depression, a lot of healthy people also use deprenyl to improve their mental performance. In fact, Dr. Knoll himself takes deprenyl every day, and recommends that every sexually mature person should be doing the same.

I've personally been using deprenyl as antidepressant and

cognitive enhancer for over ten years, and I can attest to its powerful brain-boosting effects. It improves my mental performance so dramatically that I've used it before every public talk that I've given since 1995. Along with other cognitive enhancers, such as hydergine and piracetam, I think that deprenyl has incredible potential for enhancing memory, accelerating intelligence, and improving concentration. There is a good deal of scientific evidence to support these claims. For an excellent summary of the scientific studies in this area see John Morgenthaler and Ward Dean's book Smart Drugs and Nutrients II.

Many people report that deprenyl and other "smart drugs" have sexually-enhancing "side-effects", although deprenyl appears to have the leading reputation in this area. According to Dr. Dean—the coauthor of Smart Drugs and Nutrients— "anything that improves brain function is probably going to improve sexual functioning." This is probably because sexuality and health go hand-in-hand, and sexual vitality is a pretty good indicator of overall health.

Dr. Knoll and colleagues first reported indications for deprenyl's potential as a sexuality enhancer in 1983, with reports that old male rats had increased their "mounting frequency" and "intromission" when they were treated with deprenyl. This contrasted dramatically with the untreated control animals. Many anecdotal reports, from both men and women, have confirmed that these aphrodisiac-like effects apply to humans as well. Because Deprenyl inhibits MAO— the dopamine-destroying enzyme—levels of the excitatory neurotransmitter dopamine rise in the brain, which generally cause people to feel more pleasure and become more physiologically aroused.

Interestingly, unlike most other MAO inhibitor drugs (such as the antidepressant Nardil), there are usually no dietary restrictions necessary when one takes deprenyl. When taken at moderate levels (under 10 mg.), deprenyl only inhibits the action of a specific type of MAO—MAO B—which doesn't *interfere with the body's ability to metabolize the dietary amine tyramine, like a broad-spectrum MAO inhibitor does. This is why most other MAO-inhibiting drugs carry the serious danger of triggering a hypertensive reaction if one eats tyramine-rich foods, like cheese or wine. Deprenyl has been described by researchers as working with great precision in this regard and the physicians that I spoke with agreed that it was unusually safe.*

In fact, deprenyl is better than safe. This truly remarkable drug has also been shown to increase the maximum lifespan of laboratory animals by close to forty percent. This is the equivalent of a human being living to be around a hundred and fifty years of age. Giving deprenyl to animals is the only experimental treatment—besides caloric restriction—that has been shown to increase maximum life span. [Extending maximum life span—as opposed to extending average life span—means extending the maximum number of years that the longest-lived members of a particular species have been known to attain.]

To fully appreciate how significant deprenyl's life extension potential is, one has to understand the difference between maximum life span and average life span. Many factors can affect the average lifespan (or the "normal life expectancy") that an animal lives—genetics, diet, exercise, nutritional supplements, mental attitude, etc. However, even under the very best of conditions, there is an upper limit at which the longest-lived animals of a particular species can survive, and that is the animal's maximum life span.

The average life span of a human being is approximately seventy to eighty years. However, the maximum life span of a human being is around a hundred and twenty years. The laboratory animals in the deprenyl studies showed a forty percent increase in maximum life span, the human equivalent of living a hundred and fifty years. Since deprenyl's primary effects work the same in all mammalian brains, it stands to reason that deprenyl's life extension effects are likely to carry over to humans, just as the mental benefits do. Many people have certainly verified that the increase in sex drive occurs in both humans and laboratory animals.

To follow are some excerpts from the interview that I conducted with Dr. Knoll in September of 2005. Born in 1925, Dr. Knoll was eighty at the time of this interview. We spoke about how his experience with the Holocaust influenced his decision to become a research scientist, how people can utilize deprenyl for its cognitive enhancing and anti-aging benefits, and what type of anti-aging treatments might be available in the future.

David: How did your experience with the Holocaust when you were young influence your decision to become a research scientist, and what inspired your interest in neurochemistry?

Dr. Knoll: It is a horrifying fact that in Germany millions of single-minded little-men, who had previously lived an honest simple life and never belonged to extremist groups, dramatically changed within a few years after 1933 and, imbued with the Nazi ideology, became unbelievably cool-headed murders of innocent civilians during the Second World War. This phenomenon has been documented from many angles in dozens of novels, films, and so on. However, we are still waiting for an adequate elucidation of the brain mechanism responsible for this dramatic and rapid change in the behavior of millions.

As a survivor of Auschwitz, and one of the 1,300 survivors of the "Dachau death train," I had the opportunity to directly experience a few typical representatives of this type of manipulated human beings, and had more than enough time and direct experience to reflect upon the essential changes in the physiological manipulability of the human brain. It was therefore not just by mere chance that, when in the early 1950s, I finally had the opportunity to approach this problem experimentally, I decided to develop a rat model to follow the changes in the brain in the course of the acquisition of a drive from the start of training until its manifestation.

David: What are some of the disorders that deprenyl has proven itself to be an effective treatment for?

Dr. Knoll: Successful clinical studies with deprenyl were executed in depression and in the two age-related neurodegenerative diseases: Parkinson's disease and Alzheimer's disease. The first clinical study performed in depressed patients by Dr. Varga with deprenyl was published in 1965. The clinical use of deprenyl in Parkinson's disease started in 1977. The first two papers demonstrating the effectiveness of deprenyl in Alzhiemer's disease appeared in 1987. Deprenyl was originally developed with the intention to be used as a new spectrum antidepressant. Its effectiveness was first demonstrated with the racemic form of the compound by Dr. Varga and his coworkers in 1965 and 1967, and with the enantiomer in 1971. The first study that corroborated the antidepressant effect of deprenyl was published by Dr. Mann and Dr. Gershon in 1980.

The realization of the peculiar effect of deprenyl—first in Parkinson's disease and later in Alzhiemer's disease—distracted attention from its antidepressant property which remains unutilized. Even an especially interesting aspect of this problem fell into oblivion. In a depression study performed by Dr. Birkmayer and his coworkers in 1984 on a hundred and two outpatients and fifty-three inpatients, deprenyl was given together with phenylalanine. The latter is the precursor of phenylethylamine (PEA) that, in contrast to PEA, crosses the blood-brain barrier and, as it is metabolized in the brain, increases the concentration of this natural enhancer substance. Nearly seventy percent of the patients achieved full remission from depression. The outstanding clinical efficiency was equaled only with that of electroconvulsive treatment, but without the latter's side effect of memory-loss.

David: How might healthy people utilize deprenyl for its cognitive enhancing and anti-aging benefits?

Dr. Knoll: They should take one milligram of deprenyl daily from sexual maturity until death.

David: Some studies have shown that deprenyl can significantly increase the maximum life span of laboratory animals, yet some of the longevity researchers that I've spoken with told me that these findings have been difficult to replicate. Why do you think this is, and what are your thoughts about this?

Dr. Knoll: Our finding that deprenyl prolongs life was corroborated in mice, in rats, in hamsters, and in dogs. Nevertheless, variation in the extent of the prolongation of life between the longevity studies performed in different laboratories was unusually high. The reason for this variation is now clear. A bell-shaped concentration effect curve is characteristic to the enhancer effect of the synthetic mesencephalic enhancer substances. Thus, there is an optimum dose for the enhancer effect.

Concerning the optimum dose of deprenyl there are, not only species, but also strain differences. On the other hand, even the effect of an optimum dose depends on the selected experimental conditions. We worked, for example, with the long-lived, robust, Wistar-Logan strain, which seldom grows tumors. The age of rats at the start of treatment was two years in our first study and roughly eight months in our second study. In both studies, a substantial number of rats treated with deprenyl lived longer than the estimated technical life span of three and a half years.

Dr. Milgram and colleagues were the first who repeated our survival study with deprenyl. They clearly intended to hold tightly to the parameters we used in our first study, and started experiments with two year old rats and treated them with 0.25 milligrams per kilogram with deprenyl. They changed, however, an important parameter. They worked with the short-lived Fischer 344 strain of rats, thus, they started treatment too late and found only a sixteen percent marginally significant prolongation of life span. Nevertheless, they found a convincingly significant increase in the longer survival.

Dr. Kitani and colleagues, who conducted the second control survival study with deprenyl, also used Fischer 344 rats. They obviously considered that these rats are shorter living than the Wistar-Logan rats, and they started to work with one and a half year old rats. This was an advantageous change in the experimental conditions and found a satisfyingly significant, thirty-four percent prolongation of the average life span.

However, in the hope to increase the effectiveness of their treatment they doubled the dose of deprenyl. Although a higher dose is usually more effective than a lower one, the doubling of the dose was in this special case an unfavorable change. We know now that 0.01 milligrams per kilogram of deprenyl is sufficient to exert an enhancer effect. Thus the 0.5 milligrams per kilogram dose was obviously enormously high, and this explains why Kitani and colleagues found no sign of the significant extension in the longest survival which appeared in our studies and in the Milgram et al. study.

All in all, in future longevity studies with a synthetic mesencephalic enhancer substance, it is reasonable to treat the animals with a dose that in preliminary studies proved to exert a peak effect in enhancing the release of catecholamines and serotonin in the brain stem.

David: What do you think are the primary causes of aging in general?

Dr. Knoll: Various species live together on earth in a harmonious proportion. This is obviously carefully regulated. One of the seemingly principal regulatory mechanisms that produce equilibrium among living organisms is brain aging. It ultimately leads to the elimination of those individuals who have already fulfilled their duty in nurturing the new generation.

Accordingly, the period from weaning until sexual maturity is reached is the most delightful phase of life, the glorious uphill journey. The individual progressively takes possession, on a mature level, of all abilities crucial for survival and maintenance of the species. It learns to avoid dangerous situations, masters the techniques to obtain its food, develops procreative powers for sexual reproduction and copulates. This is, at the same time, the climax of developmental longevity. The sexually fully mature individual fulfils its duty.

Thus, to maintain the precisely balanced out natural equilibrium among living organisms, the biologically "useless" individual has to be eliminated. According to the inborn program, the post-developmental stage of life (aging) begins. The essence of this stage is progressive decay of the efficiency of the catecholaminergic system during the post-developmental life span until at some point, in an emergency situation, the integration of the parts in a highly sophisticated entity can no longer be maintained and "natural death", signaled by the disappearance of the EEG signal, sets in.

David: What do you think are currently the best ways to slow down, or reverse the aging process and extend the human life span?

Dr. Knoll: Regarding the quality and duration of life the most important aging process is the continuous, slow, age-related decline of the mesencephalic enhancer regulation during the post-development phase of life. This cannot be reversed, but its progress can be slowed by the prophylactic administration of a synthetic mesencephalic enhancer substance (for the time being with the daily administration of one milligram of deprenyl). The earlier this protective treatment starts, the better are the prospects to improve the quality of life in the latter decades, which necessarily goes together with an extension of life span.

David: How long do you think it's possible for the human life span to be extended?

Dr. Knoll: The average life span in the most developed countries has already exceeded the eighty year level. This change has come about due to the prevention of premature deaths owing to the development of hygiene, immunology, and chemotherapy. The human technical life span (TLSh), close to a hundred and twenty years, has remained, however, unchanged.

In my view, to extend the human life span beyond the TLSh needs the elaboration of an ultimate technique for the prophylactic, daily small-dose administration of a safe synthetic mesencephalic enhancer substance from sexual maturity until death. The attainable upper limit in the extension of the TLSh is obviously unpredictable at present. Nevertheless, if brain research could, at some time in the future, achieve just a doubling of the TLSh, this will mean for humans the most significant accomplishment that science has ever achieved, since nothing can be more important for the individual than the quality and duration of his/her life.

David: What are some of the new anti-aging treatments that you foresee coming along in the near future?

Dr. Knoll: In the developed countries the proportion of the aged is high, and the estimated number of individuals over sixty-five will increase to 1.1 billion by 2050. Accordingly, the demand on anti-aging therapy is rapidly increasing. This trend explains the already high-sounding proposals for anti-aging treatments.

My view is that since the brain alone ensures that the mammalian organism works as a purposeful, motivated, goal-directed entity, the age-related changes in the central nervous system are of particular importance. And since the enhancer-sensitive neurons in the brain stem work as the engine of the brain, the slow, continuous, post-developmental functional decline of the mesencephalic enhancer regulation is of primary importance in the maintenance of the well-balanced equilibrium among living organisms, because it helps to eliminate the individuals who already fulfilled their duty in nurturing the new generation.

For the time being the prestigious task—the maintenance of the mesencephalic enhancer regulation during the post-developmental phase of life on the enhanced level characteristic of developmental longevity—cannot be fully accomplished. However, it is already feasible to modestly slow the age-related decay of the catecholaminergic and trace-aminergic tone in the brain via the prophylactic administration of one milligram of deprenyl daily.

The development of BPAP—a synthetic mesencephalic enhancer substance that is at least hundred times more potent than deprenyl—is by itself a hint that our present knowledge about the mesencephalic enhancer regulation is in a very early stage. The high potency of BPAP indicates already that much more potent natural enhancer substances than PEA and tryptamine might exist. Better understanding of mesencephalic enhancer regulation promises to develop more efficient techniques in the future to slow brain aging and prolong human life beyond the TLSh. According to my judgment, this is the only physiologically well-founded, feasible anti-aging therapy that I foresee coming along in the future that has a chance, in the long run, to remain the method to continuously improve the quality and prolong the duration of human life.

We shall never forget that humans obviously cannot change natural laws, but by discovering their mechanisms of action they learn to make use of this knowledge. By conquering gravitation man stepped across his naturally given limit and ultimately landed on the moon. By conquering the age-related decline of the mesencephalic enhancer regulation, man might in the future step across also this naturally given limit and extend human life span beyond the TLSh.

David: What are you currently working on?

Dr. Knoll: My ambition is to develop a more efficient compound than deprenyl for slowing the age-related decay of the mesencephalic enhancer regulation, and to detect the envisioned unknown mesencephalic enhancer substances, expected to be several thousand times more active than PEA or tryptamine. Currently we are trying to clarify in more detail the pharmacological spectrum of BPAP—our newly developed, tryptamine-derived, synthetic mesencephalic enhancer substance.

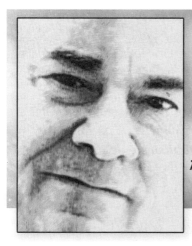

PUSHING THE HAYFLICK LIMIT

An Interview with Dr. Leonard Hayflick

Leonard Hayflick, Ph.D., is a microbiologist whose research revolutionized cell biology, and helped to provide a scientific foundation for the field of cellular gerontology (or cytogerontology)—the study of aging at the cellular level. Dr. Hayflick discovered that cultured normal human cells can only divide a finite number of times, after which they become senescent. This limited capacity for cell division is now known as the 'Hayflick limit', and this discovery has enabled other researchers to make significant progress towards understanding the molecular mechanisms of aging and cancer.

Following this groundbreaking discovery, Dr. Hayflick developed the first normal human diploid fibroblast cell strains. One of these—called WI-38—is still the most widely used normal human cell strain in the world. Dr. Hayflick was also the first to produce a vaccine (the oral polio vaccine) from these cells. WI-38 cells, or similar human-cell strains, are used today for the manufacture of most human virus vaccines throughout the world—including poliomyelitis, rubella, rubeola, adenoviruses, measles, mumps, and rabies vaccines.

Approximately a billion people have received virus vaccine doses produced on WI-38 or similar diploid cell strains, yet Dr. Hayflick makes no profit from this. In fact, he was accused by the government of stealing its' property when he asked for packaging and mailing costs from pharmaceutical manufacturers and viral research labs. Dr. Hayflick's inability to patent and profit from his development—because at the time in 1962, one could not patent living matter—became the foundation for his lawsuit against the Federal government, which, after six years of litigation he won with an out-of-court settlement. This lawsuit helped to establish the discoverers or inventors intellectual property rights that researchers in the biotech industry take for granted today.

Dr. Hayflick also discovered the cause of primary atypical pneumonia ("walking pneumonia"). Dr. Hayflick demonstrated that this illness is caused by a member of the smallest free-living class of microorganisms—which he named Mycoplasma pneumoniae—*and not by a virus, as was previously believed. Dr. Hayflick demonstrated this by growing these microorganisms in a medium that he developed.*

Dr. Hayflick earned his Ph.D. at the University of Pennsylvania in 1956. He served ten years as an associate member of the Wistar Institute and two years as Assistant Professor of Research Medicine at the University of Pennsylvania. In 1968 he was appointed Professor of Medical Microbiology at the Stanford University School of Medicine, and he is currently a professor of anatomy on the faculty of the University of California, San Francisco.

Dr. Hayflick was the Editor-in-Chief of Experimental Gerontology *for thirteen years, president of the Gerontological Society of America, chairman of the Scientific Review Board of the American Federation for Aging Research, and a founding member and chairman of the executive committee of the Council of the National Institute on Aging. He has received more than 25 major awards—including the 1991 Sandoz Prize for Gerontological research and the Presidential Award from the International Organization of Mycoplasmology. Dr. Hayflick is a fellow of the American Association for the Advancement of Science, and is one of the principal advisors for the Ageless Animals Project—which is directed by John Guerin, who was also interviewed for this collection.*

Dr Hayflick is the author of over 225 scientific papers and reviews—some of which are among the most cited scientific papers in human history. He is also the author of the popular book How and Why We Age *(Ballantine Books, 1994), which has been translated into ten languages. The story of Dr. Hayflick's distinguished and controversial career is chronicled in a book by Debbie Bookchin and Jim Schumacher called* The Virus and the Vaccine *(St. Martin's Press, 2004), and in Stephen Hall's* Merchants of Immortality *(Houghton Mifflin, 2003). Dr. Hayflick is currently working on a book about his experiences as scientist for Cambridge University Press.*

I interviewed Dr. Hayflick on April 27, 2005. Dr. Hayflick is an elegant speaker. I was excited to hear firsthand about his discoveries, and greatly appreciated his patience in answering questions that I'm sure he's answered a thousand times before, making sure that I understood every detail. We spoke about how the fetal cells that he cultured were used for viral research, vaccine production, cancer research and the causes of aging, and why he thinks that researching the causes of aging is more important than directing biomedical research efforts to the study of disease.

David: What inspired your interest in the biology of aging?

Dr. Hayflick: My interest in the biology of aging was a pure accident; it evolved from a discovery that I made in the early 1960s. The discovery that I made flew in the face of existing dogma at the time—dogma that was entrenched for more than sixty years—and because I was convinced that I had overthrown that dogma, the experiments that I did required some explanation, or at least some speculation as to what they meant. After conducting a number of experiments that excluded many possibilities that seemed reasonable, I was left with one possibility that I could not exclude, and that was that the observation that I had made was telling me something about longevity determination and/or aging.

So I speculated on that possibility in the paper that I published with my colleague Paul Moorhead in 1962.

Then I began to realize that the field of aging at that time was, to put it mildly, an impoverished field. There were perhaps a dozen people in this country, at the most, who were working in this field—or, at least, who would admit in public that they were working in this field, because at that time the climate was such that to admit in public that you were working in the field of aging was tantamount to committing professional suicide. So people that worked in the field of aging often did so in the closet. Then because of my speculation, and because of the popularity that this paper began to assume, I was contacted by one or two of the dozen people working in the field of aging to speak at some of their congresses.

One person in particular was Dr. Nathan Shock, who is generally regarded as the father of modern gerontology in the United States. We became very good friends, and it was through him that I became introduced to other people in the field, in particular members of the Gerontological Society of America. This is the professional organization that people in the field of biology of aging and geriatric medicine, as well as the social and psychological aspects of aging—indeed, every aspect of aging—are members. So I went to their meetings, initially when I was invited to speak, and I began to realize that I was becoming a biogerontologist. This was not by intention, as I mentioned at the outset, it was by accident, and I became very interested in the subject. The rest is history.

David: Can you talk a little about how the fetal cells that you cultured were used for viral research and vaccine production?

Dr. Hayflick: At the time I was working at the Wistar Institute in Philadelphia, which was directed by a man named Hilary Koprowski, who was a pioneer in polio vaccine research. (In fact, contrary to popular belief, Koprowski was the first person to develop, and actually test in humans, a live virus vaccine. It was not Albert Sabin as is popularly believed.) A fair proportion of the research activities at the Wistar Institute—by no means all of them—were conducted around virus vaccine research because of Koprowski's interest, so I couldn't help but learn more and more about human vaccine development and the problems therein.

And as luck would have it, my work with the normal human fetal cells directly impacted on the problems with human virus vaccines that emerged at that time. I suppose one could argue that was just a lucky break that I made the discovery that I did in the right place at the right time, because of what was emerging in the late '50s and early '60s with the polio vaccine. To give you some idea of the atmosphere at the time, poliovirus research was, I suppose, equivalent in the minds of scientists and the general public then as stem cell research is today. In other words, every other hour you read something about it or heard something about it.

So, first let me say what the problems were in vaccines at the time so that you'll understand how my work fitted into it. The problem that was emerging at the time was centered on the fact that monkey kidney cells were used for the preparation of the virus vaccine. As I'm sure you know, viruses can only replicate on living cells; they cannot replicate on dead material as can bacteria. So, because you need lots of viruses in order to make vaccines, you need lots of cells to make lots of viruses. The cells that were chosen by Jonas Salk and others at the time for vaccine production were primary monkey kidney cells. There were other vaccines that used other types of cells. For example, the flu vaccine was made using embryonated eggs, and it still is today.

But the polio vaccine was made in monkey kidney cells. The monkeys were obtained from various sources around the world, and people began to realize that these monkey kidney cells contain unwanted viruses, several of which were in fact lethal to humans. One of them was called the B-virus, and that killed several workers. Other viruses were found in the kidney cells themselves, and that contaminated many of the early vaccines. People sort of shrugged at the importance of this for a number of years—until the SV40 virus was discovered in the early 1960s, and that was a critical development.

I should say something parenthetically about the Marburg agent, which you may have read about in the past month. The Marburg virus is the one that's just broken out—in one of the African countries—and it's killed around two hundred people as of today. It's a cousin of the Ebola virus, and it's a huge problem. It's almost a hundred percent lethal, causing systemic hemorrhages, which is a very unpleasant way to die. I mention the Marburg agent because that was a virus that was another virus found in monkey kidneys used in Marburg, Germany for polio vaccine production in the early to mid-'70s.

Because those monkey kidneys were to be used for polio vaccine production this put a scare into everybody in this field around the world, and ended up with a conference at the National Institute of Health (NIH) in which my cells were then more seriously considered as a replacement for primary monkey kidney. But that's skipping ahead at least around ten years. Let me go back to the beginning of the story and tell you what happened in the early 1960s—1961 and 1962.

There are two parts to this story. A woman named Bernice Eddy worked at the vaccine control authority at NIH, that is, the authority that approves vaccines for use by the public. She was working with baby hamsters, which are particularly susceptible to tumors, and she decided to inoculate monkey kidney cells that manufacturers were using for polio virus vaccine production into these baby hamsters. She observed that tumors were being formed in the cheek pouch where these cells were inoculated. This puzzled her greatly, and she went to her boss, a man by the name of Joe Smadel—a very famous virologist—who pooh-poohed this observation, and essentially threw her out of his office. He didn't want to hear of any problems with polio vaccines because the whole country was celebrating the Salk vaccine and the emerging Sabin vaccine.

Okay, let's shift over to the second branch of this story and then I'll marry the two. The second branch of the story emerged because these unwanted viruses were now better known, and people were becoming more worried about them. By now we knew that there were about twenty or twenty-five of them. People began to look at monkey kidneys from other species, other than the ones that were being used at the time, namely cynomolgus monkeys and rhesus monkeys.

Enter Maurice Hilleman. Maurice Hilleman, who worked with Joe Smadel at Walter Reed Army Institute of Research years before these events occurred, was by this time vice-president for vaccine development at Merck in West Point, Pennsylvania. Maurice Hilleman is known by people in this field as one of the world's best and greatest virologists, and certainly the best vaccine maker in the world. He was a giant in this field. He died last week, and it was in most of the papers, but most people don't know his name. He was fantastic. He was, by the way, a very good friend of mine.

So Hilleman mounted a program at Merck in West Point, Pennsylvania, which is not too far from the Wistar Institute in Philadelphia. It's a suburb, and he employed a number of people who were friends of mine. So this was a fairly close-knit community. We all knew what each other was doing on a daily basis virtually. Hilleman and one of his lieutenants, a man by the name of Ben Sweet, were working with other monkey species in effort to find cleaner monkeys.

They began to work with what's called the African green monkey—*Cercopithecus aethiops*—and they added to the polio vaccine a specific antibody that prevented the polio virus from multiplying. They put that on green monkey kidney cells, expecting to find nothing because the antibody had inactivated the polio vaccine. But instead of finding nothing happening to these green monkey kidney cells, they found the cells were behaving unusually, and that many of them were dying. They pursued this and found that they had discovered a new virus, which they called SV40. It was the fortieth in a series of the thirty-nine previous ones that had been discovered. They discovered that, although SV40 was commonly found in rhesus and cynomolgus kidney cells, it didn't do any harm there, but when it was put into green monkey kidney cells it harmed those cells, which was very unusual.

Okay, now let's switch over to Bernice Eddy at NIH in Bethesda, who now knew what Hilleman and Sweet had discovered. To make this part of the story short, it was discovered that the cause of the tumors in these baby hamsters was not the kidney cells, but the SV40 virus. So here we had a virus that produced tumors in baby hamsters, that was in monkey kidneys, and indeed as was later found in the vaccines that were then being used. And it was alive.

Well, of course that created a lot of interest, to say the least, and worry. Then the coup de grace was discovered at the Wistar Institute and

Harvard, simultaneously, where it was found that if you put SV40 on my cells—namely normal human cells in culture—the SV40 would convert those cells into a human cancer cells. Now, if you can imagine anything worse than a virus doing that in a vaccine, I'd like to know what it is. There is nothing worse than that. Well, that caused a furor and it's really the basis for a book by Debbie Bookchin and Jim Schumacher called *The Virus and the Vaccine* (St. Martin's Press, 2004).

So, here I was in this climate, and by this time I had realized that my cells—which were derived from normal human fetuses—had some extraordinary properties. The cell strain that I worked on mostly was called WI-38, and I discovered that WI-38 cells had the widest human virus spectrum of any cell population then known. In fact, it not only grew all the human viruses that were known at the time, but others that were unknown. For example, I discovered a new common cold virus using those cells. So that was one major observation, and this was all reported in my original paper. The second and perhaps most critical point was that despite every effort that we could make—not only by myself but in other laboratories throughout the world (who by this time had received samples of my cells)—no one could find a hidden virus, or what we call an indigenous virus in these cells. That statement is true up to this day, forty-three years later.

So it was obvious to me that the solution to this very serious problem with monkey kidney cells—that were contaminated with the worst possible contaminants one could think of—was to substitute normal human fetal cells for those monkey kidney cells. Although that concept was embraced by Hilary Koprowski, my boss, and other people at the Wistar Institute—Stanley Plotkin in particular, who using my cells developed the rubella vaccine. Other people at the Wistar Institute developed the rabies vaccine using my cells. These vaccines are used worldwide to this day, and those people patented those vaccines without ever telling me, by the way. I do not appear on those patents. The institute realized thirty million dollars as a result of those patents, and I saw nothing, but those people saw some fraction of that money. I'm to this day unable to determine how much.

David: I interviewed Kary Mullis, who won the Nobel Prize in Chemistry in 1993 for developing the Polymerase Chain Reaction

(PCR), which revolutionized the study of genetics. He never saw a penny for his development, yet others made a fortune off it.

Dr. Hayflick: Yeah, but that's a completely different situation because he signed away—as every employee of that company did—his intellectual property rights when he was employed. I never did that. That didn't exist at the time. The intellectual property rights to a self-reproducing system became a very important problem in the mid-1970s, when I brought suit against the NIH for stealing WI-38 from my laboratory when they claimed it as their own. It's a long story that would take hours to tell. I don't know whether you know about that lawsuit or not.

David: I read about it in Stephan Hall's book Merchants of Immortality.

Dr. Hayflick: He just briefly mentioned it. It's a compelling story and has been published in "A Novel Technique for Transforming the Theft of Mortal Human Cells into Praiseworthy Federal Policy." (L. Hayflick, *Experimental Gerontology*, 1988, volume 33, pages 191-207.)

Anyhow, I'll get back to answering your question. So it was apparent to me that normal human diploid cells like WI-38 should be used for vaccine production. In fact, Stanley Plotkin, Hilary Koprowski, and I published a paper called "Preparation of Poliovirus Vaccines in a Human Fetal Diploid Cell Strain" in the *American Journal of Hygiene*, 1962, volume 75, pages 240-258, in which we showed the safety and efficacy of a polio vaccine produced in one of my human diploid cells that was fed to several infants in Philadelphia, that later included my own children. So the stage was set for the replacement of monkey kidney cells, but the political, economic, and ego forces in existence at the time prevented this from happening for approximately a decade.

It peaked when the Marburg virus, that I mentioned earlier, surfaced in the mid-'70s. Then the first country to actually license vaccines produced in WI-38 was Yugoslavia, then Germany, Russia, England, and finally in 1972, the United States, during which time several people had died from working with monkeys and their kidneys. I also have to say that approximately ten million people in this country received the polio vaccine in the early '60s, and they received at no extra charge live SV40 virus, which of course we all knew caused human cells to transform into cancer cells, and produced tumors in baby hamsters. Well, it took roughly a decade to get my cells finally approved in this country, and as it stands today approximately one billion people on this planet have received vaccines produced in my cell strain WI-38, and I haven't received a nickel from that.

David: *That's simply unbelievable.*

Dr. Hayflick: It's unbelievable also because it was not possible to patent WI-38 in 1962. We tried to patent it, but the patent office threw it out because it was impossible to patent a living thing at the time.

David: *But you can do it now.*

Dr. Hayflick: Yes, partially as a result of my lawsuit. My lawsuit played a key role in that. During the litigation that I conducted against the NIH, the FDA was defended by the Justice Department and during the litigation the ChakraBarty decision was made by the Supreme Court. The name of that decision derives from a worker at Monsanto Chemical Company, who, roughly around that period of time, discovered a species of bacteria that chewed up oil and spit out perfume or sugar, or something nice. So these bacteria could be used for bioremediation purposes—that is, oil spills. Well, if you're a company, and you discovered a species of bacteria that's going to chew up oil and produce Chanel No. 5, you got a winner. So they tried to patent it, and of course it was thrown out. But they had the bucks to appeal it to the Supreme Court, and in 1980 the Supreme Court ruled yes, you can patent living things, because by this time the pressure was mounting from the emerging biotech industry to have this happen. So that played into my lawsuit.

My lawsuit, by the way, established the fact that scientists—biologists in particular—have intellectual property rights, and that was established indirectly by my lawsuit. It was the first lawsuit in this country made in effort to establish the intellectual property rights of biologists. What happened was that many of the leaders of the biological community who branded me as a thief in public, then embraced this concept, and the thinking of the biological community turned around 180 degrees. Today, if you don't have a commercial affiliation, or aren't doing something to raise money by serving on a scientific advisory board, you're a failure in biology. When I sold my WI-38 cells to Merck for fifty bucks to pay for postage and handling I was damned as a criminal. That's the difference.

David: Things have really changed.

Dr. Hayflick: It's absolutely mind-boggling. Just one last example; If an employee of NIH, about whom everything belongs to the government— perhaps with the exception of the oxygen that she/he's breathing—ever sold anything made by them in a federal laboratory to make money in 1962 they wouldn't only put him/her in Leavenworth, they'd lower Leavenworth on top of them. Today, workers at the NIH can earn up to a hundred thousand dollars a year extra, over their salaries, for discoveries that they make in their taxpayer-owned government laboratories. The NIH even puts on an annual science fair trying to sell what they have discovered to companies nationwide, a practice that's done also by every major research university in this country, and a practice that was unthinkable in the '60s. That gives you some idea of how the climate's changed substantially as a result of my lawsuit which I eventually won. Emerging biotech companies offered amicus briefs in my defense knowing that had I lost the case the biotech industry could not have happened because the founders of those companies were taking biological material from their tax payer supported labs and opening up new companies.

David: Knowing what you know today, what sort of role do you think the limit on cell divisions that you discovered plays in the human aging process?

Dr. Hayflick: I think it plays an essential role. I think that the failure to understand its key role is based on the failure of most biogerontologists— and certainly most scientists—to understand the difference between aging and longevity determination, something that people should be aware of but they're not.

You have to understand that distinction in order to understand my answer to your question, and it's this. When you buy your Mercedes-Benz for a hundred thousand dollars, and drive it off the showroom floor you have a certain expectation about its longevity—namely, it damn well better drive well for eight or ten years without requiring major repairs, or you've been fleeced. When I drive my Yugo off of the showroom floor, and I paid five or ten thousand dollars for it, I have a completely different expectation about its longevity. I think you will intuitively understand why the longevity of your Merc and my Yugo are different—namely, different design, better workmanship, and better materials used in the Merc as opposed to the Yugo.

Now when those two machines are driven off the showroom floor the same process begins to occur, and that is the aging process, which means loss of molecular fidelity or loss of molecular integrity over time. So the aging process is going to probably start earlier, and be more profound, in the Yugo than it will be in the Merc, because the longevity determinants are completely different in both kinds of cars. Now that concept lifts over to biology, and it's just as true in biology as it is inanimate objects. This is the key to understanding the answer to your question.

The finite lifetime of cultured, normal human and animal cells is a reflection of the maximum capability of that cell lineage to replicate, which is rarely—and I would argue never—reached in real life because the aging process will kill the individual well in advance of that maximum number of divisions. There's ample evidence for that. There are literally hundreds and hundreds of papers in the scientific literature that describe the changes that occur in normal human cells as they approach their loss of replicative capacity, and many of those hundreds and hundreds of changes are similar to the changes that occur in humans as we age. So if you argue that the cells go through fifty doublings, the changes begin to appear at, let's say, the fifteenth or twentieth doubling, and become more and more apparent or emphasized up to the fiftieth doubling. Those are age changes. But the limit on the cells' capability of replication is a reflection of the longevity determining process.

David: Do you think that if we were able to stop the telomeres from growing shorter with each cell division that that might be a way of increasing human longevity?

Dr. Hayflick: No, I don't. I think that's an overly simplistic but widely held belief. First of all, cancer cells usually have telomeres that are shorter than normal cells, so the simple act of reducing the number of telomeres, or arresting them to become shorter, could be worse than not interfering with them at all. In other words, it could be that they might become cancer cells.

David: So you think that telomere loss only really becomes a problem when all the telomeres are gone, and the DNA starts to unravel?

Dr. Hayflick: Well, I don't think we know that that's happening. It's a possibility. It's speculative, but there's no evidence for that occurring.

David: One of the people that I interviewed for this collection was Michael Fossel. When I spoke with him he told me that he thought that introducing telomerase into the cell nucleus (which would prevent the telomeres from growing shorter with each division) might play a key role in human longevity.

Dr. Hayflick: I know Mike very well. He's promoted this idea for ten or fifteen years. He thought that telomere shortening and telomerase were the answer to aging and cancer, and that it would happen within a year. We're now ten years later, and it still hasn't happened. I don't think it will happen, because he's got a very overly simplistic belief.

David: One of the interesting things that Michael Fossel told me when I interviewed him was that people with progeria were born with shorter telomeres.

Dr. Hayflick: That could very well be true, but it's got nothing to do with the issue.

David: Many people believe that individuals with progeria appear to suffer from a kind of accelerated aging process.

Dr. Hayflick: That's the orthodox belief. It's a knee-jerk reaction, and I don't believe it's true. I think that the best way to describe it is as biological McCarthyism—guilt by association.

David: What do you think is happening with progeric individuals?

Dr. Hayflick: I think that there's ample evidence that it's got a genetic basis. I think that features that make it look like accelerated aging are simply coincidental with some of the aging processes, but by no means all of them. There are many pathologies known in medicine that share similar clinical manifestations but have totally different etiologies.

There are many people, who like me are reluctant to believe the symptoms of progeria are accelerated aging phenomena. They might bear on longevity determinants. They probably do, but there's no universal agreement that those clinical manifestations are absolutely aging phenomena.

David: I would imagine that many people believe it largely because of their appearance. Children with progeria look uncannily like old men and women, with balding heads and wrinkled skin, and they appear to suffer from many of the symptoms of old age. The photographs that I've seen are particularly striking.

Dr. Hayflick: Yes, but you can find photographs of two different pathologies, with two different etiologies that look similar. I mean, if a person gets hit by a bus, and their legs are crippled, and they're walking around on crutches, and I pull somebody else out of the wings who has suffered from polio that is also walking on crutches, you're not going to tell me they're caused by the same agency.

David: What do you think are the primary causes of aging?

Dr. Hayflick: It's very simple. We know the cause of aging, despite it appearing to be a mystery to most people. First of all, let me tell you what aging is and then I think the cause will be implicit. In animals that reach a fixed size in adulthood, aging is the random systemic loss of molecular fidelity that after reproductive maturity accumulates to levels that eventually exceed repair, turnover, or maintenance capacity. That's the definition. It's the progressive loss of molecular fidelity that increases vulnerability to age-associated diseases. So that's the answer.

David: What do you think causes that "random systemic loss of molecular fidelity?"

Dr. Hayflick: What causes that loss of fidelity is based on the fact that complex biological molecules are kept in a state of fidelity as a result of a variety of chemical forces and various chemical bonds—van der Waals forces and other well-known bonds that keep molecules together. It is also well known that the energetics—the energy that keeps those bonds in the state that they're in, in molecules that are functioning—do not last forever. They last for varying periods of time—from as short as nanoseconds for ATP to years for collagen—so that there's a spectrum of energy levels in biological molecules. We have elaborate maintenance, turnover, and repair systems to keep those molecules in their correct functional state.

However, after reproductive maturation molecular errors begin to accumulate and exceed repair capacity for a very simple reason. There's no need to keep those molecules in a perfect state after reproductive maturity, because the animal possessing those molecules has already done what nature intends for it to do, and that is to reproduce. The proof of that statement is that for 99.99 percent of the time that we've been human we've had a life expectancy of less than twenty years. It's only been within the blink of an eye, on an evolutionary time scale, that we've have had life expectations greater than that.

David: Do you think that aging is actually a process that evolved?

Dr. Hayflick: No, aging is something that was never intended for us to see in the first place. It is an artifact of civilization. Aging only occurs in humans, and in the animals that you and I choose to protect—like zoo animals, domesticated animals and pets. It does not happen in the wild. We were intended to die at the age of thirty, but we've learned how to deal with the causes of our death such that we have revealed, teleologically, a process that we were never intended to see in the first place. And now we've got to live with it.

David: Why do you think that researching the causes of aging is more important than directing biomedical research efforts to the study of disease?

Dr. Hayflick: Because the goal of aging research should not be—and I believe that it's simply illogical to believe that it could be—to increase human longevity. That is, I should say, the goal of aging research should not be to intervene with the aging process and thereby increase longevity. The goal of biogerontological research should be to discover why an old cell is more vulnerable to pathology than is a young cell, and that key question is not being addressed by anybody on the planet at the moment. The reason it's important should be obvious.

When every physician in the world (of course I'm exaggerating, but I'm not too far off the mark) wakes up in the morning, they say this to themselves: The greatest risk factor for the leading causes of death—that is cardiovascular disease, stroke, and cancer—is the aging process. There's no physician on the planet who will dispute that. So I have a very simple-minded question: Why is the funding for research on the fundamentals of the biology of aging microscopic when compared to funding for research on the leading causes of death?

David: That's a very good question.

Dr. Hayflick: It's such a good question that whenever I show it on a slide [during a lecture] the physicians become slack-jawed and have no answer. But I think I know what the answer is.

David: What do you think it is?

Dr. Hayflick: Misunderstanding, greed, and power. Researchers in the fields of cardiovascular disease, stroke, and cancer require funding—after all this is one of our major industries. They don't want to undermine that industry or change careers to become biogerontologists. Now they might not know this consciously, or realize consciously that that's what's happening, but it is. You can't sell a senator or a representative on funding for the aging process. You can sell them on funding for cardiovascular disease, stroke, and cancer because either they or someone they know has one of them. They don't know that the underlying process that makes them vulnerable to those leading causes of death is the aging process, because of a huge failure to educate them.

David: I recently interviewed John Guerin, the director of the Ageless Animals Project. What do you think we can learn from studying animals that don't appear to age, like rockfish and turtles?

Dr. Hayflick: Well, I would hope that we could learn what the longevity determining processes are at the molecular level, and how the energetics of key molecules are maintained for periods of time in those animals that are unattainable in mammals.

David: What do you think is some of the most important aging research that is currently going on?

Dr. Hayflick: I rather think that the most important aging research is not being done today. I think a lot of the research being done today is misleading, especially the large area of work being done with invertebrates, namely worms and flies. There's almost a weekly announcement by one of the workers in the field that they discovered a new gene for aging, and I think that's absolute nonsense. There are no genes for aging. Most people don't understand the difference between aging and longevity determinants. Genes control development and indirectly longevity. They do not control aging. I would defend that position by another simple analogy, and that is to ask people who believe that genes cause aging to show me in the blueprints for their automobile where it is written, telling their automobile how to age. There are no such directions in blueprints. Why?—because the process is a spontaneous process. It requires no instructions, and the same is true in biological material. The only reason that animals of different species live longer than others is because of the differences in the longevity determinants. That is, the characteristics of molecules at the time of reproductive maturation including the level of repair turnover and maintenance systems to operate.

David: Do you think that maximum life span of human beings can be extended?

Dr. Hayflick: Oh yes. I think it has been, and it will continue to be on an evolutionary time scale. There's every reason to believe that. We have fairly good evidence that the present human life span was established about a hundred thousand years ago, based on brain weight/body weight ratios. There's no reason to believe that it's not increasing, but we have no evidence for it, and in fact we have one amusing bit of evidence against it. The world's oldest human being was a French lady named Jeanne Calment. She was born in 1875 and died in 1997. She was 122 and a half years old. The day that she died the world's oldest person was,

I think, 118, which means that in that instant human longevity dropped four years, right? Now we know that's wrong because we're dealing with exceptions to the enormous body of the population. So what the death of Jeanne Calment told us was that at the moment of her death human longevity dropped by four years, and this is the problem in making these kinds of determinations. So it's really guesswork, but I think it's safe to accept the fact that human longevity is increasing on an evolutionary time scale. This means that we're not going to detect an increase, if it's occurring—and if we keep proper records, which is doubtful—for the next 10,000 years or more.

David: But do you think that through our own research, and our own medical advancement, that we'll be able to intervene in the aging process and extend the maximum human life span?

Dr. Hayflick: No, I don't. Let me tell you why. If you resolved all of the leading causes of death currently written on death certificates for older people—namely, cardiovascular disease, stroke, and cancer—you could not possibly add more than fifteen years on to human life expectation. So even if we put every hospital, medical center, and the NIH out of business, and drive every physician on to an unemployment line, the maximum increase in human life expectancy would be fifteen years, period. That's something that many people simply don't understand, but it's an incontrovertible truth. So there's no way that we are going to reduce the age-specific mortality rates in the next century to the extent that we reduced them in the Twentieth Century. That happens only one time and one time only, and it has already happened. That resulted in an increase of life expectancy at birth during the Twentieth Century from approximately 47 to approximately 78 years. To increase human life expectancy by even two years today would necessitate the resolution of cancer as the cause of death. I don't think that's going to happen in the next fifty years, frankly, and not very many other people do either.

David: I interviewed Aubrey de Grey for this collection and I would like to create some dialogue between the people that I'm interviewing. Aubrey's response to what you said above was:

"Len is absolutely right—for the sorts of "resolutions" of the leading causes of death that he allows himself to imagine. Another way of

saying what he's saying is that geriatric medicine—combating the
pathologies of aging but not the underlying, accumulating molecular
damage that makes those pathologies happen—is a short term
approach because the damage continues to accumulate and the
pathologies (or other ones) become more and more difficult to hold
back. However, if we do combat that underlying damage—obviating it
(stopping it from being pathogenic) or else periodically removing most
of it—then we will resolve not only the major age-related diseases
but also all the other things that older people are more susceptible
to than the young, whether it be infections, accidents (due to weak
muscles, fragile bones or slow reactions), etc., and that will reduce the
mortality rate at all ages to around what it is for today's young adults.

How would you respond to Aubrey's comment?

Dr. Hayflick: Aubrey is assuming that our scientific knowledge has
reached such a degree of sophistication and understanding that we
presently have (or soon will have) the tools and the fundamental
understanding to intervene in either the aging or longevity determining
processes. This same belief has been held for centuries. Even sixty years
ago, and before we knew the structure of DNA, this belief was held by
several prominent scientists. They were wrong. Fifty years from today
scientists will look back on early Twenty-first Century biology and be
astonished to think that we could have had the chutzpah to believe that
we were knowledgeable enough to believe that we could interfere with
the aging process. Aubrey's belief that in fifty years we will know how
to make some humans live to be two hundred has been fifty years in the
future for the last 3500 years.

David: What type of anti-aging research would you like to see going
on?

Dr. Hayflick: I don't want to see any anti-aging research being
done because I think anti-aging research is like doing research on
antigravity.

I would like to see research done on answering one of the questions I posed
earlier, namely: Why are old cells more vulnerable to pathology than are
young cells? The second thing I would like to see done is something

that a layman like John Guerin is doing, and that even the professionals are not doing because they don't understand its importance—namely to answer the question, What is the reason why there are animals that either age negligibly or not at all? There's no research being done in that area, despite John Guerin's heroic efforts. So it's really neglect. The problem, in my view, is that it's in the hands mostly of medical professionals who think only of disease and pathology, and mix it up with aging. They don't understand that there are four aspects of the finitude of life: longevity determination, aging, age-associated diseases, and death. They don't understand the difference between those four, and they especially don't understand the difference between aging and disease. Many people think that aging is a disease. I don't think it's a disease at all.

David: In your book How and Why We Age *you discuss the possibility of building an orbiting "Noah's Ark" containing the preserved vital germ plasm of important plant seeds and the cell lines of human and animal species in order to safeguard our survival in the event of a global ecological disaster. I thought that was a pretty great idea. Has there been any interest from NASA in doing this?*

Dr. Hayflick: No. I proposed it to NASA back in the '60s but it fell on deaf ears. I have recently seen it surface actually. There are a lot of science fiction stories that incorporate it. But I think I've seen recently somebody suggesting it again, but I don't recall where. It was several years ago.

David: What are you currently working on?

Dr. Hayflick: I'm doing a lot of theoretical work, because I no longer have a wet lab. I've accumulated so much data, and I'm working on many of my theoretical aspects, some of which I've already discussed with you. I'm also preparing to do another book. I've been asked to do a book by Cambridge University Press on my experiences as a scientist, because I've had some unique experiences—a couple of which I mentioned to you only briefly. The book is going to be sort of a memoir, but built around three subject areas, which I was fortunate enough to be either a pioneer, or was witness to, and these are: the emergence of tissue culture or cell culture as a scientific discipline, the emergence of vaccine technology, and the emergence of the field of aging. Since I happened to be present at all three births, roughly, and know a lot of scandalous stories, it should be fun.

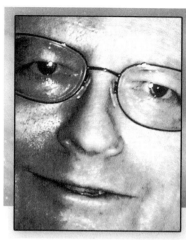

LEARNING FROM AGELESS ANIMALS

An Interview with John Guerin

John Guerin is the founder and director of the AgelessAnimals Project—also known as the Centenarian Species and Rockfish Project. This long-range research project involves investigators at fourteen universities around the world who study animals that don't seem to age.

There are certain species of rockfish, whales, turtles, and other animals that are known to live for over two hundred years without showing any signs of aging—a phenomenon known to biogerontologists as "negligible senescence." No one knows for sure how long these animals can live, but to date there have not been any observed increase in mortality or any decrease in reproductive capacity due to age. Striking examples are a 109 year old female rockfish that was captured in the wild while swimming around with fertilized eggs, and a hundred-plus year old male whale that was harpooned while it was having sex. The purpose of the AgelessAnimals Project is to understand why these animals don't seem to age and then to apply that understanding to human longevity.

Guerin is an experienced project manager who conceived of the AgelessAnimals project and orchestrates all of the studies. The two principal advisors to this project are Dr. Leonard Hayflick and Dr. Aubrey de Grey, both of whom were also interviewed for the Mavericks of Medicine *collection.*

Dr. Hayflick, discoverer of the "Hayflick limit" of cellular senescence, states that "Guerin's project is not only unique, but probes an area of almost total neglect in biogerontology, yet an area with more promise to deliver valuable data than, perhaps, any other."

When I asked Dr. de Grey about the importance of studying ageless animals he said, "All organisms with organs that rely on the indefinite survival of individual non-dividing cells (such as neurons in the brain) should age, though some, including humans, age very slowly. Some species do even better—we cannot yet measure their rate of aging at all—and studying them may well reveal ways to slow our own aging."

In addition to coordinating and orchestrating the AgelessAnimals project, Guerin lectures regularly on the subject of ageless animals. To find out more about Guerin's work and the AgelessAnimals Project visit their Web site: www.agelessanimals.org.

I interviewed John Guerin on March 14, 2005. John seemed eager and excited to discuss his project with me. We spoke about some of the latest research that's going on with long-lived animals, why this type of research has been neglected for so long, and how studying ageless animals might help us to understand the aging process better and extend the human lifespan.

David: What inspired the AgelessAnimals Project?

John: Back in 1995, I began looking into biotech, biogerontology, and the studies of aging. I read many different books, articles, and scientific papers. The turning point came when I read Dr. Leonard Hayflick's book *How and Why We Age*. Dr. Hayflick had a chapter called "Some Animals Age, Some Do Not," and I thought, Wow, now that's interesting. I'd heard rumors and old wives' tales about how some animals live for an extraordinarily long time, but this was the first time that I had come across that information from a scientific source. So, I started researching the literature on long-lived animals, and I found out that there's very little known. On my Web site I have some references on what I found.

I met Dr. Hayflick at a Gerontological Society of America meeting in November of '95, and I told him about my project management background. I said, I'd like to join whoever is working in this area, and I asked him who is. His answer was, "Nobody is, but they should be." So I tried to get something going on my own. I did a lot of research on different animals. I spent about a year looking at Koi—the fancy Japanese carp—and it's very likely that they do live quite a long time, at least over fifty years. They were reputed to live over two hundred years, but the readings were based on scales, and those are not accurate. So they didn't turn out to be a good candidate to study.

Then in 1997, I got some data from the Alaska Fish and Game. There's a chart at the bottom of my Web page with a rockfish on it that shows ages for different rockfish that were caught off the coast of Alaska, and the range is between twelve and 107 years. Now, that's a randomly caught sampling—it wasn't like they were trying to get older individuals. Those were the ones that fishermen caught and were going to people's dinner tables that evening. So when I realized that individuals at those ages were available I became very interested. We got samples from the Alaska Fish and Game in 1997. I say "we" because by then I had a couple of researchers at Oregon State University, including the Linus Pauling Institute interested in looking at the rockfish. So the Alaska Fish and Game sent us five older rockfish. After we got the aging results, it turned out that the youngest rockfish that they sent us was 79 years old, and the oldest was a 109 year old female that still had eggs.

David: That's extraordinary.

John: Yeah, and kind of sad. How long would this fish have lived if it wasn't caught? It didn't die of old age. It was fertile and still going strong in the ocean at 109 when they caught it. So that helped us to focus the project on rockfish. We have had one study on turtles. Whales are a very fascinating subject too, because they're warm-blooded mammals like we are, and they've now been documented to live over two hundred years of age.

David: How does one determine the age of these animals?

John: The most common technique for aging rockfish is the analysis of annual growth rings in the otolith, or ear bone. Basically, rockfish have incremental growth, so under a microscope their growth rings can be counted. There has been independent validation of this, and two recent international symposia have focused entirely on the importance of otolith measurement in fish life history studies. In turtles, the determination of minimum age is relatively straightforward using tag and recapture methods. Dr. Jeffrey Bada at UC San Diego Scripps did the aging analysis for the whale study. For this study the whales' ages were determined by using the aspartic acid racemization technique. In this technique, age is estimated based on intrinsic changes in the isomeric forms of aspartic acid in the eye lens nucleus. The references for these studies are on my Web site.

David: What is the goal of the Ageless Animals Project?

John: Quite simply, the goal is to understand the genetic and biochemical processes that long-lived animals use to retard aging. These long-lived animals have what's technically called "negligible senescence," as defined by Caleb Finch at the University of Southern California in Longevity, Senescence, and the Genome (1995).

David: What is negligible senescence?

John: Basically, this refers to an animal species that doesn't show any significant signs of aging as it grows older. Unlike humans and mammals other than whales, there's no decrease in reproduction after maturity. There's also no notable increase in mortality rate with age, but that's a little harder to prove. I've been talking with a statistician and he's asking, how do you know? To do a study of this type would take a couple of hundred years to complete. But compared to us there's no noted increase in mortality rate. I mean, if you are ninety years old, you're much more likely to die next year then you are if you're only twenty years old. But we don't seem to see any increase in mortality with rockfish and several of these other animals over time.

David: Why do you think these animals can live for so long without showing any signs of aging?

John: The purpose of the project is to understand why, and how to apply it to extending the healthy lifespan of humans. My background is in business project management; I have a project management professional certification. I'm not a bioresearcher, biochemist, or a biogerontologist—but I'm the one who organizes it all, and gets everyone involved. I get the researchers the samples and all that.

Actually, I thought I had a better idea about why these animals have negligible senescence when I started this project ten years ago. But it's hard to say. Back then we didn't know whales lived that long. That whales can live for over two hundred years was just discovered in the last five years. Up until then we thought that humans lived longer than any other mammal. So why certain animals would live much longer than others, and much longer than we do as a matter of fact—pretty much double what we've known humans to live—we don't understand.

There are some people who think that this can't be so, that this would violate the evolutionary theory of senescence, because nature doesn't select for longevity. But that's not necessarily true, because what's commonly seen is that there's just such a high mortality rate in nature. Even for humans, probably before two thousand years ago, we didn't live very long. We were hunted by tigers and wild animals, and traits of longevity, presumably, weren't selected for. But if these animals, like the rockfish, can be 109 years old and still be reproductive, nature is going to allow those genes to keep contributing to the gene pool, so that it won't select against longevity.

David: So we don't know if these animals are simply aging more slowly or not at all? Since we haven't found any rockfish or whales that live for three or four hundred years, that might suggest that there is a certain limit on how long they can live.

John: Well, we just do not know. We honestly do not know. It really is unfortunate that there is so little known in this field. Ecologists have never thought of this in the terms that gerontologists are now thinking of it in. To give you an idea, let's say you have a sample of a species, and you see they live to twenty years. That's the oldest you sample out of several hundred. Ecologists then assume that's their maximum longevity. That's really the basis of their thinking in most cases. Mice, as you probably well know, don't live for more than a couple years, even in the best laboratory environment, with all the optimum nutrients and food. They don't live very long. They just can't. They'll start having all sorts of age-related pathological functions, and they'll die of old age.

But this other group of organisms, those that possess what Finch termed "negligible senescence," they don't seem to be showing the classical signs of aging that we're used to. So, who is to say the longest they could live? As an example, in Finch's book that was published in 1990, at that time the longest lived whale was—I believe it was a blue whale—something like 108 years old. That's not so startling. Humans live longer than that. We're mammals. They're mammals. We live longer. Then a study was done on bowhead whales, and they found that out of forty whales sampled, four of them were over a hundred years old, and one of them was over two hundred years old. And they didn't die of old age either—they were harpooned. I have a reference on the Web site.

David: How might studying ageless animals help us to understand human aging better?

John: By understanding how other animals are naturally able to live a lot longer than we are, we can ask: What is genetically different? What is biochemically different? There are two major problems with studying long-lived animals. One is that nobody knows what causes aging. If we were able to say what causes aging, then we could target that same factor in animals that are living a very long time—whales, rockfish, sturgeon, lobsters, and several other animals—and then study it. If you looked on our Web site you've seen that we did studies in everything from lysosomes to microarrays to telomerase activity, because you just don't know what to look for. That's one problem. The other is that these animals live so long that you have to ask: How do you do an experiment? Let's say we think a certain gene's involved in longevity, so we were going to do a knockout gene. Then instead of living two hundred years a rockfish lives seventy-five years.

David: It would take quite awhile to run the experiment.

John: Yeah, it would be somebody else finishing it up, and it certainly wouldn't be of much practical benefit. So the direction we're taking in the project is we're looking at the difference between long-lived rockfish and short-lived rockfish. The other approach is basically identifying genetic differences, and going at it that way, because there's no practical way you could run an experiment that would go on for decades.

At first rockfish just seemed to be a good model, or a handily available model. They're commercially caught, go to the dinner table, and we were able to get lots of samples of them. Then, of course, the news about whales came out, which is very intriguing, and there are a lot of other animals that are either known or suspected to live a very long time. But the really intriguing thing about rockfish is that in the same genus—which is *sebastes*—there are rockfish that have not been noted more than about twelve to twenty years maximum longevity, and these are essentially cousins. They are rockfish, and some of these at least have been caught in thousands of samples, so it's not just an aberration of a small sample size.

One of the key issues people have raised to me at meetings is that you have to have something to compare these long-lived animals to in order to try and understand why they're successfully retarding aging. So what better model can you have than another species within the same genus that doesn't live a very long time? In all the meetings I've gone to I haven't had anybody come up and say, oh here's another species that has a really diverse longevity. Actually there is perhaps one other instance— the naked mole rat. In the last few years it's gotten a lot of publicity. It's a rodent and most rodents—like mice and rats—live maybe two to five years maximum. The naked mole rat has been documented to live at least into its twenties. So it's on quite another order of magnitude different than other rodents. The bat is another exception that lives way longer than other small mammals, and birds, of course, are their own interesting exception.

So comparing long-lived and short-lived rockfish is our focus, which is almost out of necessity, because how do you design an experiment to test for longevity when you've got such long-lived animals? Whatever tests we're going to do to the long-lived rockfish in the future, like a micro-array, we want to do with the short-lived ones too.

David: Could you talk about some of the principal investigators for the AgelessAnimals project, and can you summarize some of the latest research that's going on with long-lived animals?

John: There are fourteen principal investigators at fourteen different universities, such as Dr. Judd Aiken at the University of Wisconsin, Madison. He's very well-known and respected in the field. He does mitochondrial mutation studies, and this could be one of the more important areas because of what we know about free radical damage. The oxidative theory seems to be one of the more important theories of aging, so I'm encouraged, even though at this point he hasn't gotten results yet. His lab is working on amplifying the primers. So that could be a very important study. I think the microarray study is an important one too.

Dr. Ana Maria Cuervo, who's at Albert Einstein College of Medicine in New York City, did the most complete study. Her study was on lysosomes and proteolytic activity, and she actually has done more than is posted on the Web site. She added some more tests that she didn't have available a couple of years ago, and she told me about a month ago that she intends to publish her manuscript. So that would be the most extensive study. Also, there's Glenn Gerhard, an M.D. who was at Dartmouth who then took a full-time research position at a research institute in Pennsylvania. He did a SOD (superoxide dismutase) study and then also the microarray study.

David: Why do you think that the study of long-lived animals has been neglected for so long?

John: I have thought about it, and partly I have to say I don't understand why. I think that's why somebody like me got involved, because I have a project management background and I can see the big picture. There's more than one reason I can see as to why people in the field wouldn't have gotten involved. It's risky to put your career on the line to look at animals that haven't been studied very well and that do not have cultures available, whereas, with other species strains are easily available. For instance, with any mouse you want you could get a strain, and you could have it under the identical conditions you need.

But this hasn't been done with any of these long-lived animals. For me, the biggest question really is: Why hasn't the National Institute of Aging taken a lead? This is a perfect opportunity for government to get involved, where there is no profit motive. This is basic research that we're doing with these animals, and basic research doesn't necessarily have a pay-back. Now, let's say we find something like we did with the SOD study. We had a very interesting finding that SOD went up with age in rockfish, and as you may be aware, SOD is the strongest antioxidant in our bodies, and in most animals. So that it goes up with age is a very intriguing finding. That's something we hope to look into more, but in general all of the things we've done are just basic science. We're just laying the groundwork.

David: Has anybody done any studies to see if whale cells, rockfish cells, or turtle cells reach a Hayflick limit in the number of times that they can divide? Are their telomeres growing shorter with each cell division?

John: In terms of the Hayflick limit, you very well may be aware that most gerontologists don't consider that to be a limitation of aging. At some point, maybe about ten years ago, it was a much bigger topic. Nowadays, telomeres and telomerase is much more of a cancer issue, because most cancer cells keep producing the enzyme telomerase that allows cells to keep dividing.

David: When I interviewed Michael Fossel for this collection he thought differently.

John: I would have to say that the majority of gerontologists don't believe telomere length is important in aging. I remember at a meeting a couple of years ago, somebody just making an offhand remark that we used to think telomerase and telomeres were important. I think if you do a survey you would find that the majority of gerontologists don't believe they are. The telomerase limit and the Hayflick limit doesn't seem to necessarily be what it once was thought to be, because even older people have continued replication of the cells that do divide. There's a bunch of reasons that it doesn't seem as important now in aging as it once did.

David: Yes, I understand that, but I'm still curious. Do you know if these animals that have negligible senescence, if their cells reach a Hayflick limit? Is there a limit to how many times the cells from these animals can divide?

John: We have fourteen studies—twelve in the U.S. and two in Europe. One of the European studies is in Germany by Guido Krupp, who looked at telomerase levels in nine different rockfish. He looked at three samples from each rockfish—one of heart, liver, and brain—all the way from teenage years up to a 93 year old rockfish. All of the three tissues showed expression of telomerase, and there was no age-dependent change of expression of telomerase in the tissues. There were individual differences. Some were higher and some were lower. One of the higher levels of telomerase was found in the 93 year old, but the primary finding was that there was no trend with age.

As far as whales go, the only other person I know outside our group and Caleb Finch at USC, who actually is studying these long-lived animals, is Jerry Shay at the University of Texas in Dallas. He got some samples of bowhead whales, and he's basically doing these cell replications to see how many replications he gets out of them. Apparently, it's pretty hard to get the samples—they had to go through the Canadian government, and it was quite an ordeal. Jerry Shay is the only one I know of who's done bowhead whale studies, but in the ecological study I mentioned earlier four of the whales out of forty were documented to be over a hundred years old, and one of them was over two hundred years old. They reach that longevity without the assistance of doctors. Although this was not in the paper, we know that at least one of the hundred-plus year old male whales was reproductive, because when he was harpooned he was caught in the act.

David: Wait a minute. This hundred-plus year old whale was harpooned while it was having sex?

John: Yes. When I talked to the researcher, who is an ecologist, I said, "Gerontologists want to know how you know that the whales weren't about to keel over, that they weren't on their last legs, so to speak?" And then he has an example like this. I ask, were they reproductive? And he says, well, one of the males sure was.

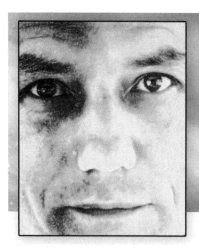

**COUNTDOWN
to
TELOMERASE THERAPY**

An Interview with Dr. Michael Fossel

Michael Fossel, Ph.D., M.D., is a clinical physician and neurobiologist with a strong interest in the human aging process. He is currently the Clinical Professor of Medicine at Michigan State University, and Attending Physician at St. Mary's Hospital Emergency Department in Grand Rapids, Michigan. Dr. Fossel is the author of Reversing Human Aging, *and the recently published* Cells Aging, and Human Disease. *He believes that we are only around a decade away from a truly remarkable form of anti-aging therapy that holds the promise of perpetually renewable youth.*

Dr. Fossel has dedicated years to studying progeria and other accelerated aging syndromes. Children with the progeric disease Hutchinson-Gilford syndrome die at an average age of twelve or thirteen. They usually die of heart disease, strokes, cancer, and other illnesses that often strike the elderly. Children with progeria look uncannily like old men and women, with balding heads and wrinkled skin, and appear to suffer from many of the symptoms of old age.

Dr. Fossel believes that the evidence from these diseases (combined with the fact that germ cells and cancer cells do not age) indicates that aging is largely a regulated process; i.e., a function of gene expression. According to Dr. Fossel, the key to understanding, and possibly reversing, human aging lies at the tips of our chromosomes. He thinks that one of the best places to intervene in the genetically-wired clock that determines our biological age is in the intracellular process of telomere replication.

Telomeres are the base pairs located at the end of our chromosomes that hold the DNA molecule together. With the exception of germ cells (sperm and eggs) and cancer cells, each time a human cell divides the telomeres become a little bit shorter. This is why, no matter how optimum a cell's environment is, after a certain number of cell divisions, the telomeres become too short, gene expression changes, down regulating cell repair and maintenance, and the cells age. The progeric disease Hutchinson-Gilford syndrome is caused by having telomeres that are too short at birth, so it doesn't take too many divisions before the cells begin to show early aging.

The reason that germ cells and cancer cells don't age—and can potentially divide forever—is because they produce an enzyme called telomerase, which keeps the telomeres intact when the cell divides. Dr. Fossel predicts that telomerase therapy could extend human life indefinitely by resetting the genetic clock in healthy somatic cells, and turning it off in runaway cancer cells. He imagines that very soon everyone will have the potential to live for centuries in a body that looks and functions like its about twenty years old.

Dr. Fossel earned his master's degree in psychology at Wesleyan University. He then earned his Ph.D. in neurobiology, and an M.D. from Stanford University. In 1998, Dr. Fossel won the Achievement Award in Preventive Medicine from the American College for Advancement in Medicine. He was the founding editor of the Journal of Anti-Aging Medicine *(now* Rejuvenation Research*), and served as its Editor-in-Chief for six years. Dr. Fossel is a widely published author of dozens of scientific papers and articles and a popular international lecturer. He has also appeared on numerous radio and television shows, and in many science documentaries.*

I spoke with Michael on July 3, 2004. Michael speaks fast, yet somehow manages to say every word clearly and distinctly. He radiates a sense of warmth and humor. In a message that he sent me, he described himself by saying, "On the whole, I prefer data to fame, accuracy to eminence, and gardening to tenure." I spoke with Michael about what he's learned from working with progeric children, how telomeres are related to human aging, and the possible medical, societal, and psychological consequences of telomerase therapy and biological age reversal.

David: How did you first become interested in medicine, and what lead you to study the human aging process?

Michael: I think that, to a degree, both of these questions have the same answer. All of us have certain bents to our personality. For me, I suppose you could say, there is need to help people—and I don't mean that in a naive, puppy-dog sense. I just get a certain amount of pleasure out of having people around me feel better, work better, live better, and enjoy themselves more.

As an example, I work clinically doing predominantly emergency medicine. The practice of emergency medicine, per se, does not have a lot of intellectual interest for me. Not none—just not a lot. On the other hand, I can derive enormous emotional benefit from it. The fact that I can leave a room, and have someone laughing, who a minute ago was terrified, is something that I need just as much I need to pay my mortgage. And I think that personality bent is what has lead me into both medicine, and in the long-run, to aging.

There's a passage in the forward to my new textbook where I talk about how easy it is for people to understand the importance of treating children, and that we often forget that, or don't understand that, when we're talking about the importance of treating the elderly. For me, that's almost self-evident. Again, I think it's a part of my personality, and it's sometimes hard for me to understand why other people don't understand the importance of that. But it's just me.

David: Can you talk a little about why you think that telomeres are so important in understanding, and possibly reversing, human aging?

Michael: That's an interesting question, because it is usually asked incorrectly, and gets answered incorrectly. There are people who have said—and it's simply not true—that I think telomeres cause aging. Not a bit. To me, there are two issues here. One is, what causes aging? And, frankly, I find that uninteresting, and I'll come back to why I say it that way. Telomeres, per se, don't cause aging. They're a piece of the entire complex cascade and process of the aging organism. But the more important question for me is, where's the most effective point of intervention?

I'll give you a couple of examples of this. I get residents who come in to work with me clinically, who feel that if they've made a diagnosis, they're done. Not a bit. Patients don't come in for a diagnosis. They come in to be made better. Now it's true that usually making a diagnosis helps you make patients better. But a patient doesn't come in for a name. If you came in with a funny melanotic spot on your arm, you don't so much care whether it's melanoma or not. You want to know if I can make it never come back and kill you, or not.

All right, now the fact is, I usually have to establish whether it's melanoma. But it's not the name, per se, that holds your interest. It's—will this kill me? Can you prevent it? That's the critical issue. The same thing's true for me in aging. The issue for me is not what causes aging, and how does the cascade work, but what can we do to intervene, to prevent age-related disease and suffering?

Now there are an awful lot of people who will start discussions with me about whether or not aging is a disease. Frankly, I don't think that's an important issue. Whatever you want to define age-related diseases as, the important issue is, can we intervene in them? For me, aging may or may not be a disease, but it certainly increases your likelihood of having a disease. So the question is, where can we intervene? Given that, my answer usually is, the most effective point of intervention is probably the human telomere—not because it causes aging, but because it's probably the most effective point of intervention.

If I'm looking at heart disease (actually, atherosclerosis, causing both strokes and heart attacks), which is the major killer worldwide, I ask myself not what causes it, but where can I intervene? There are literally dozens of critical points of intervention—everything from high blood pressure to cholesterol levels, to a number of genetic factors, to smoking, and behavioral effects. But again, while I can intervene in your risk of heart disease by lowering your cholesterol, with say Lipitor, it may be that a more effective and efficient point of intervention would be the telomere. So that's my question. Now to answer that question you really have to understand some of the processes. But it's not the process, per se, that interests me in an intellectual fashion. It's a totally concrete interest.

David: Why did you start studying people with progeria, and what have you learned about the process of human aging from studying people with accelerated aging disorders?

Michael: I started studying progeria in basically the mid-1970's. In graduate school, I think I used to have the world's literature on progeria under my bed. I found much more interest when I began to attend the annual progeric reunions for the Hutchinson-Gilford progerics. For me there are two interests here. One is what can we do for these children? The answer is, not only not much, but to the extent you'll be able to, it'll be too late for most of the children that you know. The life span is about twelve and a half years, and that's a pretty narrow research horizon.

The other question is, what can they teach us about normal aging? I find that the most effective point. The most promising way to look at almost any research question is to ask yourself, where are the outliers? Where are the anomalies? Where are the exceptions? To understand aging I think there's a certain benefit from just looking at normal human aging. But I think you learn a lot more by looking at organisms that either don't age, age slowly, age quickly, or age in a peculiar fashion.

Now, the latter two are true of progerics. They age quickly, but they age in a peculiar fashion. Not all of the body seems to age. In fact, you could reasonably ask whether this is aging at all. Is it accelerated aging? Is it aging? Does it tell us anything? I think the answer is, it does. I think what you're seeing in the arterial supplies in the skin, the joints and in the bones reflects, if not real aging, at least something that can offer us a great deal of insight into aging. Whereas, if you're looking at the immune system, or the nervous system, frankly there's very little it can offer us—except, again, as an anomaly. Why is it that the arteries of these children seem to show rapid aging, and the brain cells don't? Again, it's the anomalies, I think, that can teach us more than just the routine humdrum process.

David: How is cellular aging related to the bodily symptoms of aging that ultimately lead to disease and death?

Michael: To put it bluntly—and again, there's a certain inaccuracy in saying this, but just by saying it this way, I think it prompts a great deal of both insight and appropriate criticism—I think the answer is that all aging is cell aging. Organisms age, and if you look at an organism aging, what you're really looking at is organ aging and tissue aging. And if you look at organ aging and tissue aging, you look at cellular aging. The human body is composed of cells, and while it's appropriate to keep in mind the gestalt involved, the real process occurs not only at the cellular level, but between cells. It's like looking at society. Society isn't a thing; it's a collection of individuals. It's not only the individuals, but the way they interact. It's the same thing here. If you really want to understand a society you want to understand the individuals. If you really want to understand aging, you want to understand how the cells are affected.

David: What do you think will be the best way to reset gene expression in elderly cells and increase telomere length?

Michael: The quick answer is that the best way to reset gene expression is to increase telomere length. But the best way to increase telomere length is to use one of three processes. One is something that we're technically capable of now—although we haven't tried it yet in human volunteers—is to insert a new hTERT gene that's turned on. That can and has been done in the cells, and has been done in reconstituted tissue.

The second way, which is much more elegant, is simply to turn on and off the existing hTERT gene in human cells. That process has been looked at, and we're very close, tantalizingly close, but to the best of my knowledge it hasn't been accomplished yet.

The third approach would be to put in hTERT. That is, essentially, to put telomerase into the cells, and that was regarded as technically impossible, perhaps, as late as five years ago. Now it looks like it's probably possible, but, again, to the best of my knowledge hasn't been accomplished.

If, right now, what I wanted to do was to run a study trying to use telomerase, or telomere maintenance approaches, to correct, say, osteoarthritis, I would try insertion of a new hTERT gene into the cells of human joints. It's not the most elegant approach, but it's the process we're most able to perform right now technically.

David: Does the enzyme telomerase actually reset telomeres back to their youthful lengths, or simply prevent them from getting any shorter with each cell division?

Michael: The simple answer is both. In the hematopoietic cells in your bone marrow the latter is what happens. That is, you use recurrent and well-controlled telomerase expression to almost maintain the length of your hematopoietic stem cells. This is a very delicate, very carefully crafted process, but the end result is that over the, say, hundred years you might live, you don't lose much in the way of hematopoietic stem cell potential for division. You more or less maintain telomere length during your entire lifespan. You certainly don't shorten it as much as would be expected otherwise. Telomerase can not only be used that way, but it can be used to reset or re-lengthen telomeres.

David: What possibilities do you foresee for using some form of telomerase suppression as a treatment for cancer?

Michael: Certainly to me, I think it's probably the most interesting and tantalizing approach to controlling cancer now. The reason I say that is that it's probably the most universal approach. You remember back when I was talking about interventions in aging, and I said the question is, where's the most effective single point of intervention? With joints, for example, you could replace them, or you can try to use something to control inflammation and so forth. And the same thing in cancer. There are lots of approaches, some of which may be very effective with particular cancers, in particular patients. But if you're looking for an overall single approach, I think the most promising one is probably control of telomerase expression and function.

David: How long do you think it will be before the first telomere therapies become available?

Michael: The telomerase trials in terms of cancer are already in progress now. But if you're looking at using telomerase to, in effect, control or reverse aging pathology, I think you'll see the first human trials within ten years. We almost began that about two years ago. We had a donor who wanted to underwrite the whole process, but they pulled out, actually the night before they were to sign the final financial contracts, or we'd probably be in progress now. So it depends. It depends on the market. It depends on people's beliefs. And it certainly depends on whether this entire approach is accurate or not.

David: Is there anything that people can do now, say with nutritional therapies or caloric restriction, that can reduce telomere loss, and possibly help to slow down or reverse the aging process?

Michael: I think the answer to that parallels the question that you would have asked in 1953 or 1952 with regard to polio. What can we do to prevent our children from having polio? And you would get the same sort of answers. You need to have a healthy diet, avoid swimming pools, avoid people with polio, and keep an eye out for other risk factors. This is the same thing that you could have said in, say, 1870, with regard to tetanus. How do we prevent lockjaw (that is, tetanus)? The answers are similar. You certainly want somebody who's relatively healthy, and avoids skin breaks that are near horse manure and so forth.

But as far as therapy goes for either of those, on those two dates, the answer was pretty dismal. I think the same thing is true of aging. The best you can do is hope to ameliorate your current gene expression. If you want to avoid heart disease as an aging process there is lots of advice I could give you. Your grandmother probably gave you similar advice, just as your doctor certainly gives you advice now. But the truth of it is, that's all it does. It ameliorates the risks you have from gene expression. People who have bad genes tend to get bad atherosclerosis. That's not to say they should smoke and not exercise and so forth. No, they should certainly follow standard, appropriate medical recommendations. But the real answer is, if you want to make a significant change in the outcome of that pathology, you're going to have to do something more dramatic and fundamental like effect telomere expression.

David: Are you referring to the aging process in general or telomere loss specifically?

Michael: They're closely linked, and you're right. It sort of depends on what you're addressing, which one you want to focus on as you're answering the question. As I said before, my primary interest is the pathology. I'm not interested in wild intellectual discussions about aging and disease. No, I'm interested in people who actually have disease, and where we can intervene. So when you ask questions like that, I tend to magnetically home back to specific diseases, like osteoarthritis and so forth, and bring it back to what I see as practical intervention, rather than far-flung discussions, like aging in general. But no, in one sense, it's all one process. Aging and age-related diseases are very entangled with one another.

David: How long do you think it's possible for human life span to be extended?

Michael: I think that using the sort of approaches that we've been talking about in this conversation we can probably extend the lifespan well into the several centuries range. Could be more. My usual answer to that is the human lifespan becomes either indeterminate, or as you might say, indefinite. Again, I don't mean by that infinite. I simply mean it's indefinite. It's hard to say. I don't know any way to get a firm grasp on that question. You could say several hundred years, as I just implied, but I say that to stress that we're not dealing with just an extension of two or three years of lifespan, and partly to say that I don't how you can reasonably talk about several thousand years. But I want people to understand that it's a significant change. The prospects are enormous, as are the implications of it in all regards, socially and otherwise.

David: How do you think human societies will change when people start living for hundreds of years?

Michael: Let me start by saying that I think that the personal consequences will basically be all for the good, but that the social consequences will either be a mixed bag, or certainly less easy to pin down. The first thing to point out is that any time you have societal change, it's a societal disruption, with all that implies. It's difficult for people. I don't care what the societal change is, or how good it is, it tends to be costly to individuals. So the very fact that you're changing something already puts you at risk.

The second sort of a no-brainer is what happens to population. Most of us currently feel that the planet is overpopulated, although it's really hard to prove that. You start with assumptions about what you regard as optimal life style in optimal society, but, granting that, population will certainly go up. There's almost no way around that, unless you add in the implied risks of an increased possibility of viral transfer, war, terrorism, and so forth, all of which are possible. But the overall initial guess is the population will go up, with consequent costs to the individual, and to societies that make up the planet.

That also brings another corollary with it, which is increased risk of ecological damage. The environmental consequences are unlikely to be good. You could argue that they may be minimal, and you could argue that they may be maximal, but in any case, they're likely to be negative. I'm not sure how you can make an argument against that.

Now you get to the things that become much tougher to pin down. For example, what happens to the cost of living? That's interesting. Actually, it probably goes down, and the reason is because you end up amortizing off the cost of training individuals. For example, it works out to about fifteen years before a company breaks even on the cost that they put into training the average tool and dye maker to be good, and paying his benefits. He may work for them for about another thirty years and then retire. Now, if he works for another sixty years, you see what happens to the cost of training. It is essentially amortized off this longer period. Therefore, the cost to the company goes down, and the cost of making widgets goes down.

Also, health insurance and life insurance costs go down. Having said that, if you're actually trying to figure out those costs, you're having nightmares, because you can not figure out what those costs really are. There's nothing on which to base your prediction. If I say to you we've instituted full telomerase therapy, then you'll ask, so what's the lifespan and how do I figure out life insurance costs? You have no way of knowing. What about health costs? It's the same thing. They're bound to go down, but I don't know where they'll go to. So the cost of living tends to go down for that, and a couple of other fun reasons, but basically because labor becomes a bit more efficient in an economic sense.

On the other hand, say you're the eighteen year old looking for a job as a tool and dye maker, but the other man hasn't retired. The population is going up, so they want more widgets, and they're hiring more people. How do those balance out? Is the eighteen year old more likely to find a job as a tool and dye maker, or less? The same sort of approach goes for any profession you can think of. It takes about three years for a bank to break even on a commercial banker. As I said, it's about fifteen years for tool and dye makers, and around seven for doctors. You can see who actually matters to society, reasonably enough. Tool and dye makers are more costly.

But no matter what profession you pick, you tend to get some savings from labor costs, in terms of both of training and benefits. Disability is sort of an odd mixed bag. On the one hand, you're less likely to have a disabling condition. On the other hand, you're more likely to live with it. For example, say you've got someone like Christopher Reeves. How long is he going to live now as a quad? So what does that do to the cost of disability insurance? You see what I mean? It's very difficult. And that's even just assuming that the healthcare benefits and costs stay the same, which they're unlikely to do.

Assuming that people will be less sick, what will that do to the costs of treating a sickness they get? And what about what they expect from health insurance to get that policy? Do you add dental? Do you add increased psychiatric costs because society is now a little bit more frightening to people? What about the costs of treating a heart attack when there are fewer? Do they go up or down? What happens to the rest of medical care?

You see what I mean. It's a mess no matter what you pick, essentially, whether it's the economy, or whether it's change in social costs to people. What happens to family structures? What happens to the length of marriages? What happens to treatment of children within society? For example, what happens to the cost of child immunizations when the percentage of children in the population drops, and childbearing adults drops? This means that their political clout goes down. Do you find that people are no longer willing to pay for immunizations as a society, let alone individuals? No matter what you pick, no matter what approach you want to look at it, it becomes extraordinarily difficult to make any reasonable predictions.

David: When you speculate about how the extension of human life might affect societies in the future, have you considered the implications of advances in robotics, artificial intelligence, and nanotechnology?

Michael: No, I found making even rough guesses difficult enough just restricting myself to the effects of extending lifespan via telomerase-based approaches. Predictions tend to be linear extrapolations; technological advances tend to throw curves. Predicting (poorly) one curve is already impossible enough without adding three more curves, to say nothing of the seven others neither of us considered, but which will actually play a more central role.

David: How do you think living for hundreds of years will affect human psychology?

Michael: I think in the long run, both for society and for people, the answer is actually going to be positive. But as I've just said, it becomes almost impossible to make a firm case for that. Because people will be living so much longer, my feeling is that we're actually looking at something like the advent of civilization. Now I could easily undercut that argument in great detail, to the tune of hours, but I think, overall, the answer is that it will be good for you psychologically and it will be good for us a culture. It will actually make us a more mature culture, and I don't mean that in a bad sense. I mean that in a more civilized and kinder sense. But, boy, it's a tough argument to make.

David: In your book, Reversing Human Aging, *you compared the*

*initial market for telomerase drugs as being similar to the black
market for psychedelic drugs. Why do you think that there might be a
black market in the near future for telomerase drugs?*

Michael: Oh, you have done your homework; you actually read that
thing. I actually don't think there would be a black market, but I think
there could be. If I say I have a small company, and I can manufacture
a telomerase inducer, and you have reason to believe that it works—
never mind whether it does or not—and I'm not willing to sell it to you,
or I'm selling at a price that you can't afford, you therefore have an
inducement to either make your own, buy it black market, or find it from
some company that makes it on the sly. If you believe it works, and you
can't get it from me, you'll want to get it from someone else.

David: Can you talk a little about your recently published book Cells,
Aging, and Human Disease, *what are some of the new discoveries that
have been made since you wrote* Reversing Human Aging?

Michael: There were a couple of people who criticized the first book on
the grounds that it was speculative. That's true, but I said that. I didn't
lie about it. I said this is speculation. I don't know why they didn't
catch that. But they still criticized it, either on those grounds, or on
the grounds that it wasn't academic enough. So I decided to write the
academic book, and that's what the new book is. It's about sixty percent
text, forty percent references. It's got some 4,300 references, and it's
basically an advanced level, graduate student biology text.

The book is separated into two sections. In the first section, I discuss
age at the cellular and genetic levels. In the second section, I go through
the human body tissue by tissue. I discuss age-related pathology, how
the systems and tissue work, as well as how aging and other pathology
affect that tissue. I look at what role, if any, cell senescence plays, or
is likely to play, in that tissue, and finally what are appropriate points
of intervention, either currently or in the near future, potentially using
telomerase approaches. So, again, it basically is a textbook on how we
can use cell senescence to affect human disease. It's both very academic
and very clinical. As I implied before, it's not meant as an intellectual
text so much as a practical and clinical look at disease, with a very
strong emphasis on intervention. It's not about a pure intellectual

understanding, or just an ivory tower understanding, but rather, the focus is on intervention.

I think that the major, single advance that's been made in the last ten years really has been to show that we can reverse aging in reconstructed human tissues. In 1996, we showed that we could prevent or reverse aging in individual cells, but that was in limited cases. Since that time, not only has the work on cell types expanded, but we've shown that you can reverse aging in reconstituted human tissue. The next step we want to take would be to look at other tissues, and more importantly, a whole body approach.

The tissue that's been best looked at already has been human skin. Putting this in its simplest form, what has been shown is this. If we use young cells we can grow young skin. If we use old cells we can grow old skin. But if we take old cells and telomerase them, we can now grow young skin. So the argument that things just fall apart, that's the way it is and they can't be fixed, is not only wrong at the cellular level, but it's wrong at the tissue level. That doesn't prove that we can use it clinically, but it does prove that the blanket assertion that aging can't be changed or reversed is simply wrong, at least with regard to a couple of tissues that we've looked at. So that's very promising.

David: Where do you think humanity should be focusing its scientific efforts right now?

Michael: Most people, and my temptation, would be to answer that from a very self-serving or personal approach. Obviously, as most researchers would say, you should be putting your money where I tell you, which is where I do my research. But the truth is you don't know. The United States, and in fact most developed cultures, have a faith these days in the upstarts of small businesses. Not everyone does, but a lot of people do. They look at small businesses, and say, my God, look at the things that happen. For example, Microsoft started in a garage and look what happened. The truth is that most small businesses fail, depending on how you want to define failure, and an extraordinarily small number of them succeed spectacularly. But if you look at it in retrospect you see the success stories not the failures.

The same thing is really true scientifically. If we look back at things like quantum theory, or any number of other scientific approaches, whether they're conceptual or practical, we see the success stories. But we miss the extraordinarily large number of foolish notions that, at the time, were looked at seriously. So the answer I think has to be that, not only can't you just make an assertion and say, well, this is exactly where you should put your money, but, in fact, it's very hard to do so rationally—because, frankly, it's hard for human beings to be rational, logical, careful, and not let their own silliness, in a sense, or fashions intervene.

It's like phrenology. If we were right now back in Europe a hundred years ago we'd be considering putting money into phrenology perhaps. Well, most of us these days regard that as the height of foolishness. But the lesson we need to take from that is that the things that we think are very promising, may in fact be foolish. So it's hard to answer that question. I think that we have to do the best we can, and I don't like the procedures we use now to decide what we're going to do with scientific funds, but I don't have a better idea. It's like capitalism, which is a very bad system, but it's hard to find a better one. I think that's true here too. We try to figure out where's the best place to put scientific funding, and we probably don't do a very good job, but for the life of me, I'm not sure how we can do a better job—except to continue to try to be rational, fair, balanced, and logical, knowing that we're likely failing, but not having a better alternative.

David: What do you think happens to consciousness after death?

Michael: I have to tell you something odd. Given my druthers, I would prefer to talk about my sex life over my religious views on the world, and that comes perilously close. I find my views of religion, metaphysics, or life after death, as remarkably personal, in a sense, as to not make them public. But given a quick answer to that, I have to say I don't think that death is final, and leave it at that.

David: I wonder how you're going to feel about this next question then. What is your perspective on the concept of God?

Michael: You've already heard my perspective on our inability to be logical, reasonable, and unbiased—historically and scientifically—and

I suspect that in spades is the problem we have in trying to conceptualize God. I don't think we're capable of it in any but almost laughable ways. So, much as I take religions very seriously—religions plural and my own personally—I suspect that they're a far, far distance from anything that reflects reality.

David: Do you see any sort of teleology in the evolutionary process, or do you see evolution as being a blind chance process?

Michael: That's like trying to say to me, is God infinitely wise? It brings up all sorts of questions about what is God, and what is wise? And I think the same thing bears on questions of blind chance, teleology, evolution, and frankly again, my own inability to come to grasp with these things, or my own distrust of my ability to conceptualize these things in any accurate way. I tend to act as though evolution was a blind chance, while always wondering.

David: Is there anything that we haven't talked about that you would like to add?

Michael: Yeah, let me give you this, just because I suppose it interests people. Sometimes people ask me—and you sort of got at this, but you didn't follow up—when will we reverse human aging? That's it asked in its most bald-faced sense. It's like asking, are we interfering with God's will? People like to ask these things. When will we reverse human aging? The answer to me is kind of interesting. If you had asked me, when did we step on the moon, we can answer to the second. In fact, with a little research, we can answer to the millisecond, as close as you want, even allowing for the time delay between here and the moon.

If you asked me, when did we cure polio, the answer gets curiously slippery, and yet definite. If I ask most people on the street they'll say, well, it was 1954 wasn't it? And they're very right. That's when the commercial vaccine was released, then taken back, and then released again, at least in the U.S. But if you asked anybody who has a little more knowledge, they'll first point out immediately that we haven't cured polio. It's still around in this world, and we have high hopes.

They might also go on to point out that in the theoretical, or the research sense, we cured polio sometime in the early 1950's, before the release of the vaccine, because that's when we (meaning Salk) first had a grasp of how things worked in polio. So, in a conceptual sense, we cured polio in 1951 or '52 perhaps. But leaving that aside, one, you notice it's really hard to pin it down, and two, probably the best we can do is ask the man on the street, and that's not a bad way of asking the question, as long as you understand limitations.

The same thing pertains here. If you ask, when will we reverse human aging, there's no way we could answer anyway. Even looking back from the future, I think you wouldn't be able to answer it anymore than you can about when we cured polio. But what you could do is you could go forward a hundred or two hundred years and poll the person on the street, and say, when do you think we reversed human aging? I think that if you took the mean of those answers, in the same sense that polio was "cured" in 1954, that the answer will be a date sometime in the next decade.

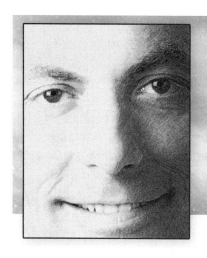

THE TECHNOLOGY
of
IMMORTALITY

An Interview with Dr. Michael West

Michael D. West, Ph.D., is a geneticist, a stem cell pioneer, and an entrepreneur. He has extensive academic and business experience in age-related degenerative diseases, telomerase molecular biology, and human embryonic stem (ES) cell research. Dr. West founded the first biotechnology company focused on controlling the aging process in human cells, and he has spent the last twenty years researching the cellular and molecular mechanisms of human aging. He is the founder of Geron Corporation, a biotechnology firm in Menlo Park, California, and is currently the President and Chief Scientific Officer of Advanced Cell Technology (ACT) in Alameda, California. Geron funded the research that isolated human embryonic stem (ES) cells, and ACT is at the forefront of therapeutic cloning. ACT cloned the first human embryos for the purpose of advancing therapeutic research.

Human embryonic stem cells—the primal cells that give rise to essentially all cell types in the body—are now routinely grown in culture. This breakthrough technology is opening the door to an astonishing array of potential medical applications. ES cells can differentiate into all types of tissue and can be used to grow new organs. With ES cells scientists can literally grow new heart cells or new kidney cells, or perhaps soon, whole organs. Since ES cells can be made using one's own DNA, the body will accept the new tissue as its own. Although

ES cell therapy is still in its infancy, our understanding about ES cells is advancing rapidly, and their therapeutic potential looks more promising every day.

Dr. West received his M.S. in Biology from Andrews University in 1982, and he earned his Ph.D. from the Baylor College of Medicine in 1989, concentrating on the biology of cellular aging. Dr. West's research into the cellular and molecular mechanisms of human aging during the early 1990s led to his founding Geron. From 1990 to 1998, Dr. West was a Director and Vice President at Geron, where he initiated and managed research programs in telomerase therapy. Telomerase is an enzyme which allows cells to divide indefinitely. Inhibiting the production of telomerase in cancer cells kills them, and turning on telomerase production in healthy cells makes them essentially immortal. Dr. West also organized and managed the program at Geron from 1995 to 1998 which, in collaboration with Dr. James Thomson and Dr. John Gearhart, led to the first isolation of human embryonic stem and human embryonic germ cells.

Dr. West's current biotechnology company, ACT, is applying human ES cell technology in the emerging field of regenerative medicine. ACT's research is focused on the use of stem cell therapy in treating age-related disease and nuclear transfer technology, which allows for the production of stem cells to be genetically matched to the patient. They own or license over three hundred patents and patent applications related to the field of stem cell therapy, and a library of stem cells for acute clinical applications. In November 2001, researchers at ACT announced that they had cloned the first human embryos for the purpose of advancing therapeutic research. The results were limited in success. Although this process was carried out with eight eggs, only three began dividing, and only one was able to divide into six cells before stopping. Nonetheless, this was a dramatic demonstration that human cloning is indeed possible.

Dr. West currently serves as Chairman of the Board, President, and Chief Scientific Officer of ACT, and is Adjunct Professor of Bioengineering at the University of California, Berkeley. He is also the author of the book The Immortal Cell, *and the story of Dr. West's quest to solve the mystery of human aging is chronicled in Stephen Hall's book* Merchants of Immortality.

When I spoke with Dr. West, I got a strong sense that he is truly excited by his research. We spoke about the potential therapeutic uses of ES cells, telomerase therapy, and the future of biotechnology.

David: What do you think are some of the biggest problems with modern medicine, and what do you think needs to be done to help correct the situation?

Dr. West: I'm a gerontologist. Speaking from the standpoint of gerontology, the biggest mistake that I see medicine making today is in not adequately planning for the future, for what is called the "age wave" or the "graying of America." The aging of America, and other industrialized countries, is the most profound demographic trend of our time. It's going to greatly strain our resources to adequately care for the elderly. For the first time in the history of the United States, we face the risk that we will discriminate against a group of our citizens based on a biological characteristic—their age. We may have to simply say, "You've reached a certain age and we're no longer going to provide medical services for you because we won't be able to afford it." That's not the kind of country that I want to live in. I don't think that's the kind of country that those of us who are entering this age bracket want to live in either. I don't think it's the kind of future that we want to see. So it's not an exaggeration to say that we have a crisis of epidemic proportions here with the aging population and its associated healthcare costs.

David: How did you get involved in embryonic stem cell research?

Dr. West: It goes back to the fundamental interest that I've had in the cellular basis of what's called the "immortality of species." As you know, life continues generation after generation, in an apparently immortal fashion. This is because germ-line cells (our sex cells) come from the previous generation of germ-line cells, and there's an immortal lineage of these cells that connects the generations of all living beings on the planet. That lineage of cells is immortal in the sense that they have no dead ancestors and have survived all of the insults of life—free radical damage, cosmic rays, and everything else that can injure living things.

These cells have survived all those sources of injury and, according to some estimates, have been evolving for over four billion years as a continuous life form. Of course, this immortal lineage of cells that connects the generations, and causes babies to be born young, is of great interest to gerontologists. This is because the cells that make up the rest of our body—what's called the somatic lineages of cells—clearly do not share in the immortality of the germ line. Our goal has been to learn from the immortality of the germ line and transfer these characteristics to somatic cells.

Telomerase was the first attempt to do that. Telomerase is an enzyme, a critical piece of which is a protein made by a gene commonly called the "telomerase gene." The actual name for it is human telomerase reverse transcriptase, or hTERT for short. But that particular gene is turned "off" (it's inactivated) in mortal cells that age, and it's turned "on" (activated) in cells that are immortal. The gene is turned "on" in our germ-line cells and is turned "off" in most somatic cells.

David: And, unfortunately, our bodies are basically composed of somatic cells.

Dr. West: Yes. You probably know that back around 1992, we began trying to track down the telomerase gene, and we eventually managed to clone it. Having done that, we found that telomerase is useful for preventing somatic cells from aging. There are clearly cells in our body that don't age, simply because they don't divide. Heart muscle cells and neurons in the brain are two examples. It could be that they age as a consequence of other cells that are aging.

For instance, heart muscle cells do not divide and therefore do not age. But damage to heart muscle can occur due to a heart attack, arrhythmias, or other heart disease. Damage to the heart muscle could also be the result of the aging of cells of other biological structures, such as the cells that make up the vessels to the heart, or some other cells that have a finite life span and upon which the heart muscle is dependent for healthy functioning. When that tissue becomes diseased and the blood vessel can no longer feed the heart muscle, the heart muscle is damaged secondarily. But however you think about it, the point is that there are aging or damaged cells and tissues in our body that need to be replaced.

The ES cell research is an attempt to find a novel way of treating age-related disease. It's essentially a transplant therapy, replacing damaged cells and tissues, by going back to this immortal germ line. These ES cells are so primitive that they are still in the immortal germ line. So when you make a somatic cell from an ES cell, the cells that result are born young, as a baby is born young. We are creating a technology to replace damaged cells and tissues with young cells as a therapy for aging.

David: Are ES cells currently being used to help repair damaged tissue?

Dr. West: No. It's a brand-new technology. It's so new that the first report of isolated ES cells is only a few years old.

David: What are some of the future applications that you foresee?

Dr. West: The ES cell is, as we say, "totipotent," which literally means "total power." These cells have the ability of becoming any cell or tissue type in the body, so the applications are endless. The Director of the National Institutes of Health, Dr Harold Varmus, has said that there is not a single area of medicine that these new technologies will not potentially impact. I think that's probably an accurate statement, because they can potentially be made into anything.

David: How long do you think it will be before we'll be able to use ES cells to grow any type of tissue or organ that we need?

Dr. West: I think it's going to be a spectrum of opportunities. Some things will be relatively easy to do, and then other things are going to be harder to do. I guess some of the early applications of ES cells may be things like cartilage for arthritis, and blood cells for leukemia or other blood disorders; maybe neurons for neurological disorders.

David: Like Parkinson's disease?

Dr. West: Parkinson's disease, certainly, is a classic disease where you simply need those cells back. But any disease where there is a loss of cell or tissue function is a clear target for this sort of thing. There are all kinds of other possible applications. In heart disease, when you lose heart muscle, you need to replace it. A lot of arrhythmias could be treated this way. With just a little imagination, you can see there are literally thousands of applications. Until last year, we never had the ability to make any cell type in the laboratory. So it's obviously a very exciting development.

David: The discovery that the tips of our chromosomes—telomeres— become shorter with each somatic cell division may have important implications for our understanding of how we age. What sort of potential for extending human life do you foresee as being possible by preventing telomeres from being shortened during cell division?

Dr. West: We still do not know the real answer to that question. It's amazing. I would put the blame for our lack of knowledge of this as simply the lack of funding that goes into aging research. As you know, Geron has been able to raise a fair amount of capital to promote aging research. Now, here at Advanced Cell Technology, we've been able to raise some money. The National Institute on Aging sponsors some research into aging.

But if you put all the biotech together, along with the federal government, it's still a small fraction of what's spent on AIDS, and, of course, the budget on AIDS is too small. We probably spend more in a week bombing foreign countries than we ever spent on aging research. That's where I put the blame. We simply do not know. What we do know is that telomerase abolishes aging on a cellular level—what we call "cellular aging." So, for cells at least, we've solved the problem of aging. The lack of telomerase is what causes cells to age. When the immortalizing telomerase gene (hTERT), which directs the synthesis of telomerase, is turned off, cells become mortal.

Since we're made of cells, this should have an application to human medicine. I would bet that it does, but we simply don't know what percentage of human aging is caused by cellular aging. If you pinned me down on it, I would say somewhere between five and a hundred percent of human aging. I don't know whether it's closer to five or a hundred, but it's somewhere in that range. Recent studies point toward the higher end of that range. But even if it's only five, it's noteworthy that here we've tracked down the fundamental molecular cause of at least a part of human aging and have found a means of intervening in it and changing it. So even if it's just a small piece of human aging, at least it's some advancement.

David: Have you found that any genes trigger the release of endogenous enzymes that may be able to benefit us now through some type of supplementation?

Dr. West: No, I don't know of any. There are some genes that have been reported that induce telomerase, but none of them give us any clues as to any supplementation that would help—and that may be what you would expect. There are literally billions of people on the planet eating many different types of foods and supplementing their diet in many different ways. As of today, however, there's no known case of anyone who has dramatically affected their life span—maybe because there is no dietary means of fundamentally altering this biology.

The reason that we think this biology is in place is that it may be a powerful antitumor mechanism. Cancer is a runaway cell—a cell that's inappropriately growing without limits, like a runaway car that doesn't stop for stop signs. But all of the cells in our body can only divide a finite number of times. So the "car" has only an eighth of a tank of fuel. That way, if it becomes a runaway car, it can't go too far. Our bodies are actually littered with cells that have started to run away. If you look at your skin, you'll see little moles and splotches, which often represent some of the pigmented cells, where you can see the cells starting to run away in uncontrolled growth. But the mole, or the pigmented blotch on your skin, you'll notice, grows to a certain size and then stops.

We believe that this is a reflection of the mortality of cells—that they have a finite life span. If there were a simple dietary means of unlocking a replicative immortality, it might allow those cells to just continue to grow. So the repression of telomerase may be an antitumor mechanism. Now that's not the same as to say that telomerase would induce cancer. The ability to refuel the gas tank of a car doesn't make it a runaway car. But it may be that allowing all the cells in our body to be immortal would raise the risk of cancer. Over the eons, natural selection has tended to "mortalize" the body, since in ancient times we rarely lived very long anyway. The average human being lived maybe 20 years in ancient times. So why would you need your cells to divide forever, when cancer or being eaten by a lion was much more of a risk?

David: Can you talk a little about the cloning research at Advanced Cell Technology?

Dr. West: What we've been working on here more recently is nuclear transfer or cloning. Having ES cells is great, but they're not you— they're somebody else.

David: I thought the whole idea was to use your own DNA?

Dr. West: Right, that's what the nuclear transfer idea is. The ES cells that exist today came from embryos made during in vitro fertilization. That's from taking a sperm and an egg and then making this little microscopic ball of cells we call a blastocyst. This contains the ES cells that can become anything. They're sort of like a raw material for life in some respects. They can be grown in a dish and made into the cells and tissues in the dish. But those cells that exist today are not you. Your body will reject cells that are not your own.

So any cells or tissues that are made from an ES cell that's not your own, your body would reject. But your body doesn't have any ES cells— they're long gone. So what we're working on is a cloning technology to make ES cells for you. We just scrape some cells off your skin and put them back into an egg cell whose DNA has been removed. What you then get is this little ball of cells—ES cells that have your DNA. So what you're doing there is cloning, but you're not making an embryo that would be put in a woman. That would lead to a cloned copy of yourself.

Rather, we're proposing cloning stem cells.

You're just making cells, not people. That's called "therapeutic cloning," as distinct from "reproductive cloning." So we're trying to make that work. The wonderful thing about this—which isn't widely known—is that we've actually shown that you can take an old cell that's at the end of its life span, and if you put it into an egg cell, it's like taking the cell back in a time machine. The cell is actually made young again.

Dolly, the sheep that was cloned, was made from an adult animal but was obviously born young. In the same way that she wasn't prematurely old (despite starting out as an old cell), we've shown that we can take old cells in a dish, and when we do this cloning technique, the cells we get are young: they have their whole life span ahead of them again. We believe that somehow, that step of putting the cell back into an egg cell winds the clock up again and takes the cell back to the beginning of life. So, theoretically, it looks as though we should be able to take a very old person and make new, young, transplantable tissue for that person, just like their own tissue when they were born.

David: And give them a new heart?

Dr. West: Potentially. Under certain conditions, we've observed ES cells actually forming complex tissues, such as intestines.

David: I read in Science *that a dog's bladder had been engineered.*

Dr. West: That bladder was made using tissue engineering, which is a little different: it was manufactured. But the ES cells will actually form complex tissues themselves. They self-assemble into tissues like intestine that are obviously young. No matter how you think humans age, here is a technique that will allow us to create young, transplantable tissue. We honestly believe that we will be able to make new liver tissue, or maybe even young whole organs that are composed of your own cells, to replace the old worn-out ones. It's a long-term project, and it's years away from being available for most applications. But it's an exciting prospect.

David: What are your thoughts about the rate at which our

understanding of ES cells is progressing?

Dr. West: I'm happy to say that the field is advancing at a fast pace, despite the fact that there's been very little federal funding for the research, and this is largely a result of just simple scientific ingenuity. I'm aware of numerous remarkable advances that have taken place in field, and we're actually ahead, I would say, of where I thought we would be as of today. Of course, we could be much further if the federal government were funding this research. As you know, the state of California voted for the allocation of three billion dollars to fund precisely this area of research—called Proposition 71—and it's anticipated that the funding will eventually materialize. So, despite the fact that we have not had a lot of federal funding, which is the normal way medical research is undertaken, I'm happy to say we've made some rather remarkable progress.

David: What do you think are the primary causes of aging?

Dr. West: I've believed for some time that aging has multiple facets and components, but it is not as complex or difficult to understand as many people have proposed. In the early days, for many people diabetes looked to be a very complex disease. You have sugar in your urine. You have problems in your eye, retinal disease. You get ulcers on your skin, heart disease, and you have all these complications associated with the disease. It looks very complicated and difficult to solve. Well, we now know, of course, that diabetes is caused by the simple loss of a single protein—insulin—and the regulation of that insulin. That is the sole cause, and all those other complicated manifestations of the disease are now largely explainable, likened back to that single cause.

Diseases like progeria and Werner's Syndrome are what we frequently refer to as premature aging syndromes. Although not exactly like human aging, they are very similar in many ways. You see grey hair, wrinkled skin, cataracts, coronary disease, osteoporosis—and many of these manifestations of aging we know are caused by a single genetic mutation. So what I believe is the case is that much of what we call human aging is due to the damage of DNA. In particular, I'm an advocate of the idea that much of that damage is at the telomeric region of the DNA. I think that in the future we will look back to these days, and we'll see this as time when we came to understand that at least much of what we call human aging is due to damage to the DNA, that that's a large percent of human aging.

I mentioned earlier that it's somewhere between five and ninety-five percent of human aging, and that recent data suggests that telomeres are more up toward the higher end of that percent, closer to the ninety-five percent. There are studies now in rodents, where human telomeres are inserted into those rodents. The Werner mutation has been put into those rodents and now, for the first time, rodents tend to age like humans. They have age-related diseases like humans. That strongly suggests that we're beginning to understand some of the fundamental biology of human aging. Scientists are quick to point out that I'm not saying a hundred percent of human aging, but much of what we call human aging.

David: What are your thoughts about the future of Western medicine in general, and what sort of new medical breakthroughs do you foresee coming over the horizon?

Dr. West: I believe in science and in the scientific method. Despite what I notice as being a widespread distrust of traditional scientific medicine, I believe that scientific medicine is going to deliver beyond anyone's expectations in the coming decade. I can't express the amount of enthusiasm I have over new developments like embryonic stem cells, and the rapid increase in power in our ability to work with DNA and see all the molecular biology. As I'm speaking to you here just now, I have in front of me a spreadsheet with forty thousand genes on the vertical axis and many of the cell lines that we're working with on the horizontal axis. In a matter of seconds, I can tell you the expression level of any gene in any of these cell lines.

The analytical abilities that I now have allow me to do research at somewhere between a hundred and a thousand fold faster than I could ten years ago. This helps me to answer fundamental questions. I'm interested in the collagen gene, the gene that makes the protein from which a lot of skin tissue is composed. If I want to know what the collagen gene does as embryonic stem cells differentiate, I can have that answer in about five seconds now. That would have taken me weeks or months worth of work in the past. So the rapidity at which we answer fundamental scientific questions today is so much faster that we wonder how we were even able answer scientific questions like this in the past. Without the public knowing it, medical research has so dramatically changed from what it was ten years ago that it's just hard to even compare.

David: What are you currently working on?

Dr. West: Regenerative medicine. I'm interested in the immortality of the germ line cells and learning lessons from them. I'm also interested in using nuclear transfer and other techniques to wind back the clock of aging and make young cells for old people. The medical toolbox that gerontologists of the future will bring to the patient, and to the problems of aging, will have several tools in it. There's not going to be one tool that fixes it all. So, in some cases, we're going to need to put young cells into old people that can rebuild tissues and restore function lost as a result of age. There are going to be some approaches where regenerative medicine, as it's been dubbed, is applied, and they'll probably be some approaches where traditional drugs are applied. So there will be several tools in the toolbox.

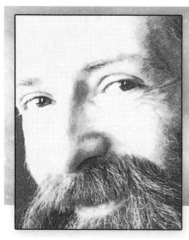

THE SEVEN LIVELY SENS
(Strategies for Engineered Negligible Senescence)

An Interview with Dr. Aubrey de Grey

Aubrey de Grey, Ph.D., is on a search for the Holy Grail of medicine—the ability to stop and reverse the human aging process. Although this ambitious biogerontologist at the University of Cambridge in England was trained as a computer scientist, he is also a self-taught biologist with a strong interest in why organisms age. After marrying a geneticist in 1991, Dr. de Grey became so interested in biology that he began teaching himself the subject. In 1996, he had progressed far enough to make a significant contribution in molecular biology by identifying previously unknown influences that affect the mutations that occur in mitochondria (the intracellular structures that provide cells with energy), after only reviewing the relevant literature on this for several months.

Dr. de Grey received his M.A. in computer science at the University of Cambridge, and has been working there as a computer scientist in the Department of Genetics since 1992. His insights into mitochondria earned him a Ph.D. in biology from the university, although Dr. de Grey is not a laboratory researcher. He does no biology experiments. Rather, he is purely a theoretician in the realm of biology, and he prefers to see the Big Picture. By studying the literature from different scientific disciplines, he has assembled a master plan for how to "cure aging." Although controversial, he has outlined what many experts believe are feasible engineering solutions to the seven basic consequences of prolonged metabolism that accumulate as what we call "aging."

These seven factors involved in aging, and Dr. Grey's proposed solutions, will be discussed in the interview, but briefly they are: (1) The loss of cells that we need; (2) The accumulation of cells that we don't need; (3) DNA mutations inside the cell nucleus; (4) DNA mutations inside the cell's mitochondria; (5) The accumulation of "junk" inside of cells; (6) The accumulation of "junk" outside of cells; and (7) The formation of cross-linked proteins outside cells.

For each of these seven problems Dr. de Grey has a solution. These solutions are organized as part of a project he has masterminded, which he calls "Strategies for Engineered Negligible Senescence," or SENS. Two of these strategies are ideas of his own, while the other five came from colleagues. The strength of Dr. de Grey's ideas are in his engineering approach—which is goal-directed to find practical solutions— and his interdisciplinary perspective. What may be most important about Dr. de Grey's work is that he has brought together many experts from different fields that normally wouldn't be interacting and sharing ideas. It is through this cross-fertilization of ideas that so much excitement and controversy has resulted from his work.

Dr. de Grey is currently the Chairman and the Chief Science Officer of the Methuselah Foundation, which offers financial prizes to researchers who can break previous records of lifespan in mice. He is on the scientific advisory boards for the Maximum Life Foundation, Legendary Pharmaceuticals, Centenarian Species and Rockfish project, and the Alcor Life Extension Foundation. Dr. de Grey is also on the Board of Directors of the International Association of Biomedical Gerontology and the American Aging Association, and he is editor-in-chief of the journal Rejuvenation Research. *To find out more about Dr. de Grey's work visit his Web site: www. sens.org*

I interviewed Dr. de Grey on February 3, 2005. Aubrey is extremely attentive, mentally energetic, and eloquent with words. We talked about the reasons for aging, the obstacles that stand in the way of reversing the aging process, and the social and psychological consequences of having a population that lives for hundreds or thousands of years.

David: How did you first become interested in biogerontology?

Aubrey: This is one of the most common questions that I get asked, of course, but it's actually one of the ones I find hardest to answer. I've been wracking my brain for years about this, because, you see, it was very gradual. I'm sure that from the dawn of time—from when I was a kid—it was obvious to me that aging was not a good thing, but that didn't really count as being interested in gerontology because I never regarded it as my problem. I was not a biologist back then. My main interests in school—as a kid and as a university student—were in math and computers. I guess I took the view that while it's obviously hard to do anything about aging, there are professional biologists who must doubtless be hammering away at this, and they'll make their breakthrough in the fullness of time.

So it was really only after I met my wife that I became interested in biogerontology. My wife is a geneticist, and she's quite a lot older than me. She was already forty-five when we met. She was a full professor at UC San Diego and was on sabbatical here in Cambridge. It was really through, first of all, learning a lot of biology, just by accident, by just talking to my wife, that I began to reawaken this interest. I began to think about the question, what is actually so hard about postponing aging? And the more I thought about it, the more I'd find I couldn't really understand what was so hard.

So I started to talk about this to my wife and to other people of her generation, and it became apparent that they didn't really know either, but that they regarded it as not an interesting problem, which was scandalous to me. I mean, I understand why they thought that, because, you see, scientists are interested in understanding things. They're interested in knowledge for its own sake, whereas engineers are more interested in knowledge as a means to an end, and I think that I'm very much an engineer at heart.

So I was scandalized by this. Eventually, I was sufficiently scandalized that I went off and actually taught myself some of the relevant areas of biology that were not ones in which my wife herself was an expert— like biochemistry, for example—so as to be able to understand what was known about the biology of aging, and what people might actually try to do something about. I got very lucky. I was able to make an interesting contribution in one area of gerontology after I'd really only been reading the literature extensively for a month or two. That contribution was published and well-received in 1997. Since then, I've basically been going without stopping.

David: Can you describe how you arrived upon your initial insight— your "aha" moment—of how the aging process can be reversed, and why you think that the key to longevity is basically an engineering problem?

Aubrey: I don't think there was a real moment when I realized that it's an engineering problem. It was obvious to me that it was an engineering problem. Bodies are just machines. They're very complicated, but they are just machines. The big breakthrough I made—that you may be referring to, and which has been talked about a little bit in other publications—is that in the summer of 2000, I realized something about how to approach the problem. This was not to approach the general concept of aging as an engineer, but actually how to break the problem down, how to subdivide it into parts that could each—with reasonable plausibility—be, not just slowed down, but actually repaired and reversed without too much risk of side-effects and things spinning out of control in ways that one couldn't predict. That was in the middle of the night in Los Angeles in July of 2000.

David: What do you think are the seven primary causes of aging?

Aubrey: It's probably not really quite correct to call them "the causes of aging." What they are is the early manifestations of aging. These are intrinsic side-effects of metabolism, of being alive in the first place, and they are things that build up throughout life. Although these side-effects are not the cause of aging, they start to become harmful once they get to a certain level of abundance. Once there are enough of them around, the body starts to suffer from them and eventually it suffers seriously. But the point is that initially they are completely inert. So this is really why a twenty year old, and a thirty or forty year old, are more or less equivalent in terms of functionality—in as long they've looked after themselves reasonably well. You can run as fast, you can think as fast, and so on, more or less, because the things haven't reached a pathogenic level.

So the seven areas are as follows. First of all, there is a loss of cells. There are certain tissues in which, when the cells in that tissue die, the tissue doesn't know how to replace them, not at the adequate rate anyway. For example, in the heart, or in certain areas of the brain, cells die and are not replaced.

The second one is the opposite of that. It's having too many cells of a certain type. This includes cells that really ought to have either not come into being in the first place, or they ought to have died and for whatever reason they haven't. An example would be in the fat, in the abdominal cavity, which is important for bringing on diabetes.

Number three is mutations in our chromosomes. This, of course, is very important in the cause of cancer, and, in my mind, that's almost certainly the only thing that mutations in our chromosomes actually matter for.

Number four is mutations in a special part of the cell called the mitochondrion. It's the only part of the cell that has its own DNA apart from the chromosomes, but that DNA matters as well, and mutations there don't give us cancer, but they do other stuff.

Then number five is that, in our arteries and other tissues there are structural proteins that give them the shape and elasticity that they have, and these biomechanical, biophysical properties degrade with time, largely because of chemical reactions that cause extra chemical bonds between proteins that shouldn't be there. These bonds build up and cause hardening of the arteries, for example.

Number six is, again, in the space between cells. But here it's not changes to the structural proteins; it's just the accumulation of aggregates of protein material that the body is incapable of breaking down. In other words, it's the accumulation of garbage. The best known example of this is the formation of a substance called amyloid, which is the material found in the brains of people with Alzheimer's disease.

And then, finally, the seventh one is, again, the accumulation of garbage, but this time the accumulation of garbage inside cells. This is usually in a specific component of the cell called the lysosomes, although sometimes—especially in the brain—it is in other places in the cell. So these are the seven things that we need to fix.

David: And you have ideas for how to fix each one of them?

Aubrey: That's right, although it would be wrong to call them all my ideas. For two of these things I have made very specific and very new and radical proposals for how we should go about this, which I think are pretty feasible, and are likely to be much more effective than anything else that's on the table at the moment. But, for the others, all I've really done is read the right literature and talk to the right people, because all the ideas that I've brought in are ideas that other people have been working on already. In general, they have not been working on them within gerontology though. This is why I was the first person to come along and actually create this grand scheme, with all these components of a unified whole. I was able to do this because most gerontologists don't know what's going on in these areas well enough to know how close they are to being successful.

It's because biology is a very big field. So, just as most biologists don't know much gerontology, most gerontologists don't much of other things. It's much easier if you're a theoretician like me and you don't do experiments, because experiments, of course, are very time-consuming. Even writing the grant applications to get money for your students for the experiments is very time-consuming. So most gerontologists, like most biologists, don't really have much time to read—and this is a major failure of biology in general, I have to say. The comparison with physics is very instructive here.

In physics, you don't have this problem at all. In physics, there are lots of people who do experiments, and there are also lots of people, like me, who are theoreticians—people like Stephen Hawking, just to name a famous example. They become experts in a much wider range of disciplines than you can if you're spending all your time doing experiments. They have new ideas for new experiments to do, and new things to try that result from bringing concepts together from far apart. And there's virtually nobody in biology doing that. There's certainly nobody except me in gerontology doing that, and that's a large part of why biology goes so slowly.

David: So you think that's the main reason why we haven't made more progress in reversing the aging process, despite such remarkable achievements in molecular biology as the successful completion of the human genome project?

Aubrey: I think that's a large part of it, yes. The human genome project, of course, was a bit over-hyped. The media made it out to be the most important thing since the wheel or whatever. But completing the human genome project certainly was a very good thing. It's made a lot of experiments go much faster than they would have otherwise done. But yes, that's a large part of the reason. It's simply the absence of people bringing ideas together. To solve a very complicated problem, you generally need a fairly complicated solution.

David: While we're waiting for the SENS project to reach escape velocity, what do you think are currently the best ways to slow down, or reverse the aging process and extend the human life span?

Aubrey: We basically don't have anything. We certainly don't have anything to reverse the aging process, and I'm not very optimistic about anything to actually even slow it down very much. Of course, if you're the sort of person who has an unusually short life expectancy in the first place—either because you have dodgy genes of one sort or another, or because you just have a very bad diet, you smoke or whatever—then there are obviously lifestyle things that you can do that will make you live longer. But if we factor all them out, and we say, what can you do over and above simply living and eating the way your mother told you to? Then I take the view that there's more or less nothing that can give you more than a couple of years.

Some of my colleagues feel that caloric restriction might extend human life. As you probably know, if you feed mice or rats somewhat less than they would like you to, then they live a bit longer, and some of my colleagues think this might also work in humans. I think it'll work—but I think it'll work much less well in humans than in most shorter-lived organisms. If you do this with rats and mice, then you can probably get a thirty or forty percent extension of lifespan. So that's a healthy amount. In a human lifespan that would be great. Even if you got twenty percent, that would be very nice. But I think it's very unlikely that we'll get even as much as five percent. The reasons I think this are partly because of a whole bunch of data that exists that I feel my colleagues have actually really been sweeping under the carpet, and secondly because there's very good evolutionary theoretical reasons to believe that longer-lived organisms will not have the genetic machinery to make them live proportionately as long in response to starvation as shorter-lived organisms would have.

I have a paper that's actually coming out tomorrow in a Swiss journal called *Gerontology*. It's coming out online tomorrow and then in print version a week from then, which explains this in a lot of detail. It's already caused quite some waves, and I expect it'll cause quite a few more after it comes out.

David: Everyone that I interview is aware of how caloric restriction increases maximum lifespan, but few people are aware of the deprenyl studies that have been shown to extend maximum lifespan. Are you aware of these studies, and do you know if anyone has ever replicated them?

Aubrey: I'm surprised that people you've spoken to are unaware of these studies—they're quite well-known. Unfortunately, as you fear, they have not been readily reproducible, at least not in terms of magnitude. A top Japanese gerontologist, Kenichi Kitani, has worked with deprenyl a lot over the past decade or more and you should look him up in PubMed if you want more detail. The bottom line is that deprenyl is one of half a dozen substances, including growth hormone, DHEA, melatonin etc., that have occasionally been reported to extend maximum mouse lifespan, but do not seem to do so reliably, or at least not by a significant extent.

David: What are some of the new anti-aging treatments that you foresee coming along in the near future?

Aubrey: A lot of my colleagues are working on things on the basis that calorie restriction may actually give us maybe fifteen or twenty years of extra life.

David: You mean working on ways to mimic caloric restriction?

Aubrey: That's right—tricking the body into thinking it's on calorie restriction when it's not. I think that's marvelous, because, you see, even though I'm pessimistic given what we know already about calorie restriction. I might be wrong in my interpretation of it, and it may be that we will actually get a lot more life extension from it, so I definitely think it ought to be tried, and these products may not be very far away. We have learned a great deal in the past five or ten years about the genetic basis for the life extension phenomena of calorie restriction in rodents. We ought to be able to use pretty realistic pharmacological and genetic tricks as therapies to elicit the same sort of response in humans as they do in mice. These ideas, and the experiments to see whether this works, have been taken forward by a number of my senior colleagues. They managed to get all the venture capital that they need to support the work, so this will be tried fairly soon.

When it comes to the components of the actual SENS initiative, some of the components are even further along than that. For example, there is a drug being produced by a company called Alteon in New York that actually breaks these extra chemical bonds that I was talking about that cause hardening of the arteries. And there's another company in California that has been working on immunization against Alzheimer's plaques to get rid of the garbage that accumulates between cells in the brain, by causing cells to actually internalize this stuff and break it down.

Both of those drugs have been in clinical trials already. The Alzheimer's one was aborted because the vaccine had bad side-effects, but they're working really hard to produce better vaccines, and they will do so pretty quickly. The cross-link breaker one doesn't even have any side-effects, so that's going really well. But, in terms of life extension, the point is we're probably going to have to get all of these things—or at least most of them—working simultaneously in order to actually get a significant deferment of aging, so half of them working just won't cut it.

David: Could you briefly explain what your strategies are for reversing each of the seven factors involved in aging?

Aubrey: Okay. I've mentioned two of them in the last answer. We've got these new drugs that break the chemical bonds that cause hardening to occur in structural proteins, and we've also got systems for stimulating the immune system against garbage outside of cells. So the other one that everyone knows about is the ways to replace cells in tissues that don't replace their own cells well enough, and that's what stem cell therapy is mainly for. So stem cell therapy is being explored very heavily in, for example, type 1 diabetes, where you lose the ability to make insulin because you lose the islet cells in the pancreas.

But it's also being used for various age-related problems; in particular the one that's got furthest is Parkinson's disease, where people have been putting neural stem cells into the brain to differentiate into the particular type of neuron that's lost in Parkinson's disease. So there's a long way to go with stem cell therapy of course. There are many things that we certainly can't do yet with stem cell therapy, but that's an area which can be approached incrementally. It's an area which has got a lot of work going on, and little steps are discovered, little tricks, of how to treat and manipulate your cells in the laboratory, so they get into a state where they will do the right thing after you put them into the body. There are a lot of things like that going on.

Then the one that's sort of in an intermediate stage of development, I suppose, is the one about getting rid of cells that we've got too many of and we wish would just keel over. So there are various systems being developed to make such cells keel over, or else to put them into state where they're not harmful after all. In the case of visceral fat—the fat of the abdominal cavity that seems to be largely responsible for diabetes—people have tried, in rats, just surgically removing the stuff, and that has had marvelous effects on reversing diabetic complications in rats.

There are also drug therapies being looked at that will make these cells transform into benevolent cells. Some people are looking at somewhat more high-tech approaches involving some sort of gene therapy that puts new genes into cells that kill those cells, and specifically only kills the cells that are in this bad state. Again, of course, this is a situation where the immune system can be activated to engulf and destroy cells that we want to get rid of. There are various ways of doing that, and most of these things are some way along in mice at this point.

The other three are all a lot further off, and we haven't really got to the mouse stage even. We're only at the cell culture level. So one of them is, I mentioned, the mutations in the mitochondrion. It turns out that we've only got very little DNA in the mitochondrion—DNA that only encodes thirteen proteins, as opposed to tens of thousands of proteins encoded in the nucleus. It's rather interesting that we have any genes in the mitochondrion, because the mitochondrion itself is a big complicated machine made of about a thousand different proteins. All the others, apart from these thirteen, are already encoded in the nucleus, and the proteins that they encode are constructed in the cell, outside the mitochondrion. Then they're imported into the mitochondrion by a very special and really sophisticated system.

So you'd think you could do the same with the other thirteen. Then you wouldn't need mitochondrial DNA. It turns out that there are pretty good reasons why these things are encoded in the mitochondrial DNA, but these reasons are not complete show-stoppers. They have been show-stoppers for evolution, but we have different tools than evolution has, and so it's looking very good now. There has been very important progress in that area recently that indicates that we ought to be able to put copies of these genes into the nucleus, and that would solve the problem, because the nuclear DNA is enormously better protected and better maintained than the mitochondrial DNA. So if you had working copies of the mitochondrial DNA in the nucleus, then it wouldn't matter whether you had mitochondrial mutations any more. The proteins that had been constructed by the mitochondrion would be coming in from the outside, so it'd be okay.

David: The mitochondria are almost like organisms unto themselves, aren't they?

Aubrey: Well, they used to be organisms. They were originally free-living bacteria. That's right. But they are very much not organisms unto themselves anymore. They're wholly integrated into their hosts now.

All of the strategies that I've discussed so far are not my own ideas. The idea that I just explained, for example, was first discussed twenty years ago, and it was first discussed as a therapy more than fifteen years ago. People have been working on it for most of that time. One of their big breakthroughs will actually be coming out in a paper in my journal *Rejuvenation Research* in the next issue in a month or so, with the results of a study that began in 1991. So we've been working on this for awhile, and I believe that we'll crack it.

The other two that I haven't dealt with are the ones where, basically, I have completely identified a new approach from scratch that no one else has done before. The first one deals with the junk that accumulates inside cells. I have a really crazy idea here. I realized that this junk is energy-rich. If you go to a graveyard, for example—somewhere that's enriched in human remains—you probably won't find this stuff, because anything that energy-rich is not going to be sitting in the ground for very long if it's worth eating. If you're a bacterium, a microbe in the soil, you can eat this stuff and live off it. I didn't come up with this principle myself by any means; this is the principle behind a field that's been flourishing for fifty years called bioremediation, which is basically a part of the environmental decontamination industry.

People are interested in getting rid of contaminants in the soil to build houses on the soil, for example, and this works. If you have any chemical in the soil that you want to get rid of that's energy-rich, and it's organic, then you can find bacteria that will break it down. Even explosives like TNT are no problem. You can find bacteria than can break down TNT, dioxins, and PCBs. It's ridiculous, and it's simply because evolution is very, very clever. If you give evolution a reason to evolve the machinery to do something, it'll do it eventually.

So I reckon this ought to work for the junk that accumulates in our human bodies when we're alive that we don't know how to break down. There will be bacteria in the soil that do know how to break it down, and this idea has gone down very well. I've discussed it extensively over the past few years, and pilot studies have already been done to demonstrate that it really works, so this is likely to be developed fairly soon. But it is difficult to say how soon as there is only early data at this point. We don't even have it actually working in cell cultures yet, so I would expect that it will be the best part of ten years before we see a serious improvement and it is functioning well in mice. Then, of course, it will be longer to get it working in humans.

The final one is mutations in chromosomes. I mentioned earlier that I think that the only mutations in our chromosomes that actually matter are those that cause cancer. Other mutations just don't accumulate fast enough to do us any damage in anything like a normal life time.

So I came up with a really complicated, really ambitious therapy for cancer which I felt one needed in order to really avoid the fact that cancer is so insidious. Cancer is insidious because it has the advantage of natural selection. Cancers are a seething mass of genetic instability. They're basically doing experiments all the time to try to work out how to evade all of the things that the body throws at them to kill them, and the things that the doctors throw at them to kill them for that matter. That's why we've made so little progress over the past thirty years, since Nixon announced the war on cancer. Cancer is by far the hardest aspect of aging to fix.

So I came up with an idea than involved essentially removing—from the whole body, not just the cancer—the ability to extend the telomeres, the ends of the chromosomes, which one has to extend in order for the cells to divide indefinitely, which, of course, is what cancers do. It would take me another half hour to explain the whole thing. It's a complicated therapy, but, again, I have discussed this extensively with people who are expert in the various components of the therapy. We had a whole meeting to discuss it.

David: This book will include an interview with Michael Fossel, who went into great detail describing how telomeres influence cell division and the possibility of telomerase therapy in the future.

Aubrey: Oh, that's interesting. Michael Fossel and I are good friends, but he thinks that the main key to actually fixing aging is to reinvigorate the ability of cells to maintain their telomeres, and I think that's crazy. I think that what we want to do is actually eliminate the ability of cells to do that so that we won't die of cancer. This is actually an area in which I am in the gerontological mainstream, and Michael isn't.

David: Why do you want to live forever?

Aubrey: It's not that I really want to live forever, but rather, it's just that I don't want to die any time soon. Furthermore, I don't expect that, in due course, when I have not died any time soon, I will want to die any time soon then either. If you live a year, and you're still healthy, young, vibrant, and enjoying life, then you're not going to want to die that year, and you'll want to live another year. Then you won't want to die that year either. So you don't live to a thousand all in one go. You live to a thousand one year at a time.

David: Why do you think so many people are resistant to the notion of physical immortality?

Aubrey: I think that people are resistant because it would be such a dramatic change in everything about society and how we think about each other. Now people are scared of change, even if it's obviously good. I think that's really what it comes down to.

David: Why do you think the aging process evolved, and do you think that there might be an evolutionarily advantageous reason for genetically-programmed death?

Aubrey: That's an easy question. It didn't evolve. It's just that the absence of aging hasn't really evolved. Aging is what happens by default.

David: So you don't think there's an evolutionary advantageous reason for it?

Aubrey: That's right. There's no advantageous reason not to age. It's just that it's disadvantageous to work too hard not to age. Evolution doesn't care about the life spans of individual organisms. It cares about the survival of individual genes, or genetic information, and how many organisms you have to get through per unit of time—how many generations—is irrelevant. There are certain evolutionary pressures that do alter life span; so of course, evolution does sometimes evolve longer-lived organisms from short lived ones, in the same way that we evolved from apes that don't live as long as we do, for example. But that's a secondary thing. Evolution would never evolve aging away completely because it's too hard, and there's no point. There's a certain amount of maintenance that it's worth carrying around the genetic machinery to do, and beyond that it's just not worth it. You might as well just get on with reproducing more.

David: What sort of relationship do you see between aging and predation?

Aubrey: Oh, plenty. This is the major reason why different organisms have different life spans, and this has been understood for about forty years now, actually. The rate at which you are killed for reasons other than aging determines how much effort it is worth putting into not dying of aging. The rate at which your species is killed is not due just to predation, of course. You can include here things like starvation and hypothermia, but predation is a really important one.

So, for example, if you're a highly predated organism—an organism that doesn't live very long because you get eaten—then you'd darned well better get on and breed before you get eaten, because you won't get another chance. So it's worth putting your effort into breeding, and there's not much point in spending a lot of energy on a lot of genetic machinery in heavy duty molecular maintenance, whereas if you are a low predation organism, like a bird for example, that can fly away from predators, then it's not the same at all. It's better to put a lot of effort into not aging, so that you can live a long time and choose which summer to have a lot of offspring, like when there's lots of food around, for example.

David: I read that you signed up with Alcor, the cryonic suspension facility in Arizona. How long do you think it will be before we have developed nanotechnology sufficiently to revive people in cryonic suspension?

Aubrey: Oh, it's going to be a very, very long time indeed. My hunch is that it's not going to be in the next hundred years. But, of course, anything that far out is complete guesswork, so it's only a hunch.

David: Can you talk a little about your interest in cryonics, and what sort of potential you see for cryonic suspension as a form of life extension?

Aubrey: I think cryonics is now an absolutely valid biomedical strategy. Until a few years ago one could argue—not conclusively, but strongly— that the damage done to someone's brain when they are cryopreserved is so extensive that the possibility of resuscitation, even with arbitrarily advanced technology, is basically nil, because the information necessary to reconstruct the brain has gone. But we now have cryoprotectants that are so good that a brain can be taken down to liquid nitrogen temperature without any formation of crystalline ice at all—it becomes a glass. That means there is hardly any structural damage—and we know that if the structure is preserved, then function should be restorable too, even though electrical activity was suspended, because that's what happens when people fall into frozen lakes and are resuscitated after minutes (over an hour in some cases) of cardiac arrest.

For me, this is even more realistic to think about than for most biologists, because I focus on life-extension technologies that repair pre-existing molecular and cellular damage. Thus, in a very real sense, resuscitation from cryonic suspension is a natural extension of the range of therapies that I work on for people who are not yet legally dead. Once you understand that the legal definition of death is just a convenience, and has virtually no biological meaning, it's easy to see that restoring someone from a state that is legally dead but biologically almost intact is not science fiction at all. It might not work, to be sure—not least because it is a tricky business making sure that you get the best cryopreservation possible—but for those of us who won't live long enough to make the "escape velocity" cut, it's our best bet.

David: How long do you think it's possible for human life span to be extended?

Aubrey: You mean in the absence of cryonics? You mean continuously alive?

David: Yes.

Aubrey: Oh, I think it's more or less certain that we can do so indefinitely, but not all at once. I think that the therapies that I talk about—which ought to be possible to develop within the next twenty-five or thirty years if we get good funding soon—will probably give us a few decades of extra lifespan. That's not forever. That's not living indefinitely at all. But a few decades is a long time, especially since these therapies will be ones that will be applicable to people who are already in middle age at the time those therapies arrive.

So you can imagine someone who's sixty, for example, benefiting from these therapies and basically staying physiologically sixty or less, physiologically in their early middle age, shall we say, for another thirty years. After those thirty years, if nothing else has come along to make the therapies better, then other stuff will start catching up with them. Little imperfections and incompleteness in the therapies will build up and aging will happen just as now. It just will happen later on. But, of course, as I said, that's only the case if nothing else comes along in those thirty years, and that's not what's going to happen.

In those thirty years, people will be banging away feverishly to improve these therapies in terms of cost, and in terms of convenience and safety of course, but also in terms of comprehensiveness. So, well before these thirty years are up, therapies will be coming along that will confer another thirty years, a half century, or whatever. Basically people who are young enough and fit enough at the time these first generation therapies come along to benefit from them (let's say they're in their sixties or less) will, by and large, have no reason to die of old age at any age, because we will keep ahead of the game. I've been calling this "life extension escape velocity" that we will be exceeding. We'll be solving problems before they arrive.

David: How do you think human societies will change when people start living for hundreds or thousands of years?

Aubrey: There will probably be pretty big changes, enormous changes actually. One of the most important ones of course is that there will be a requirement to have very few children around. Now, this may of course be a make or break thing. It may be that society decides that children are really important to have around, and it's actually better to carry on having people age, or not using these aging therapies, so that we can have lots of children around and not have ridiculous overpopulation. But that's a decision that society is entitled to make for itself, so it's definitely not a justification for our hesitating now. If we hesitate now, then we're denying future society the choice whether to age or whether to not have many kids around. We have no right to make that choice for them.

David: Do you see space migration playing a role then?

Aubrey: No. It's very possible and it would be a good idea to have some space migration happening. In principle, it's not completely impossible to suppose that we could have a rate of immigration into space that would allow the population of the Earth to be stabilized, even if we carried on having kids at the rate we have them now, but unfortunately, that's not good enough, because then space fills up. And I really mean space fills up. Think about this mathematically. If we want to maintain a demographic of society, of the whole of humanity overall, including what's in space, that's the same as it is now—in other words the same proportion of the human race that is now under the age of eighteen—then that means that the human population has to grow exponentially forever.

Now the problem with growing exponentially is the space we take up. We can't increase exponentially because we have to get to it. The amount of space we can take up a thousand years from now is at most a sphere of radius as far as we can actually fly a thousand years from now. That doesn't sound very difficult, does it? But, in fact, it is difficult. If you work out the numbers on this you discover that in only a few thousand years of continuous exponential growth—even making quite generous assumptions about how dense the population can be—we end up having to increase this sphere that we occupy by a rate that's greater than the speed of light. No kidding.

Actually, we would hit problems considerably before that. We would hit problems more or less around the time that we got to the edge of the solar system, simply because we would run out of matter. We wouldn't have enough material around to build ourselves, to actually constitute human beings, or even to build all the space ships. In principle, of course, it would make a difference for a few hundred years, but as an indefinite solution, it definitely doesn't work.

David: Since our brain and nervous system can only store a finite amount of information, how do you envision the future development of human memory storage, if people are living for indefinite periods of time? Do you think that we'll develop brain implants and technological means to increase our brain's data storage capacity, or do you think that we'll just have to learn to live with the fact that we're going to forget most of what we experience over time?

Aubrey: People often bring this up, but it's really a non-issue, because it'll be the same as it already is. We forget things already, so the amount of actual information that we have at our fingertips in our sixties—whether it's memories, personality or whatever—is really not much different from what we had in our forties, because we've been forgetting things as fast as we've been learning them, and that's natural. That's how the brain works. Memories are stored in a holographically distributed way in the brain. We don't know the details of how they are stored, of course, but we do know that much. So memories that are not recalled, or not used, gradually fade away, and eventually they're not there anymore, whereas memories that are used and recalled reasonably frequently are reinforced by that process, and we don't forget them. Now that reinforcement will carry on happening. So things that happened when you were ten, you'll still remember them when you're ten thousand, if you've been reminded of them, or you've thought about them for whatever reason every so often in the meantime.

David: But there would be a much higher percentage of what one has forgotten.

Aubrey: Yeah, the total amount forgotten would be a much higher proportion of the stuff that you ever knew. So what?

David: I guess we'd just have to learn to live with the fact that most of what we experience will be forgotten, or else we could develop some type of nanotechnological brain implant to increase memory storage.

Aubrey: Well, think about how much it would bother you. I mean, I can't remember half the names of the people who were in my school class when I was sixteen, and that doesn't bother me in the slightest.

David: How do you think living for hundreds of years will affect human psychology? How do you think it will change our consciousness and the way that we think?

Aubrey: I really don't think it will change it very much at all. I think we'll just carry on enjoying life the way we do now, except we'll enjoy it rather more because we won't have to worry about aging and looking out for our parents, because our parents won't be frail.

David: What do you think happens to consciousness after death?

Aubrey: I have absolutely no opinion on that, and furthermore I don't intend to do the experiment.

David: Do you see any sort of teleology in the evolutionary process, or do you see evolution as being a blind chance process?

Aubrey: Oh, evolution is definitely blind chance, but teleological ways of thinking about processes—whether it's evolution or other things— are very useful for our understanding. It is sort of anthropomorphizing, but anthropomorphizing is sometimes useful for understanding things. It's just that you have to remember to go back and check later on when you come up with some interesting explanation for something. You have to go back and actually check that it really works if you think it through chronologically as well, so cause and effect is definitely a one-way street.

David: Can you talk a little about the Methuselah Mouse Prize?

Aubrey: The Methuselah Mouse Prize is a really great success. It was an idea that had been batted around within academia, among gerontologists, for a few years before it got going. I got involved in the summer or spring of 2001. Just in talking about things I came up with some ideas, but it was still just talk, nothing was actually happening. Then, in 2002, I accidentally bumped into this guy, David Gobel, who is an entrepreneur and businessman, now based in the D.C. area. Gobel has all the things that scientists don't have. He has business experience. He understands public relations. He knows how to set up a 501C-3. Things like that. And he had been very excited about the possibility of prizes for health-related accomplishments, and he certainly put thought into the possibility of a prize that was related to life extension.

So, basically, he and I ran with this and made it happen pretty quickly. We gave the inaugural Methuselah Mouse Prize in the summer of 2003, and since then, we've given two other inaugural prizes for other competitions that we started out with different rules, encouraging different types of research, but still on mouse life extension. Financially this has been an enormous success, and we now have well over 120,000 dollars in the actual prize fund, and in addition to that, we're getting close to a million dollars that's actually been pledged for the prize, to be given in aliquots of a thousand dollars a year by the various benefactors. So it's really an enormous success, and the P.R. value is great. The idea of the whole thing, of course, is to do something that people can identify with. People turn off when they listen to science quite often, but they understand a world record, which is what these prizes are for, of course. The prizes are for producing unprecedentedly long-lived mice. People understand competitions and prizes, so it's just been enormously successful, and continues to be so.

David: What's the conference that you're organizing in Cambridge this September going to be about?

Aubrey: The conference that I'm going to be running in Cambridge in September this year is the second one of these that I've done. I ran a similar conference in September of 2003, which was a massive success. Basically, the purpose of this conference is to do on a comprehensive scale the same thing that I've done on a much smaller scale four times now, which is to bring scientists together whose areas of expertise are rather wide-ranging—but which all relate to a particular area or a general concept that I want to explore. So, for example, the conference that I ran last summer was on this business of using bacterial genes to get rid of junk inside cells. It's a complicated concept, and it needs people who understand the things that this junk does in the body, how it contributes to age-related diseases, and so on.

It needs people who know how to manipulate genes, and who can get the proteins to go to the right places in cells. It also needs people who know how to find bacteria that can do a particular thing, and who can then find the genes that are responsible for the bacteria doing that thing. So these are people who would never normally be talking to each other, and I got them all together in a room for a day. We published a paper on this. Similarly, the previous year, I did the same sort of thing for the idea I had for curing and preventing cancer.

So, basically, the conference this September is going to be doing that on a much bigger scale, with maybe fifty or sixty speakers, covering all areas of my whole anti-aging scheme. It's a marvelous way of getting people to educate each other about what's possible, because even when scientists are working on something that's going really well, they'll tend to appreciate that their own part is going pretty well, but their instinct will be that everyone else's work is probably not going so well. So when people hear about each other's work this way it makes a big difference.

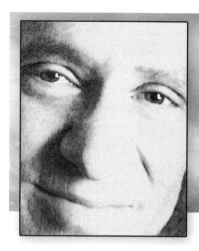

REPROGRAMMING YOUR BIOCHEMISTRY FOR IMMORTALITY

An Interview with Dr. Ray Kurzweil

Ray Kurzweil is a computer scientist, software developer, inventor, entrepreneur, philosopher, and a leading proponent of radical life extension. He is the coauthor (with Terry Grossman, M.D.) of Fantastic Voyage: Live Long Enough to Live Forever, *which is one of the most intriguing and exciting books on life extension around. Kurzweil and Grossman's approach to health and longevity combines the most current and practical medical knowledge with a soundly-based, yet awe-inspiring visionary perspective of what's to come.*

Kurzweil's philosophy is built upon the premise that we now have the knowledge to identify and correct the problems caused by most unhealthy genetic predispositions. By taking advantage of the opportunities afforded us by genomic testing, nutritional supplements, and lifestyle adjustments, we can live long enough to reap the benefits of advanced biotechnology and nanotechnology, which will ultimately allow us to conquer aging and live forever. At the heart of Kurzweil's optimistic philosophy is the notion that human knowledge is growing exponentially, not linearly, and this fact is rarely taken into account when people try to predict the rate of technological advance in the future. Kurzweil predicts that at the current rate of knowledge expansion we'll have the technology to completely conquer aging within the next couple of decades.

Part of what makes Kurzweil's upbeat vision of the future so appealing is his impressive track record as an inventor and engineer, as well as the success of his past predictions. Kurzweil is a leading expert in speech and pattern recognition, and he invented a vast array of computer marvels. He was the principal developer of the first omni-font (any type font) optical character recognition software, the first commercially marketed large vocabulary speech recognition system, the first print-to-speech reading machine for the blind, the first CCD flatbed scanner, the first text-to-speech synthesizer, and the first music synthesizer capable of recreating the grand piano and other orchestral instruments.

Kurzweil has successfully founded and developed ten businesses in speech recognition, reading technology, music synthesis, virtual reality, financial investment, medical simulation, and cybernetic art. In 2002, Kurzweil was inducted into the U.S. Patent Office's National Inventors Hall of Fame, and he received the Lemelson-MIT Prize, the nation's largest award in invention and innovation. He also received the 1999 National Medal of Technology, the nation's highest honor in technology, from President Clinton in a White House ceremony, and has received twelve honorary Doctorates and honors from three U.S. presidents.

In addition to coauthoring Fantastic Voyage, *Kurzweil wrote* The 10% Solution for a Healthy Life, *and several best selling books on the evolution of intelligence—including* The Age of Intelligent Machines, The Age of Spiritual Machines, and The Singularity Is Near, When Humans Transcend Biology. *Kurzweil's books on the evolution of intelligence read like mind-bending science fiction, but are based on a scientific analysis of technology trends. Kurzweil predicts that computer intelligence will exceed human intelligence in only a few decades, and that it won't be long after that before humans start merging with machines, blurring the line between technology and biology.*

For more information about Kurzweil see his Web site: www. kurzweilai.net, where one can subscribe to his free newsletter. Web sites on his books include www.Fantastic-Voyage.net and www.Singularity.com

Kurzweil works in Wellesley, Massachusetts. I spoke with Ray on February 8, 2006. Ray speaks very precisely and he chooses his words carefully. He presents his ideas with a lot of confidence, and I found his optimism to be contagious. We spoke about the importance of genomic testing, some of the common misleading ideas that people have about health, and how biotechnology and nanotechnology will radically affect our longevity in the future.

David: What inspired your interest in life extension?

Ray: Probably the first incident that got me on this path was my father's illness. This began when I was fifteen, and he died seven years later of heart disease when I was twenty-two. He was fifty-eight. I'll actually be fifty-eight this Sunday. I sensed a dark cloud over my future, feeling like there was a good chance that I had inherited his disposition to heart disease. When I was thirty-five, I was diagnosed with Type 2 diabetes, and the conventional medical approach made it worse.

So I really approached the situation as an inventor, as a problem to be solved. I immersed myself in the scientific literature, and came up with an approach that allowed me to overcome my diabetes. My levels became totally normal, and in the course of this process, I discovered that I did indeed have a disposition, for example, to high cholesterol. My cholesterol was 280 and I also got that down to around 130. That was twenty-two years ago.

I wrote a bestselling health book, which came out in 1993, about that experience, and the program that I'd come up with. That's what really got me on this path of realizing that—if you're aggressive enough about reprogramming your biochemistry—you can find the ideas that can help you to overcome your genetic dispositions, because they're out there. They exist.

About seven years ago, after my book *The Age of Spiritual Machines* came out in 1999, I was at a Foresight Institute conference. I met Terry Grossman there, and we struck up a conversation about this subject—nutrition and health. I went to see him at his longevity clinic in Denver for an evaluation, and we built a friendship. We started exchanging emails about health issues—and that was 10,000 emails ago. We wrote this book *Fantastic Voyage* together, which really continues my quest. And he also has his own story about how he developed similar ideas, and how we collaborated.

There's really a lot of knowledge available right now, although, previously, it has not been packaged in the same way that we did it. We have the knowledge to reprogram our biochemistry to overcome disease and aging processes. We can dramatically slow down aging, and we can really overcome conditions such as atherosclerosis, which leads to almost all heart attacks and strokes, diabetes, and we can substantially reduce the risk of cancer with today's knowledge. And, as you saw from the book, all of that is just what we call 'Bridge One'. We're not saying that taking lots of supplements and changing your diet is going enable you to live five hundred years. But it will enable Baby Boomers—like Dr. Grossman and myself, and our contemporaries—to be in good shape ten or fifteen years from now, when we really will have the full flowering of the biotechnology revolution, which is 'Bridge Two.'

Now, this gets into my whole theory of information technology. Biology has become an information technology. It didn't used to be. Biology used to be hit or miss. We'd just find something that happened to work. We didn't really understand why it worked, and, invariably, these tools, these drugs, had side-effects. They were very crude tools. Drug development was called drug discovery, because we really weren't able to reprogram biology. That is now changing. Our understanding of biology, and the ability to manipulate it, is becoming an information technology. We're understanding the information processes that underlie disease processes, like atherosclerosis, and we're gaining the tools to reprogram those processes.

Drug development is now entering an era of rational drug design, rather than drug discovery. The important point to realize is that the progress is exponential, not linear. Invariably people—including sophisticated people—do not take that into consideration, and it makes all the difference in the world. The mainstream skeptics declared the fifteen year genome project a failure after seven and half years because only one percent of the project was done. The skeptics said, I told you this wasn't going to work—here you are halfway through the project and you've hardly done anything. But the progress was exponential, doubling every year, and the last seven doublings go from one percent to a hundred percent. So the project was done on time. It took fifteen years to sequence HIV. We sequenced the SARS virus in thirty-one days.

There are many other examples of that. We've gone from ten dollars to sequence one base pair in 1990 to a penny today. So in ten or fifteen years from now, it's going to be a very different landscape. We really will have very powerful interventions, in the form of rationally-designed drugs that can precisely reprogram our biochemistry. We can do it to a large extent today with supplements and nutrition, but it takes a more extensive effort. We'll have much more powerful tools fifteen years from now, so I want it to be in good shape at that time.

Most of my Baby Boomer contemporaries are completely oblivious of this perspective. They just assume that aging is part of the cycle of human life, and at 65 or 70 you start slowing down. Then at 80 you're dead. So they're getting ready to retire, and are really unaware of this perspective that things are going to be very different ten or fifteen years from now. This insight really should motivate them to be aggressive about using today's knowledge. Of course, all of this will lead to 'Bridge Three' about twenty years from now—the nanotechnology revolution—where we can go beyond the limitations of biology. We'll have programmable nanobots that can keep us healthy from inside, and truly provide truly radical life extension.

So that's the genesis. My interest in life extension stems primarily from my having been diagnosed with Type 2 diabetes. I really consider the diabetes to be a blessing because it prodded me to overcome it, and, in so doing, I realized that I didn't just have an approach for diabetes, but a general attitude and approach to overcome any health problem, that we really can find the ideas and apply them to overcome the genetic dispositions that we have. There's a common wisdom that your genes are eighty percent of your health and longevity and lifestyle is only twenty percent. Well, that's true if you follow the generally, watered-down guidelines that our health institutions put out. But if you follow the optimal guidelines that we talk about, you can really overcome almost any genetic disposition. We do have the knowledge to do that.

David: What do you think are some of the common misleading ideas that people have about health and longevity?

Ray: One thing that I just alluded to is the compromised recommendations from our health authorities. I just had a lengthy debate with the Joslin Diabetes Center, which is considered the world's leading diabetes treatment and research center. I'm on the board, and they've just come out with new nutritional guidelines, which are highly compromised. They're far from ideal, and they acknowledge that. They say, well, we have enough trouble getting people to follow these guidelines, let alone the stricter guidelines that you recommend. And my reply is, you have trouble getting people to follow your guidelines because they don't work. If people followed your guidelines very precisely, they'd still have Type 2 diabetes. They'd still have to take harsh drugs or insulin.

If they follow my guidelines, the situation is quite different. I've counseled many people about Type 2 diabetes, and Dr. Grossman has treated many people with it, and they come back and they have completely normal levels. Their symptoms are gone, and they don't have to take insulin or harsh drugs. They feel liberated, and that's extremely motivating. In many ways it's easier to make a stricter change. To dramatically reduce your high glycemic index carbs is actually easier than moderately reducing them, because if you moderately reduce them you don't get rid of the cravings for carbs. Carbs are addictive, and it's just like trying to cut down a little bit on cigarettes. It's actually easier to cut cigarettes out completely, and it's also easier to largely cut out high glycemic index starches and sugars, because the cravings go away and it's much easier to follow. But, most importantly, it works along with a few supplements and exercise to overcome most cases of Type 2 diabetes.

However, this doesn't seem to be the attitude of our health authorities. The nutritional recommendations are consistently compromised. There's almost no understanding of the role of nutritional supplements, which can be very powerful. I take two hundred and fifty supplements a day, and I monitor my body regularly. I'm not just flying without instrumentation. Being an engineer, I like data and I monitor fifty or sixty different blood levels every few months, and I'm constantly fine-tuning my program. All of my blood levels are ideal. My homocysteine level many years ago was eleven, but now it's five. My C-reactive protein is 0.1. My cholesterol is 130. My LDL is about 60, and my HDL—which was 28— is now close to sixty. And so on and so forth.

I've also taken biological aging tests which measure things like tactile sensitivity, reaction time, memory, and decision-making speed. There are forty different tests, and you compare your score to medians for different populations at different ages. When I was forty, I came out at about thirty-eight. Now I'm fifty-seven—at least for a few more days— and I come out at forty. So, according to these tests, I've only aged two years in the last seventeen years. Now you can dispute the absolute validity of these biological aging tests. It's just a number, but it's just evidence that this program is working.

David: Why do you think that genomic testing is important?

Ray: Our program is very much not a one size fits all. It's not a one-trick pony. We're not saying that if you lower your carbs, lower your fat, or eat a grapefruit a day then everything will be fine. In fact, our publisher initially had a problem with this, but they actually got behind it enthusiastically, because it fundamentally differs, as you know, from most health books that really do have just one idea. We earnestly try to provide a comprehensive understanding of your biology and your body, which does have some complexity to it. Then we let people apply these principles to their own lives.

It is important to emphasize the issues that are concerns for yourself. We use an analogy of stepping backwards towards a cliff. It's much easier to change direction before you fall off the cliff. But, generally, medicine doesn't get involved until the eruption of clinical disease. Someone has a heart attack, or they develop clinical cancer, and that's very often akin to falling off a cliff. One third of first heart attacks are fatal, and another third cause permanent damage to the heart muscle.

It's much easier to catch these conditions beforehand. You don't just catch heart disease or cancer walking down the street one day. These are many years or decades in the making, and you can see where you are in the progression of these diseases. So it's very important to know thyself, to access your own situation. Genetic testing is important because you can see what dispositions you have. If you have certain genes that dispose you to heart disease, or conversely cancer, or diabetes, then you would give a higher priority to managing those issues, and do more tests to see where you are in the progression of those conditions. Let's say you do a test and it says you have a genetic disposition to Type 2 diabetes. So you should do a glucose-tolerance test. In fact, we describe a more sophisticated form of that in the book, where you measure insulin as well, and can see if you have early stages of insulin resistance.

Perhaps you have metabolic syndrome, which a very substantial fraction of the population has. If you have these early harbingers of insulin resistance, that could lead to Type 2 diabetes, so obviously the priority of that issue will be greatly heightened. If you don't have that vulnerability then you don't have to be as concerned about insulin resistance, and so on. But if you do have insulin resistance, or you have a high level of atherosclerosis, then it really behooves you to take important steps to get these dangerous conditions under control—which you can do. So genomic testing is not something you do by itself. It's part of a comprehensive assessment program to know your own body—not only what you're predisposed to, but what your body has already developed in terms of early versions of these degenerative conditions.

David: What are some of the most important nutritional supplements that you would recommend to help prevent cancer and cardiovascular disease?

Ray: We spell all that out in the book. Coenzyme Q10 is important. It never ceases to amaze me that physicians do not tell their patients to take coenzyme Q10 when they prescribe statin drugs. This is because it's well known that statin drugs deplete the body of coenzyme Q10, and a lot of the side-effects such as muscle weakness that people suffer from statin drugs are because of this depletion of coenzyme Q10. In any event, that's an important supplement. It is involved in energy generation within the mitochondria of each cell. Disruption to the mitochondria is an important aging process and this supplement will help slow that down. Coenzyme Q10 has a number of protective effects including lowering blood pressure, helping to control free radical damage, and protecting the heart.

A lot of research recently shows that curcumin, which is derived from the spice turmeric, has important anti-inflammatory properties and can protect against cancer, heart disease, and even Alzheimer's disease.

Alpha-Lipoic acid is an important antioxidant which is both water and fat-soluble. It can neutralize harmful free radicals, improve insulin sensitivity, and slow down the process of advanced glycation end products (AGEs), which is another key aging process.

Each of the vitamins is important and plays a key role. vitamin C is generally protective as a premier antioxidant. It appears to have particular effectiveness in preventing the early stages of atherosclerosis, namely the oxidizing of LDL cholesterol.

In terms of vitamin E, there's been a lot of negative publicity about that, but if you look carefully at that research, you'll see that all of those studies were done with alpha-tocopherol, and vitamin E is really a blend of eight different substances—four tocopherols and four tocotrienols. Alpha-tocopherol actually depletes levels of gamma-tocopherol, and gamma-tocopherol is the form of vitamin E that's found naturally in food, and is a particularly important one. So we recommend that people take a blend of the fractions of vitamin E, and that they get enough gamma-tocopherol.

There are a number of others that are important to take in general. If you have high cholesterol, Policosanol is one supplement that is quite effective, and has an independent action from the statin drugs. Statin drugs actually are quite good. They appear to be anti-inflammatory, so they not only lower cholesterol but attack the inflammatory processes, which underlie many diseases, including atherosclerosis. But as I mentioned it's important to take coenzyme Q10 if you're taking statin drugs.

There are others. Grape seed proanthocyanidin extract has been found to be another effective antioxidant. Resveratrol is another. We have an extensive discussion of the most important supplements in the book.

David: What sort of suggestions would you make to someone who is looking to improve their memory or cognitive performance?

Ray: Vinpocetine, derived from the periwinkle plant, seems to have the best research. It improves cerebral blood flow, increases brain cell TP (energy) production, and enables better utilization of glucose and oxygen in the brain.

Other supplements that appear to be important for brain health include Phosphatidylserine, Acetyl-L-Carnitine, Pregnenolone, and EPA/DHA. The research appears a bit mixed on Ginkgo biloba, but we're not ready to give up on it.

We provide a discussion in the book of a number of smart nutrients that appear to improve brain health. There are also a number of smart drugs being developed, some of which are already in the testing pipeline, that appear to be quite promising.

David: What do you think are the primary causes of aging?

Ray: Aging is not one thing. There are a number of different processes involved and you can adopt programs that slow down each of these. For example, one process involves the depletion of phosphatidylcholine in the cell membrane. In young people the cell membrane is about sixty or seventy percent phosphatidylcholine, and the cell membrane functions very well then—letting nutrients in and letting toxins out.

The body makes phosphatidylcholine, but very slowly, so over the decades the phosphatidylcholine in the cell membrane depletes, and the cell membrane gets filled in with inert substances, like hard fats and cholesterol that basically don't work. This is one reason that cells become brittle with age. The skin in an elderly person begins to not be supple. The organs stop functioning efficiently. So it's actually a very important aging process, and you can reverse that by supplementing with phosphatidylcholine. If you really want to do it effectively you can take phosphatidylcholine intravenously, as I do. Every week I have an

I.V. with phosphatidylcholine. I also take it every day orally. So that's one aging process we can stop today.

Another important aging process involves oxidation through positively-charged oxygen free radicals, which will steal electrons from cells, disrupting normal enzymatic processes. There are a number of different types of antioxidants that you can take to slow down that process, including vitamin C. You could take vitamin C intravenously to boost that process.

Advanced glycation end-products, or AGEs, are involved in another aging process. This is where proteins develop cross-links with each other, therefore disrupting their function. There are supplements that you can take, such as Alpha Lipoic Acid, that slow that down. There is an experimental drug called ALT-711 (phenacyldimenthylthiazolium chloride) that can dissolve the AGE cross-links without damaging the original tissues.

Atherosclerosis is an aging process, and it's not just taking place in the coronary arteries, of course. It can take place in the cerebral arteries, which ultimately causes cerebral strokes, but it also takes place in the arteries all throughout the body. It can lead to impotence, claudication of the legs and limbs, and like most of these processes, it's not linear but exponential, in that it grows by a certain percentage each year.

So that's why the process of atherosclerosis hardly seems to progress for a long time, but then when it gets to a certain point it can really explode and develop very quickly. We have an extensive program on reducing atherosclerosis, which is both an aging process and a disease process. We cite a number of important supplements that reduce cholesterol and inflammation—such as the omega-3 fats EPA and DHA—as well as the statin drugs. Supplements like curcumin [turmeric] are helpful. Supplements that reduce inflammation will reduce both cancer and the inflammatory processes that lead to atherosclerosis. There are a number of supplements that reduce homocysteine, which appears to encourage atherosclerosis. These include Folic Acid, vitamins B2, B6, and B12, magnesium, and trimethylglycine (TMG).

So you can attack atherosclerosis five or six different ways, and we recommend that you do them all, so long as there aren't contraindications for combining treatments. But generally these treatments are independent of each other. If you go to war, you don't just send in the helicopters. You send in the helicopters, the tanks, the planes, and the infantry. You use your intelligence resources, and attack the enemy every way that you can, with all of your resources. And that's really what you need to do with these conditions, because they represent very threatening processes. If you are sufficiently proactive, you can generally get them under control.

David: What are some of the new anti-aging treatments that you foresee coming along in the near future, like from stem cell research and therapeutic cloning?

Ray: It depends on what you mean by "near future," because in ten or fifteen years, we foresee a fundamentally transformed landscape.

David: Let's just say prior to nanotechnology, and then that will be the next question.

Ray: The next frontier is biotechnology. We're really now entering an era where we can reprogram biology. We've sequenced the genome, and we are now reverse-engineering the genome. We're understanding the roles that the genes play, how they express themselves in proteins, and how these proteins then play roles in sequences of biochemical steps that lead to both orderly processes as well as dysfunction—disease processes, such as atherosclerosis and cancer—and we are gaining the means to reprogram those processes.

For example, we can now turn genes off with RNA interference. This is a new technique that just emerged a few years ago—a medication with little pieces of RNA that latch on to the messenger RNA that is expressing a targeted gene and destroys it, therefore preventing the gene from expressing itself. This effectively turns the gene off. So right away that methodology has lots of applications.

Take the fat insulin receptor gene. That gene basically says 'hold on to every calorie because the next hunting season may not work out so well.' That was a good strategy, not only for humans, but for most species, thousands of years ago. It's still probably a good strategy for animals living in the wild. But we're not animals living in the wild. It was good for humans a thousand years ago when calories were few and far between. Today it underlies an epidemic of obesity. How about turning that gene off in the fat cells? What would happen?

That was actually tried in mice, and these mice ate ravenously, and they remained slim. They got the health benefits of being slim. They didn't get diabetes. They didn't get heart disease. They lived twenty percent longer. They got the benefits of caloric restriction while doing the opposite. So turning off the fat insulin receptor gene in fat cells is the idea. You don't want to turn it off in muscle cells, for example. This is one methodology that could enable us to prevent obesity, and actually maintain an optimal weight no matter what we ate. So that's one application of RNA interference.

There are a number of genes that have been identified that promote atherosclerosis, cancer, diabetes and many other diseases. We'd like to selectively turn those genes off, and slow down or stop these disease processes. There are certain genes that appear to have an influence on the rate of aging. We can amplify the expression of genes similarly, and we can actually add new genetic information—that's gene therapy. Gene therapy has had problems in the past, because we've had difficulty putting the genetic information in the right place at the right chromosome. There are new techniques now that enable us to do that correctly.

For example, you can take a cell out of the body, insert the genetic information in vitro—which is much easier to do in a Petri dish—and examine whether or not the insertion went as intended. If it ended up in the wrong place, you discard it. You keep doing this until you get it right. You can examine the cell and make sure that it doesn't have any DNA errors. So then you take this now modified cell—that has also been certified as being free of DNA errors—and it's replicated in the Petri dish, so that hundreds of millions of copies of it are created. Then you inject these cells back into the patient, and they will work their way into the right tissues. A lung cell is not going to end up in the liver.

In fact, this was tried by a company I'm involved with, United Therapeutics. I advise them and I'm on their board. They tried this with a fatal disease called pulmonary hypertension, which is a lung disease, and these modified cells ended up in the right place—in the lungs—and actually cured pulmonary hypertension in animal tests. It has now been approved for human trials. That's just one example of many of being able to actually add new genes. So we'll be able to subtract genes, over-express certain genes, under-express genes, and add new genes.

Another methodology is cell transdifferentiation, a broader concept than just stem cells. One of the problems with stem cell research or stem cell approaches is this; If I want to grow a new heart, or maybe add new heart cells because my heart has been damaged, or if I need new pancreatic islet cells because my pancreatic islet cells are destroyed, or need some other type of cells, I'd like it to have my DNA. The ultimate stem cell promise, the holy grail of these cell therapies, is to take my own skin cells and reprogram them to be a different kind of cell. How do you do that? Actually, all cells have the same DNA. What's the difference between a heart cell and pancreatic islet cell?

Well, there are certain proteins, short RNA fragments, and peptides that control gene expression. They tell the heart cells that only the certain genes which should be expressed in a heart cell are expressed. And we're learning how to manipulate which genes are expressed. By adding certain proteins to the cell, we can reprogram a skin cell to be a heart cell or a pancreatic islet cell. This has been demonstrated in just the last couple years. So then we can create in a Petri dish as many heart cells or pancreatic islet cells as I need, with my own DNA, because they're derived from my cells. Then inject them, and they'll work their way into the right tissues. In the process, we can discard cells that have DNA errors, so we can basically replenish our cells with DNA-corrected cells.

While we are at it, we can also extend the telomeres. That's another aging process. As the cells replicate, these little repeating codes of DNA called telomeres grow shorter. They're like little beads at the end of the DNA strands. One falls off every time the cell replicates, and there's only about fifty of them. So after a certain number of replications the cell can't replicate anymore. There is actually one enzyme that controls this—telomerase, which is capable of extending the telomeres. Cancer actually works by creating telomerase to enable them to replicate without end. Cancer cells become immortal because they can create telomerase.

As we're rejuvenating our cells, turning a skin cell into a kind of cell that I need, making sure that it has its DNA corrected, we can also extend its telomeres by using telomerase in the Petri dish. Then you got this new cell that's just like my heart cells were when I was twenty. Now you can replicate that, and then inject it, and really rejuvenate all of the body's tissues with young versions of my cells. So that's cell rejuvenation. That's one idea, or one technique, and there are many different variations of that.

Then there's turning on and off enzymes. Enzymes are the work horses of biology. Genes express themselves as enzymes, and the enzymes actually go and do the work. And we can add enzymes. We can turn enzymes off. One example of that is Torcetrapib, which destroys one enzyme, and that enzyme destroys HDL, the good cholesterol in the blood. So when people take Torcetrapib their HDL (good cholesterol levels) soar, and atherosclerosis dramatically slows down or stops. The phase 2 trials were very encouraging, and Pfizer is spending a record one billion dollars on the phase 3 trials. That's just one example of many of these paradigms: manipulating enzymes. So there are many different ideas to get in and very precisely reprogram the information processes that underlie biology, to undercut disease processes and aging processes, and move them towards healthy rejuvenated processes.

David: How do you see robotics, artificial intelligence, and nanotechnology effecting human health and life span in the future?

Ray: I mentioned that we talk about three bridges to radical life extension in *Fantastic Voyage*. Bridge One is aggressively applying today's knowledge, and that's, of course, a moving frontier, as we learn and gain more and more knowledge. In Chapter 10 of *Fantastic Voyage*, I talk about my program, and at the end I mention that one part of my program is what I call a positive health slope, which means that my program is not fixed.

I spend a certain amount of time every week studying a number of things—new research, new drug developments that are coming out, new information about myself that may come from testing. Just reading the literature I might discover something that's in fact old knowledge, but there's so much information out there, I haven't read everything. So I'm constantly learning more about health and medicine and my own body and modifying my own program. I probably make some small change every week. That doesn't mean my program is unstable. My program is quite stable, but I'm fine-tuning at the edges quite frequently.

Bridge Two we've just been talking about, which is the biotechnology revolution. A very important insight that really changes one's perspective is to understand that progress is exponential and not linear. So many sophisticated scientists fail to take this into consideration. They just assume that the progress is going to continue at the current pace, and they make this mistake over and over again. If you consider the exponential pace of this process, ten or fifteen years from now, we will have really dramatic tools in the forms of medications and cell therapies that can reprogram our health within the domain of biology.

Bridge Three is nanotechnology. The golden era will be in about twenty years from now. There'll be some applications earlier, but the real Holy Grail of nanotechnology is nanobots, blood cell-size devices that can go inside the body and keep us healthy from inside. If that sounds very futuristic, I'd actually point out that we're doing sophisticated tasks already with blood cell-size devices in animal experiments.

One scientist cured Type 1 diabetes in rats with a nano-engineered capsule that has seven nanometers pores. It lets insulin out in a controlled fashion and blocks antibodies. And that's what is feasible today. MIT has a project of a nano-engineered device that's actually smaller than a cell and it's capable of detecting specifically the antigens that exist only on certain types of cancer cells. When it detects these antigens, it latches onto the cell, and burrows inside the cell. It can detect once it's inside and then at that point it releases a toxin which destroys the cancer cell. This has actually worked in the Petri dish, but that's quite significant because there's actually not that much that could be different in vivo as in vitro.

This is a rather sophisticated device because it's going through these several different stages, and it can do all of these different steps. It's a nano-engineered device in that it is created at the molecular level. So that's what is feasible already. If you consider what I call the Law of Accelerating Returns, which is a doubling of the power of these information technologies every year, within twenty-five years these computation-communication technologies, and our understanding of biology, will be a billion times more advanced than it is today. We're shrinking technology, according to our models, at a rate of over a hundred per 3-D volume per decade.

So these technologies will be a hundred thousand times smaller than they are today in twenty-five years, and a billion times more powerful. And look at what we can already do today experimentally. Twenty-five years from now these nanobots will be quite sophisticated. They'll have computers in them. They'll have communication devices. They'll have small mechanical systems. They'll really be little robots, and they will be able to go inside the body and keep us healthy from inside. They will be able to augment the immune system by destroying pathogens. They will repair DNA errors, remove debris and reverse atherosclerosis. Whatever we don't get around to finishing with biotechnology, we'll be able to finish the job with these nano-engineered blood-cell sized robots or nanobots.

This really will provide radical life extension. The basic metaphor or analogy to keep in mind is to ask the question, How long does a house last? Aubrey de Grey uses this metaphor. The answer is that a house lasts as long as you want it to. If you don't take care of it, the house won't last that long. It will fall apart. The roof will spring a leak and the house will quickly decay. On the other hand, if you're diligent, and something goes wrong in the house you fix it. Periodically you upgrade the technology. You put in a new HVAC system and so forth. With this approach, the house will go on indefinitely, and we do have houses, in fact, that are thousands of years of old. So why doesn't this apply to the human body?

The answer is that we understand how a house works. We understand how to fix a house. We understand all the problems a house can have, because we've designed them. We don't yet have that knowledge and those tools today to do a comparable job with our body. We don't understand all the things that could wrong, and we don't have all the fixes for everything.

But we will have this knowledge and these tools. We will have complete models of biology. We'll have reverse-engineered biology within twenty years, and we'll have the means to go in and repair all of the problems we have identified.

We'll be able to indefinitely fix the things that go wrong. We'll have nanobots that can go in and proactively keep us healthy at a cellular level, without waiting until major diseases flare up, as well as stop and reverse aging processes. We'll get to a point where people will not age. So when we talk about radical life extension, we're not talking about people growing old and becoming what we think of today as a 95 year old and then staying at a biological age 95 for hundreds of years.

We're talking about people staying young and not aging. Actually, I'm talking about even more than that, because in addition to radical life extension, we'll also have radical life expansion. The nanobots will be able to go inside the brain and extend our mental functioning by interacting with our biological neurons. Today we already have computers that are placed inside people's brains, that replace diseased parts of the brain, like the neural implant for Parkinson's disease. The latest generation of that implant allows you to download new software to your neural implant from outside the patient—and that's not an experiment, that's an FDA approved therapy.

Today these neural implants require surgery, but ultimately we'll be able to send these brain extenders into the nervous system, noninvasively through the capillaries of the brain, without surgery. And we'll be using them, not just to replace diseased tissue, but to go beyond our current abilities—to extend our memories, extend our pattern recognition and cognitive capabilities, and merge intimately with our technology. So we'll have radical life expansion along with radical life extension. That's my vision of what will happen in the next several decades.

David: What are you currently working on?

Ray: I spend maybe forty or fifty percent of my time communicating—in the form of books, articles, interviews, speeches. I give several speeches a month. Then there's my Web site: KurzweilAI.net. We have a free daily or weekly newsletter; people can sign up by putting in their email address (which is kept in confidence) on the home page.

Then I have several businesses that I'm running, which are in the area of pattern recognition. I've been in the reading machine business for thirty-two years. I developed the first print-to-speech technology for the blind in 1976, and we're introducing a new version that fits in your pocket. A blind person can take it out of their pocket, snap a picture of a handout at a meeting, a sign on a wall, the back of a cereal box, an electronic display, and the device will read it out loud to them through an earphone or speaker.

We're developing a new medical technology, which is basically a smart undershirt that monitors your health. There will be a smart bra version for women. It takes a complete morphology EKG and monitors your breathing. So, for example, if you're a heart patient it could tell you whether your atrial fibrillation is getting better or worse. When you're exercising, it can tell you if you're getting into a problem situation. So it gives you diagnostic information. It can also alert you if you should contact your doctor. So basically your undershirt is sending this information by Bluetooth® to your cell phone, and your cell phone is running this cardiac evaluation software. So that's another project.

Then we have Ray and Terry's longevity products at RayandTerry.com, which goes along with *Fantastic Voyage*. We have about 20 products available now, and we'll have about fifty within a few months. Basically, all the things we recommend in the book will be available. We also have combinations. So, for example, if you want to lower cholesterol, we have a cholesterol-lowering product, and you don't have to buy the eight or nine different supplements separately. We put all of our recommendations together in one combination to make it easy for people to follow.

There's a total daily care that has basic nutritional supplements, like vitamins and minerals, and coenzyme Q-10, and so on. We have a meal-replacement shake that is low carbohydrate, has no sugar, but actually tastes good, which is actually very unique, because if you've ever tasted a low-carb meal-replacement shake you know that in general the taste is not desirable. This might sound promotional but that was the objective, and it's actually made up of the nutritional supplements that we recommend. So that's another company, and those are the companies that we're running.

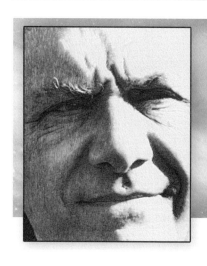

UNLOCKING THE SECRETS
of
MIND-BODY MEDICINE:

An Interview with Dr. Bernie Siegel

Bernie S. Siegel, M.D., helped to create a revolution in modern medicine. He is the author of Love, Medicine, and Miracles, *the groundbreaking best-selling book that sold more than two million copies and went to number one on* The New York Times *bestseller list.*

In his practice as a general and pediatric surgeon, Dr. Siegel began recognizing common personality characteristics in those patients who did well and those who didn't. Studying these personality patterns helped Dr. Siegel to understand the important role that thoughts and emotions play in our health, and he began incorporating what he learned into how he treated his patients. In so doing, he helped to create a paradigm shift in clinical medicine that paved the way for what is now commonly known as mind-body medicine.

Dr. Siegel earned a medical doctorate from Cornell Medical College, and he received his surgical training at Yale University. In 1978, Dr. Siegel and his wife, Bobbie, founded the Exceptional Cancer Patients (ECaP) program in New Haven, Connecticut. This highly regarded and successful program—which incorporates a combination of group and individual therapy—is based upon what Dr. Siegel calls "carefrontation" or "a loving, safe, therapeutic confrontation that facilitates personal change, empowerment, and healing."

Dr. Siegel's book, Love, Medicine, and Miracles, *was published in 1986. As a result of this book's enormous popularity, Dr. Siegel appeared on numerous television shows, including* Oprah, Donahue, *and* 20/20. *Some of Dr. Siegel's other books include* Peace, Love and Healing, How to Live Between Office Visits, Prescriptions for Living, Help Me To Heal, *and* 365 Prescriptions for the Soul. *Dr. Siegel also produced a series of popular audio cassettes, including* Meditations for Enhancing Your Immune System, *and* Humor and Healing.

Since retiring from clinical practice in 1989, Dr. Siegel has focused his energies on humanizing medical care and medical education. He is especially interested in teaching other health care professionals about how the mind-body connection affects health. Dr. Siegel travels extensively to speak and lead workshops. He recently completed a new children's book, and is working on a book about how dreams and drawings can be used to reveal the somatic aspects of disease and healing. To find out more about Dr. Siegel's work visit his Web site: www. ecap-online.org

I interviewed Dr. Siegel on November 12, 2004. I found Bernie to be extremely warm and charismatic. He's very funny and playful, curious and open-minded, and I immediately felt comfortable with him. We spoke about how beliefs and emotions affect our health, how dreams might offer insights and clues as to how to treat a particular illness, what he thinks needs to be done to help improve the Western medical profession, and he offered a few prescriptions for how to slow down or reverse the aging process.

David: What inspired your interest in medicine, and why did you choose to become a surgeon?

Bernie: When I look back at my life, the number one reason that I come up with has to do with being artistic as a child, and having talented hands, but not realizing you could earn a living as an artist. I know that may sound silly, but as a kid I just didn't know that. So I thought it would be good to use my hands because they're skillful. I liked people, science fascinated me, and I liked fixing things. When I looked at what could accomplish all of those things, I realized, hey, you could be a surgeon and do them all.

I can remember taking care of a lot of children with various deformities back in medical school at what's called the Hospital for Special Surgery. I was initially doing orthopedic work, and the funny thing was I realized that my personality was not to be an orthopedic surgeon—because it took too long for a bone to heal. I couldn't wait. (*Laughter*) So I became a general and a pediatric surgeon. In other words, I began taking care of children, but with congenital anomalies and other different things, as well as adults, because we had a practice partnership. So I took care of all ages, but I cared for all the children, and I really let the children teach me how to take care of adults.

But I always say that the reasons I became a physician were healthy. They're not normal for a surgeon, because a lot of psychologists contacted me years ago saying, you're not a normal surgeon, and please fill out these personality profiles. Then they'd call back and say, we were right—you're not normal. And yes, I understand that, but I think that's also what got me into people's pain. Many students today don't have anything to do with people in their reasons for wanting to go to medical school. When they're filling out the form, it says, why do you want to be a doctor? They'll say the human body fascinates me. When I say to them, draw yourself working as a doctor, they'll draw pictures with no human beings in them.

It's just unbelievable to think that you can say to a student, draw yourself working as a doctor, and they hand you a picture with diplomas, computers, instruments, prescriptions, bottles of drugs, and things of that sort. There are no people in the picture. So it's because I cared about people, as I say, that I got into pain—because you ultimately realize that you can't fix everything, and you can't save everybody. It got to be very painful, and none of that is dealt with in your training. They don't prepare you for loss, and that's a part of the problem. There's nowhere to discuss the pain, or share your feelings and help heal.

David: Can you talk a little about how you think our thoughts and beliefs affect the health of our bodies?

Bernie: You can't separate thoughts and beliefs from your body. In other words, what you think, and what you believe, literally changes your body chemistry. So, if you have a pessimistic, hopeless outlook, you'll change your body, your immune function, and you can die a lot faster. I have literally seen this. I hear these stories from people, when someone's hope is taken away. Let's say they're told they have a few months to live, but they can go home, climb into bed, and be dead in a week. So it's really like turning off the "live switches". When you study survivors you find that relationships, connections, hope, and meaning all relate to people staying alive. For instance, just on simple terms, women live longer than men with the same cancers, and this has more to do with the men saying, I can't work, so what's the point of living? And the women seeing all the connections in their family, and reasons for being here.

So, as I say, your thoughts, beliefs, all relate to the health of your body, and many doctors literally can kill people with their words or, in a sense, heal them and cure them with words, and give them hope. This was something that I got into years ago, and everybody would yell at me, oh you're giving false hope. But hope can't be false. (*Laughter*) If you have hope, it's real. So there's no such thing as false hope. Hope is a memory of the future. What they're talking about is, that you're supposed to tell people what day they're going to die. But who knows that? If the statistics say there's six months average survival that doesn't mean there aren't people walking around ten years later, you see, who had that disease, and some who died in a week. So you're coming up with an average. But individuals are not affected by an average. Yes, I might use it to make therapeutic choices. If something can improve your chances of surviving, you'd say, okay, let's have an operation, let me have chemotherapy, whatever—but it doesn't say where you'll be next year or five years from now.

David: How do you think multiple personality disorder sheds light on the process by which the mind affects the body?

Bernie: If you look at the case histories of people with multiple personality disorder, one of the things that you see is that there are people who are allergic to something in one personality but not in another. There was one case where somebody was diabetic in one personality and not in another. So, you see, when you change personalities your physiology can change with it. Now, a study was done that shows this operating on a simpler basis. If I give you a role or a script to play, and if it's a depressing one, it will adversely affect immune function and stress hormone levels. However, if I give you a comedy it will enhance them. You see, it's like the multiple personality—you're changing your character. But what impresses me is that in a play it's not even you or your life. You're just acting. But still, when you act that part, your body responds to it, and that's what people have to remember. This is what I always say to them—rehearse and practice who you want to be. As a physician I see myself as a coach. I try to help people be survivors. I point out to them what the qualities are of those who do better than I expect, so that they can imitate them, and rehearse and practice being a survivor. One doctor wrote of how his patients survived in a concentration camp when being sick and unable to work meant they were put to death.

David: Why do you think that the expression of emotion is important for our health, and why do you think that love has such powerful healing potential?

Bernie: If you don't get your anger out and express it, then you turn it inward, and it builds into resentment and hatred. It stays in you, and really breaks you down. You start attacking yourself. A lot of people with autoimmune diseases have issues with anger that they have held in. As a matter of fact, one doctor did a study with twin sisters that sheds light on this. If you ask this of an audience people always have the right answer. You say, one girl is very sweet and she does everything to make her parents happy. She pleases everyone, and internalizes her anger. Then her twin sister is a little devil. Who do you think develops breast cancer? Everybody votes for the good girl. So when you deny your needs and your feelings, you're hurting and attacking yourself.

Ashley Montagu, the anthropologist, has written a lot on love. Love changes you. The touch, the relationship, the connection changes you. When you're loving, every cell in your body is getting a very significant message about how wonderful life is, so it does its best to keep you alive and healthy, because it knows you're enjoying life. Some of that is simple chemistry. Studies have been done that show if you pet your dog your oxytocin and serotonin levels go up. Now these are hormones and brain chemicals that make you feel good and help you to connect. It's the kind of feelings that a woman who delivers a baby experiences, how she connects with that infant. So when you're loving, you are connected to everything and everybody.

I don't know if you saw *Time* magazine a couple of weeks ago, but the cover story was about a "God gene". See, I think that's mislabeled. It should be a "love gene". Some people are literally born with what this man calls a "God gene", and in his description of what this means, he poses twenty questions to see whether you might have it or not. But the questions are about how you see yourself connected to the universe, and to other people, and a lot of other things that are more about love than God. So if you're born with a "love gene" it enhances your life and connection to others.

But, I have to say, this is where our parenting enters in, and all our life experience. My next book is about how to be a healthy and loving parent. You could have the gene and have abusive parents who destroy everything that's in you—all your meaning and divinity, and make you into a total failure—or, I think, you can be born without the love gene and have incredibly loving parents who, in a sense, instill it in you. The majority of the world has neither. So what we see is that those who grow up with love take better care of themselves, because they can accept themselves for who they are, and work at becoming a better person. Rather than saying, "You're a failure. God is punishing you. You're terrible," they can say, "Okay, let me use this pain and learn from it. Let me use criticism to change and grow, and to become a better person."

But those who don't grow up with that kind of self-acceptance and love have a lot of trouble with life. One study with Harvard students showed that those who didn't feel their parents loved them had a significantly higher chance of suffering from a major illness later in life—and this was regardless of parents smoking, committing suicide, or being mass murderers. It really focused on the love issue. If they said, "my parents loved me", thirty-five years after graduation, one out four had suffered a major illness. And of those who said, "My parents didn't love me", I think ninety-eight percent had suffered a major illness.

So again, what I always see is, we take better care of our pets than we do ourselves. People smoke outdoors and tell you they do it to protect their animals. Because their pets had asthma and lung cancer they now smoke outdoors so they're not killing their pet, and they don't say a word about the fact that they're killing themselves.

David: What are some of the personality characteristics that exceptional cancer patients have?

Bernie: In a broad perspective, I'd say that they express their emotion, including appropriate anger. They seek knowledge, and they combine the knowledge with their willingness to take action, so that the inspiration and the information go together. I'm always saying knowledge isn't power if you don't have inspiration. Let me put it simply; you don't smoke because you're stupid, okay. You know it isn't good for you, but you do it anyway. So when the inspiration and the meaning come into your life, then you might put the cigarette out. And last but not least, they have a spiritual support basis. Now this is not about religion or theology as much as it is faith that a god, or a support, is out there. It's not about being punished for breaking the rules of your religion, but rather a constant support.

In terms of specific questions to help determine who will be a long-term survivor, Dr. George Solomon, a psychiatrist, came up with the following questions when AIDS first broke out. Briefly, the questions he used are: Do you have a sense of meaning in your life? Are you able to express anger appropriately? Can you ask for help from friends and family when you need it? Can you say "no" when someone asks you to do something you don't want to do? Are you in charge of what is prescribed for you versus letting others tell you what to do? In other words, you make the decisions.

Do you have enough play in your life? I define play as things that make you lose track of time, which become very meaningful and healthy for you. Do you use your emotions and feelings to help guide you and direct you? Or do you become depressed about being depressed, and just have a downward spiral, so that you're living a role in your life to the detriment of your own needs? See, because some people give up their lives to please everybody else, and then when they learn they have a life-threatening illness, they stop doing what others wanted them to do, and start living their own life. And my way of saying it is, how would you introduce yourself to God? It isn't about whether you have kids, a job, or whatever. It's about identifying with that divine source, which you're made of the same thing.

David: What are some of the suggestions that you would make to help improve the Western medical profession?

Bernie: (laughter) One simple suggestion would be to put every doctor into a hospital bed for a week as a patient. Put them in a hospital where they are not known, and have them admitted with a life-threatening illness as their diagnosis. Then let them stay there.

Another suggestion is to teach doctors how to communicate. If you take the word "words", as one of our children did, and repeat it in an art project, with no space between the words, you realize that words becomes wordswords, swords. Just today I got a phone call from somebody who was waking from surgery and being told how bad things were. From the minute that she woke up, they started telling her how terrible her diagnosis was and what's going to happen to her. That really destroys the patient. Most doctors aren't aware of what they're doing, because they haven't been lying in that bed.

So many doctors think differently after they get sick, or after their loved ones get sick. Then they say, whoops, it's not a diagnosis, it's an experience. And, again, that's what I try to teach doctors—people are living an experience. They're not living a diagnosis. You have to deal with the person and their life, and what they're going through. Those are the things that I think we should work on in our training—how to deal with our emotions and how to express them—and not just have meetings about "what do you think?" and "how do we classify this death or complication?" Rather, we would discuss how it feels to have a patient that you're taking care of die, or what it feels like to have someone come into your office that you can't cure. I mean, we can't even use the word death. You go to a hospital, and everybody talks about "failures", "passing", and "loss", and nobody says so-and-so died, because that word just carries too much emotion for people.

See, what changed me was a patient saying, "I need to know how to live between office visits." That's what doctors have to do. The word "doctor" is derived from the word "teacher", and we have stopped teaching people how to live. Doctors of the past did because they didn't have all this technology and they had to care for people that they also knew. Today we don't even know the patients we're taking care of. That's why there are all these mistakes in the operating room, and all these medical errors—because we're taking care of diseases, room numbers, and diagnoses, and not people. So that's important.

David: What do you think a conventional Western doctor can learn from an indigenous shaman?

Bernie: Again, it's about the person—seeing him or her as a total unit, so that you look at their life. It's something I learned to do—to ask what are you living? What are you experiencing? The words that popped out of people always amazed me, because they always related to their life. Somebody might say words like "failure", "roadblock", "draining", or "burden" to describe his or her life. These are words that people use. They were always about their life. So then I would work at, let's heal the burdens, remove the roadblocks, and why you're feeling like a failure. By helping these people heal their lives, I realized I was also helping them to find a way often to be cured.

See, these were not people avoiding their mortality. I think shamans understand that too—we're all going to die. So if you help people live, they might not die because they're enjoying life. I know that may sound crazy, but I've watched people refuse treatment, go home to do what they wanted to do before they died, and then they lived for decades without any treatments and no sign of a disease. This is because they were home loving every day and they felt that they were contributing to the world. I have a wonderful letter that ends with, "...and I didn't die, and now I'm so busy I'm killing myself." And that's from a lady who went home, made out a will and gave away her treasure. In other words, she was not denying that she was likely to be dead in a short amount of time. So these are not people who go home and deny—although I may add, "deniers" do better than people who feel hopeless and helpless. The fighting spirit, that survival behavior, gives you the best results.

David: How do you think dreams can offer insight into the symbolic meaning of one's illness and help us to heal?

Bernie: I often ask the question, why do we sleep? I was just reading a magazine called *Cerebrum*, and I notice other scientists are beginning to ask that too. Why do why sleep? Why does our body have a rhythm? It's called our circadian rhythm, so that we're active and awake in the day, and then we quiet down and go to bed at night. You can throw away clocks and people still live that way.

To me, dreams represent what I call the universal language, how creation or God speaks to us through universal symbols. My true sense is that one of the reasons we sleep is to allow ourselves to be in touch with this inner wisdom and knowledge that present themselves to us through dreams. I use drawings literally to communicate with lots of people, and help them make decisions, because then they can put the symbols on a piece of paper which are largely coming from their unconscious. I say to people, draw your self—like I mentioned I did with doctors, asking them to draw themselves at work. Those are simple instructions and a hundred people hear the same thing, but you get a hundred different images, because it's coming from an intuitive place within them. Then we can interpret the drawings, and interpret the dreams, and help them be in touch with that.

But it really is fascinating to me because most living things don't sleep. I didn't know that, but most animals don't sleep. When you think about it, a fish can't go to sleep, and I learned that horses sleep on their feet because they're afraid of predators. When you think about it, sleeping is a dangerous thing. We lock ourselves in houses and have alarm systems now, so we're safer, but why should we do it in the first place? I'd say yes, it lets our body rest. I think there are certain physical parts of our body that need to rest. As a matter of fact, one study showed if chemotherapy was given at night the patient could tolerate far more with no side affects and the response was much better. The body was at rest while the cancer cells were not. But I think also, while they're quiet, there's this other wisdom that comes forward.

Here's the reason I call it a wisdom. There are people whose intellect tells them—don't have an operation. Don't have chemotherapy. Don't this, don't that, and they may make a decision that comes from their intellect. Then the drawing that they do will show them that the decision is either right or wrong. Again, it's their inner wisdom—intuitive wisdom, heart wisdom, whatever you want to call it—saying no, this is not good for you or it is good for you. And believe me, that other wisdom knows more. Drawings can answer all kinds of questions, like where should I live? Or what job should I take? It doesn't have to be about medicine.

So I help them to either change their belief systems, their ways of thinking, or I help them make different decisions, but to try to help them put these two things together and reprogram their mind and body. At other times people will say no, I don't want that, and the drawing will be beautiful. I say your inner wisdom knows it's good for you and I suggest you go and do it, and don't worry about it. So it helps them find a harmony through that. But the trouble is most of us are busy thinking, and we forget how to use this inner wisdom, which comes from the body, from feelings, as well as this intuitive aspect.

David: What do you mean when you say that a disease is more than "just a clinical entity; it is an experience and a metaphor, with a message that must be listened to"?

Bernie: It's easiest just to give you examples, and these aren't necessarily all about life-threatening illness. One is a lady with cancer who said that her disease is a failure after I asked her what it was like to experience the cancer. She had been yelling at her doctor for making her ugly with a scar—yet the incision was in her upper thigh, and nobody even knew it was there, unless she was wearing a bathing suit. So her physician said to me, "It's something more, maybe you can talk to her and figure this out."

When she came in I said, "How would you describe what you're experiencing?" She said, "It's a failure." I said, "How does failure fit your life?" See, that's my question then. And her first answer was, "Oh, my body failed." I said, "No, you're not answering my question. How does failure fit your life?" And she said, "Oh, my parents committed suicide when I was a child, so I must have been a failure as a child."

Then her life poured out. See, what she had decided was not to ever develop a relationship with anybody because it's just going to hurt her again, like her parents did to her. So she's living a life of pain because of that childhood experience, and then, because of the cancer, and that word, she changed totally. She set out to change herself and her entire life, and stop being afraid of the world, relationships, and everything else.

Another was a lady with a severe migraine headache that was sent to the hospital because she was vomiting and in pain. I was in another doctor's office while she was there, so I walked over to talk to her for a minute. She was lying in a room with all the lights out. I walked over and said, "How would you describe your headache?" She said, "It's a burden." And I thought, that's a weird word for pain. So I worked with her on burdens. She wasn't my patient, so I didn't plunge into her life, but we talked about burdens, and how you can deal with them and live with them. After about fifteen minutes I left her. Then the nurse walked in a few minutes later to say to me that her pain was gone and she's going home. And by the way—the burden's her marriage. (*Laughter*)

When I asked a woman with a urinary tract infection how she would describe it, she laughed and she said, "Oh, it's very draining." Then she looked at me and said, "Okay, thank you," and walked away. See, she knew that she's got to deal with all the things that are draining her. So for some people, it becomes very obvious, and they look at me and say, thank you. For others, yes, you can help them a little bit to define what that word means in their life and why. As a matter of fact, I just received an email from a friend of mine who's having problems, and one of the things that he said to describe the situation was that he felt like he was hitting his head against the wall. So I said, Okay, let's look at the barriers in your life that you're banging your head against. People send me pictures, and these descriptions, and they say, Okay, what does it mean? How can you help me? Then I ask them to think about why they use these expressions, and how it applies to their life. I also use this process in my own life.

I was once training for a marathon. I was really doing a lot of running in hot weather, and I began to have dizzy spells, particularly in the morning. It became just so hard to get out of bed. So I said, "Hey, what would I ask a patient? How would I describe this?" And I said, "The world is spinning around." Then I said, "Yep, right. Slow down." (*Laughter*) It was very obvious to me that my body was trying to keep me in bed and get me to rest, and I'm out there pushing, pushing, pushing. So I listen to those words myself.

David: What do you think are currently the best ways for a healthy person to slow down, or reverse the aging process and extend their life span?

Bernie: I think if you want to reverse the aging process, the number one thing that every doctor agrees upon is to exercise. Keep moving and keep active. Also, have some meaning in your life. What I find particularly helpful is to not think of yourself as an age. Don't let the child in you die. See things through the child's eyes, and it just makes life interesting and humorous. If you are always doing what you love and have no sense of time how can you age?

I mean, I'm a real character. What I mean by that is, if I see a contract that says "sign here", I write "here" on it. (*Laughter*) See, that's the kid in me. Every time I see a sign that says "Depressed Drains", I say let's stop and try to cheer up the drain. (*Laughter*) It's this little kid inside that keeps me laughing and seeing the world differently. I think when you do that you don't age. Studies show that if you live in an environment that you lived in twenty years ago, you feel younger. In other words, if I took and secluded you, and only gave you newspapers, movies, and media from twenty years ago, you'd come out feeling younger, and healthier if I examined you.

So those are things people need to do. To keep the child alive, and not say I'm a certain age, I'm getting older. No, do what you feel like doing. Keep yourself active and moving, and again, have meaning, connections, and relationships. You'll stay alive a lot longer. Studies have shown this. I can give you a plant to take care of, and you'll live longer than somebody across the hall from you in a nursing home to whom I say, I'm putting a plant in your room to decorate it, and then I'll take care of it. But if I go in and say, here's a plant, you're to see it gets sunshine and water it regularly, you end up living longer and being healthier than the person across the hall.

A study in Australia that was written up a few months ago in the paper showed that if you went home to a dog after your heart attack you had a six percent mortality rate that year. If you went home without a dog, it would be closer to thirty percent. You say, what has a dog got to do with it? Again, it's the relationship. The connection may be taking the dog for a walk, or whatever, but it means something to you. So those are the things I would say. Find meaning. Keep the child in you alive. Keep moving. Keep thinking. Be creative. Experiment. Do different things. It just goes on and on, and I could give you pages and pages, but I think it's just those basic things that get you started.

David: How do you envision the future of medicine?

Bernie: I think that it needs to be a combination of things. The technology is important, I would never deny that. There are people alive today because of science and what we are able to do, like transplanting organs. But at the same time, you have the awe and the wonder of somebody awakening with a transplanted organ, and then having memories of the other person's life. So it's combining the practical and the technological with the mysterious and the meaningful. Quantum physicists and astronomers, I think, understand this better than doctors, because they are living with uncertainty, and the wonder and the awe of creation. So they're in a very different place, and I always enjoy speaking to them. Doctors also need to find that place, so that they are contributing to each person's life that they see in some practical way, as well as in some spiritual way.

I also think that doctors need to allow their patients to heal them, and give them something back. One woman used the term "mutual investment society," and maybe this is the best description of the future of medicine. She said, "It ought to be a mutual investment society, so you are invested in the doctor and the doctor's invested in you."

When people ask me how to find a good doctor I often say to them, find one who is criticized by family, patients, and nurses—because they're listening and learning from the criticism. See, because what I've learned is, when somebody doesn't listen and apologize to you, you stop criticizing them. You just get somebody else or stop talking to them because it's pointless. They're always making speeches. So when we become a mutual investment society, and each of us is teaching the other, then the natives and the tourists help each other. Patients are the natives, doctors are the tourists. We have to understand each other's land, as well as what we're living and going through.

David: In your book, Peace, Love, & Healing, *you talk about using mind-altering techniques such as progressive relaxation, prayer, meditation, visualization, and hypnosis to help heal the body when it becomes ill. What are your thoughts about using medical marijuana in this way? In the controversy over the medicinal value of marijuana, the potential benefit created by the shift in consciousness that marijuana causes is rarely discussed. Have you ever encountered any patients who benefited—not so much from the anti-nausea or other symptom-relieving properties in cannabis—but rather by the changes in consciousness that marijuana caused, so that they viewed their illness from a new perspective?*

Bernie: I'm not against medical marijuana, but I think that the medicinal properties are probably exaggerated, in the sense that, if people are cared for, we already have enough medications and drugs to help them feel better. What I see is that it's so much related to the person's belief. I have watched people's nausea disappear when they took the wrong pill. But the pill had a "C" on it, so the person thought it was compazine, which is for nausea. So they stopped being nauseated even though it was another drug.

You might say, why did the nausea disappear? It's because of what the person believes. I have watched a woman stop vomiting after her husband handed her a bag with a dozen roses in it. He had been handing her a bag every day before he drove her home, and she would throw up in it the whole way. She said, "I opened the bag and there were a dozen roses from my husband in it, so I never vomited again." You see, so much of it has to do with the person's belief and mind and everything else.

So, obviously, I'm not against medications that can help, and if the marijuana helps, fine. But you were just saying how it changes consciousness, and we can change consciousness without taking the drug. You can meditate. You can use hypnosis. I can use words that create a trance state that help you not have side effects. Again, you get back the communication, and with that comes a whole host of other things. It's the power of the mind.

If someone is undergoing a form of chemotherapy that causes people to have their hair fall out, and you give them injections of saline or a placebo pill, and say it'll make your hair grow, for a third of people their hair grows. The opposite also works. People have their hair fall out when receiving a placebo. I could rub someone's skin with a swab, and if I say it'll make it numb, and a third of the people have anesthesia, but there's nothing in the swab. So again, the power of our beliefs and minds—where this started—is enormous. Doctors don't know how to use it because they're not taught how to communicate with people and enhance those beliefs.

David: You've already spoken about this a little, but could you specifically address what sort of role you think spirituality plays in the healing process?

Bernie: I think it does several things. It gives people's live's meaning. I grew up with a mother who, when we had trouble, used to say, "God is redirecting you; something good will come of this." And I bring that up because, if you grow up in religion, then you could be punished for evil or misbehaving. In that way religion could become a burden and a handicap for you. So the way I deal with this is to say to people, "If you lose your car keys, does God want you to walk home?" And people laugh. Then I say, "Okay, if you lose your health, go look for that too." For me, the word spirituality means there's a great resource, that the loving energy and intelligence that created the universe is there for us, to help us. So prayer can bring you peace when you don't know what to do. Remember how I spoke about the importance of connection? Well, if you're connected to a god or a creator, you feel like you're never alone. You always have support.

So these are things that help people. Our Father, referring to God, is always loving us. To quote a friend of mine, she said, "When I let love into my prison, it changed every negative item in it and ... turned them into something meaningful." And this love is coming from our Father. So when you have that kind of love, and that kind of connection, you get through things. And the prayer, the meditation—to me they all become almost like one, when you're willing to look within yourself. A ritual I go through every day is gratitude, which helps me focus on the nice things about the world, not just my troubles. I look at confession—what are the things about me that I need to change? Then I say prayers for others and myself. I find that as I do that, I evolve, and my prayers become much less about material needs than they do about greater needs for myself and the world.

In all the years thinking about this, I may add, I have been asking this question: What can I pray for for you? What would you answer to this? What would you ask me to pray for, if I said I want to say a prayer for you?

David: Oh, to make the world a better place.

Bernie: You're now the sixth person. I've been asking that question for roughly twenty years, and only five people have ever said, "World peace." It blew my mind that everybody else is focused on themselves. So you said it, and again, you transcended yourself. I'd say that's what the spirituality allows you to do—to transcend yourself. Then yes, you have benefits from that transcendence. Try this meditation for a few days. Repeat the word God whenever you have a quiet or troubled moment and then "Thank you for everything. I have no complaint whatsoever."

David: What is your personal concept of God?

Bernie: My definition of God is "loving, intelligent, conscious energy, Satchidananda, being, consciousness, bliss." Astronomers will tell you that the universe can't be an accident. It just took too many things happening at the right moment to make it an accident. So I think there's intelligence and consciousness, and why do I say love and energy? Because it's a world that has existed. I always say, if I cut my finger it heals, and if there was no love in it, then I would bleed to death. Ice floats, which defies the laws of physics, because when the water gets more dense it should get heavier and sink. But instead—bloop—it floats. So our planet stays alive. These are things people don't think about, but this evidence is meaningful.

I often say to people that I'm on the board of directors of heaven as an outside consultant. So I say to God, why would you make a world with all these troubles, diseases, and inflictions? See, this was very important for me as a doctor. I have to say this bothered me as a doctor, especially as a medical student. You'd watch all this suffering and wonder, *why*? Why? So I'll give you another test. (*Laughter*) Another one of my questions is, Why would you want to be God? If I said you could be God for a day, tomorrow, why would you want to be God?

David: I guess so that I could help raise consciousness and reduce suffering in the universe.

Bernie: Yes, like you, most people say that they would change things. I always say that the right answer is: *So that I would understand why.*

Now, in order to understand, I go to God and I say, "Why didn't you make a perfect world?" And the answer is: A perfect world is a magic trick. It's not creation. It has no meaning. We're here to live and to learn. Life is a school. And once we really become co-creative, compassionate, and loving, think about what a world we would have. Yes, you'll still have a world with disease and death—but those who are suffering will have compassion and love, and we won't be killing each other. One of things I've always mentioned as a surgeon is that we're all one family. As a surgeon, I know we are all the same color inside, and our external differences are for recognition, not for wars and destruction.

David: What do you think happens to consciousness after death?

Bernie: What I am sure happens to consciousness after death is that it continues on. I don't see it in a sense of saying, "Oh, I'm going to be reincarnated." No, your body is gone, but what you have experienced and are aware of will go on. So somebody will be born with your consciousness, and it will affect the life they live.

I know people who see life's difficulties as a burden and say, "Why is God punishing me and why am I going through this?" Maybe these people ought to be asking, what am I here to learn, experience, and change? Rather than sitting there whining and complaining. What can I do? What am I here to learn? Now, I don't criticize these people because I remember Elizabeth Kübler-Ross saying that if you're in high school you don't get mad at somebody in first grade. So I think we're at different levels of consciousness based upon our experience and what we are born with.

But I personally believe from my experience, for instance, that one of the reasons I'm a surgeon in this life is because I did a lot of destruction with a sword in a past life—killing people and animals. This is not conscious, like the answers I gave you earlier, but at a deeper level I chose to use a knife in this life to cure and heal with, rather than kill with. I often say to people—think about things that effect you emotionally that you have no explanation for. This may be due to some past life experience, and that is why you're acting the way you're acting. Now, whether I'm right or wrong, I have to say that, as long as it's therapeutic that's what I'm interested in.

But on a personal level, I believe that consciousness in non-local, and it can be carried on and picked up by people. I think this shows in animals too. There's a certain wisdom that they have. Oh, I forgot his name ... in England ...

David: Rupert Sheldrake?

Bernie: Yes, Rupert Sheldrake. He was here not too long ago, and I sat with him a little bit. I've always loved some of the things that he shows. I live in a house full of animals.

David: I worked with Rupert for around three years on a number of different research projects. We coauthored several papers together, and I did the California-based research for two of his books, including the one on pets that anticipate their owner's arrival.

Bernie: Oh, one personal experience. A friend of mine, Amelia Kinkade, who I met in California, is an animal-intuitive. She has written some books. But to make a long story short, we had a cat that disappeared here in Connecticut, and Amelia sat in Los Angeles and told me where to find the cat. She said "I'm looking through its eyes. I know it's not dead." And I was sure this cat, which had gotten out of the house, had been killed in the woods by some predator. But she said "No, I can see the moon," and then she went on to describe the house, the yard in detail, the other animals who were there, and where this cat was. Then I got the cat the next morning. So do I believe that consciousness is not local? You bet. (*Laughter*)

Carl Jung said a long time ago, it's not about beliefs, it's about experience. So, if you have an open mind and you experience something, you don't need to believe it, but you shouldn't dismiss it either. What I often find with physicians is after if I've told them something they say that they can't accept it. And I say, "Excuse me, this happened to a patient." And they'll say, well, I can't accept it. So I say, "Why don't you answer, I can't understand it or explain it?" But they literally block it out of their conscious system because they don't know how to deal with it. It wasn't taught to them. They have no explanation. And I'm open-minded. See, it's like saying, hey, how'd the universe get created? Well, I don't know. All right, but you don't commit suicide because of it. So I'm willing to experience things that I can't explain. That's why I hear a lot of things from patients that they wouldn't tell somebody else.

David: What are you currently working on?

Bernie: Oh, I keep writing about my experience, and all kinds of things. I've written children's stories, as well as stories for adults. One of the little stories I've written recently has to deal with loss. I use some metaphors and symbols that struck me, like each life is a candle. If we see ourselves as candles, then we see that we are each here for a certain period of time and the candle will ultimately burn out. I also see that if we grieve excessively, we put out the candles of our loved ones who have died, and are walking around with a beautiful candle in their hand. So it's constantly working on loss, and writing about that. I tend to write more books now with titles like *Prescriptions for Living or Prescriptions for the Soul*, which are about the age-old eternal messages that most people have never been truly educated about.

We get information, but we don't get an education. We're not taught how to deal with difficult situations. So I'd say more of what I work on now is to help people deal with life—not just some specific illness, but how does one get through life with all its troubles? I want people to realize that there isn't anything that I have to say that hasn't been said by the great sages of the last two thousand years. There's Buddha, Jesus, the Talmud, and the Kabbalah. There is a lot of great stuff out there you ought to read. What I find is, I keep giving them these same messages, but in modern up-to-date stories related to my life and family. So it's easy for people to say, Oh, I get it, rather than reading some mystical text that was written a thousand years ago.

Something just struck me the other day when I was reading. It said "If you meet the Buddha on the road kill him." I've read that a million times, and never really understood it. But as I continued reading it became clearer. It said, "and if you meet your parents kill them, and if you meet your teacher kill your teacher." Then it went on to say that you shouldn't give them all the credit, that all the genius and inspiration that you see in them is also in you. So honor yourself. It's okay to kill all these images and honor yourself. I think that's what I try to get people to do, and if they haven't ever been honored, to have them "re-parent" themselves. "Re-parenting" is a term I use that means that we each need to be that kind of loving parent for each other.

David: Is there anything that we haven't discussed that you would like to add?

Bernie: If you're on a radio program they always say, "Oh, we're running out of time." So I say, "You're right." I always say that most important message to people—that we're all here for a limited time. So I think death is a great, great teacher. I always say to people, don't try to not die, because it doesn't work, and you'll get very upset with yourself. But try to enjoy living. I think when you know you have limited time, you don't let a lot of things bother you, drive you crazy, or take up your time. It really empowers you to choose joy and happiness.

I was reading a book some psychiatrist wrote about how a young man had enlightened him. This was an unhappy boy, from a very wealthy family, who's trying to be successful, and he's a mess. The psychiatrist said one day the kid came in and said, "I think I got it." "What is it?" He said, "If you're successful you may not be happy, but if you're happy you are a success." It was like a light went on in the kid's head. So his job from then on was to find what makes him happy. That's something I grew up with up. Any decision that we had to make, my mother's wisdom was: What will make you happy? She was always asking you to pay attention to what felt right for you. I often say to people, this is not about personal interest, this is about choices. It wasn't, do what will be good for you and not other people. No. It was like, what job should I take? Where should I live? Well, what'll make you happy? So you contributed to the world through *your life*, not through what was imposed on you.

The reason that I stress the spiritual dimension is because: He who seeks to save his life will lose it. You become the good girl again, the good kid, and you lose your life. Then when you're willing to lose your life, you'll save it. You lose your untrue self. I find those types of stories in every religion, where someone is willing to give his life to save others. See, that's what we're here for. These myths and fairy tales are everywhere to be found, and they're teaching us the same thing. But most people never get the message until it's too late to live it. So find your way of serving and loving now!

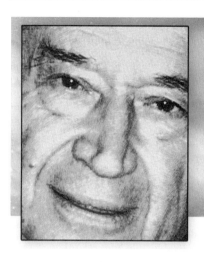

THE NEW SCIENCE
of
CANNABINOID-BASED MEDICINE

An Interview with
Dr. Raphael Mechoulam

Raphael Mechoulam, Ph.D., is the Lionel Jacobson Professor of Medicinal Chemistry at the Hebrew University of Jerusalem, where he has been working on cannabinoid chemistry (a term he coined) for over forty years. Throughout this time, Dr. Mechoulam and colleagues have made some of the most important contributions to the field of cannabinoid research. His lab was the first to identify and synthesize delta-9-tetrahydrocannabinol (THC), the primary psychoactive compound in cannabis. This discovery in 1964 (with Dr. Yehiel Gaoni), opened the door to a whole new field of medical research that began exploring, not only the therapeutic potential of THC (marketed as Marinol in America), but other natural and synthetic cannabinoids as well, and offered exciting new insights into how the brain functions.

Dr. Mechoulam, along with pharmacologist, Dr. Habib Edery and colleagues, went on to isolate and elucidate the structures of most members of the cannabinoid group of compounds in the cannabis plant. Twenty-eight years after discovering THC, in 1992, Dr. Mechoulam, along with Dr. William Devane and Dr. Lumir Hanus, identified the brain's first endogenous cannabinoid (or endocannabinoid)—the brain's natural version of THC—which they called "anandamide," from the Sanskrit word "ananda," which means "eternal bliss" or "supreme joy."

It turns out that the brain actually has a whole family of cannabinoid neurotransmitters and receptors. Just as the active compound in opium (morphine) led to the discovery of the endorphin (endogenous morphine) system in the brain, the active compound in cannabis (THC) led to the discovery of the brain's endocannabinoid system. Later Dr. Mechoulam and colleagues identified the THC metabolites and, more recently, along with Dr. Lumir Hanus and Dr. Shimon Ben-Shabat, he discovered a second endocannabinoid known as 2-arachidonylglycerol (2-AG). These findings have profoundly advanced our understanding of cannabinoid systems.

Endocannabinoids function as neuroprotective agents, they are part of the brain's reward system, and they help with the reduction of pain. Vigorous exercise stimulates the release of anandamide, and the sense of euphoric well-being that comes with a healthy workout—what jogging enthusiasts refer to as a "runner's high"—is due to elevated levels of endocannabinoids. The endocannabinoid system in the brain is also believed to help mediate emotions, consolidate memory, and coordinate movement. In fact, cannabinoid receptors are found in higher concentrations than any other receptor in the brain, and the endocannabinoid system acts essentially in just about every physiological system that people have looked into.

While the political controversy over medical marijuana continues in America, pharmaceutical companies—such as G.W. Pharmaceuticals in the United Kingdom and Sanofi-Aventis in France—are busy researching and developing a wealth of new medications based on compounds found in the cannabis plant. Controlled studies have revealed therapeutic utility of cannabinoids in the treatment of multiple sclerosis and other spasticity ailments, asthma, rheumatoid arthritis, cancer chemotherapy side-effects, glaucoma, AIDS wasting syndrome, and seizure disorders such as epilepsy. Analgesic action and tumor retardation have also been shown.

But even more exciting is the wave of new drugs that are

currently being developed from cannabinoid analogs—both agonists and antagonists, meaning drugs that both activate and deactivate cannabinoid receptors in the brain—From new types of pain killers and neuroprotective agents for head trauma and stroke victims, to appetite stimulants and appetite suppressants. Most recently, one of the synthetic compounds (HU-211) from Dr. Mechoulam's lab has completed phase 2 clinical trials against head trauma with evidence of a neuroprotective effect. The pace of cannabinoid research has certainly been accelerating over the past few years, and Dr. Mechoulam—who has been at the forefront of this research since the beginning—thinks these new drugs are just the tip of the iceberg.

Dr. Mechoulam is recognized as one of the world's experts on cannabinoid-based medicine. In addition to his groundbreaking discoveries, he has written hundreds of scientific papers on his cannabinoid research, and he is the author of the book Cannabinoids as Therapeutic Agents, *an early review of the research in this area. Dr. Mechoulam has received numerous honors and awards for his outstanding contributions to the field, and he was the president of the International Cannabinoid Research Society. Dr. Mechoulam is a member of the Israel Academy of Sciences, and among the numerous prizes that he has received for his work, is the highest national scientific prize in Israel—the Israel Prize.*

I interviewed Dr. Mechoulam on December 21, 2004. Raphael is mentally energetic, kind, and generous. We spoke about how he came to discover THC and anandamide, the role that endocannabinoids play in the brain, natural ways to increase the brain's production of anandamide, and the vast array of new cannabinoid-based drugs that are being developed.

David: What originally inspired your interest in cannabinoid chemistry?

Raphael: That was many years ago. I had completed my Ph.D. and I was back from the Rockefeller Institute (now Rockefeller University) in New York. I was a pure organic chemist at that time, and I was interested mainly in natural products—hopefully natural products with physiological activity. Now, surprisingly, I found that from a chemical point of view, cannabis was quite an unknown product. While morphine had been isolated from opium almost 150 years before that, the active compound in cannabis was actually unknown. People had never isolated it in a pure form. That was something that I realized after really reading the literature quite carefully. Of course, the structure and synthesis were unknown. So I thought it was a good idea to look at cannabis because, essentially, nobody was working on cannabis at that time. So I started working on it. We got the material, surprisingly, from the police. I got five kilograms of hashish to work on, and that was the start of the story. I thought it would be over in a couple of months, and it has been going on and on and on forever.

David: What initially motivated your search to identify the primary psychoactive component of cannabis, and could you briefly summarize how you came to discover THC?

Raphael: We were looking for natural compounds with biological activity and these were obviously compounds with important biological activity. But until we had identified the compounds, elucidated their structures, and synthesized them, it was quite impossible to do any biological work with them. There were stories about what these compounds were supposed to do. There was quite a lot of work from people in France during the previous century, and, of course, a lot of historical literature, but this is not science. Even in those days this was not something that could be accepted as scientific evidence, and we obviously needed a strong basis for physiological work. So the work we did at that time was in collaboration with biologists because, obviously, you cannot isolate an active compound without having something to test your fractions. You separate the materials by various chemical means, and you have to test those fractions that are active.

Now, active in those days meant that we had to give them to some kind of animal. There were no in vitro tests (no tests that we could do in the test tube) at the time—so we gave the fractions to monkeys. Then we chose those fractions that caused sedation in monkeys. The monkeys fell asleep when we gave them rather high doses. So we could fractionate the materials in this manner and, ultimately, we ended up with THC in its pure form for the first time. Then we elucidated the structure so we could work on the biology of this compound.

You see, most scientists will work in one field, such as chemistry, pharmacology, or physiology, and I think they're making a mistake because there is no such thing as one field of science. Normally, everything is connected. Nature doesn't realize the differences between chemistry, biology, physics, physiology, or whatever. We create different fields of science because we are incapable of grasping all these things together. So my idea was to start with chemistry because that area was unknown and one could not advance further. But, after identifying the chemical structure of the active compound, one could go into the other fields, which I did over the next few decades.

David: How did you come to discover the brain's first endogenous cannabinoid?

Raphael: After we had identified THC, we also had to identify the rest of the materials in cannabis. Surprisingly, it is a terrible mixture, and that was one of the reasons why it had never been isolated. The technical means for identifying THC were not available in the nineteenth century, or early twentieth century, up until the '50s, really. So once we had THC and some of the other compounds, we did some metabolic studies, and we found out what happens with the compounds in the body. Then we looked into some pharmacology, in collaboration with many friends and colleagues, all over the world actually. We looked at the effects of these compounds, particularly THC. We worked on epilepsy in Brazil. We worked with people at Oxford in England who had done various activities, and so on.

Now, in the beginning it was not clear what the basics of the action were. We knew a lot about the actual physiological effects and the pharmacology. All these things could be investigated with pure THC, and there were thousands of papers on THC. We had isolated it, and as we had a synthesis, it was not very difficult to work with it. But the basics of the metabolic action were completely unknown, and there were some real reasons for that. The reason for this lack of clarity arose when we synthesized a mirror-image of the THC molecule. The THC molecule has two asymmetric centers, and therefore, it is available in both positive and negative forms. Now, the negative form is the active one, so, supposedly, the positive form should have been inactive. But, actually, it was. People said that they had repeated our synthesis and tested the compounds, and they were active.

Now, if you have a compound which has two forms—called enantiomers—and they're both active, then chances are that it doesn't bind to a receptor, to a enzyme, or anything like that because these receptors are also asymmetric, and therefore only one of the symmetric compounds should act, or should bind to them. Well, it turned out that this was wrong, that people were mistaken. We took some THC, synthesized both compounds in completely pure form, and it turned out that only the negative form was active. So it was just a technical error by many groups who tested both enantiomers, because we found that this is not true, that only one form was active. Therefore, there was an asymmetric molecule in the body, and this led quite shortly thereafter to the discovery of the first receptor, which, of course, is asymmetric as well. That was done by Allyn Howlett at the St. Louis University Medical School in 1988. She did some excellent work, and her student was Bill Devane.

I invited Bill Devane to join my group in the late '80s, early '90s, and he came and stayed with us for about two years. He came here to study some chemistry, but I had some other ideas for him. I thought that, if there is a receptor, then the receptor is not in our brain just because there is a plant out there, but because there is, obviously, a compound synthesized in the brain which activates this particular receptor. Because Bill had experience with the receptors—it was the subject of his Ph.D. thesis—that meant that we could chemically identify a compound which will bind to this receptor in the brain.

So I had Bill, and there was a Czech fellow who joined me just about that time. He also came for six months, and he's still with me ten years later, Lumir Hanus. They worked very hard indeed. We had to separate and separate brain extracts, and test them on binding, and then we tested them in the U.K. on some physiological activities. And ultimately, we got an extremely small amount of material. But that was enough to be able to show the structure, to elucidate the structure of that. So we were glad. We synthesized it immediately, and that compound turned out to be anandamide.

David: What was the reason that you named it "anandamide?"

Raphael: We assumed it has to do with joy. After all, people normally use marijuana to feel better, to be happy—and we were certainly happy, having succeeded after so much work to identify the compound. It was completely unexpected that the compound would be a fatty acid derivative. The compound in the cannabis plant is a tricyclic compound and here we had a fatty acid, which is completely different from a chemical point of view. But they had more or less exactly the same actions, both in vitro and in vivo. We called it "anandamide" because "ananda" means "supreme joy" in Sanskrit, and "amide" comes from its structure, because it has an amide bond. So together it sounded okay. We called it "anandamide."

We also knew that there was a different type in the periphery that was not present in the brain. So we looked in the periphery, in the spleen, and we found a second compound, very closely related to anandamide, called 2-arachidonylglycerol. Anandamide is arachidonyl ethanolamide. So these are the endogenous cannabinoids—the endocannabinoids. It has turned out by the work of hundreds of groups now, including my own. Obviously there is a lot of interest in this group of compounds.

David: What do you think the function of anandamide and other endocannabinoids are in the brain?

Raphael: The endocannabinoid system acts essentially in just about every physiological system that people have looked into, so it appears to be a very central system. Actually, the cannabinoid receptors are found in higher concentrations than any other receptor in the brain, and they are found in very specific areas. They are not found all over, but rather in those places that one would expect them to be—such as areas that have to do with the coordination of movement, emotions, memory, reduction of pain, reward systems, and reproduction. So I believe that this is a very central and essential system that works together and communicates with many other systems.

David: Exercise has been shown to elevate endocannabinoid levels in the brain, and this probably accounts for what jogging enthusiasts refer to as the "runner's high." Do you think that increasing the amount of natural cannabinoids in the brain has any health benefits, and if so, what are some other ways that you think might increase the brain's natural production of endocannabinoids?

Raphael: A good friend of mine was involved in that research. The results were a little bit on the marginal side, not tremendously high. They saw a little bit more anandamide than normal. I would have expected much more. There was just this one paper, so people have not gone into that very thoroughly. It's probably true, but I think that we have to do a little bit more work on that. I talked to Dr. Piomelli, who was one of the people on that paper, and I believe he also thinks one should see a little bit higher levels.

But there are many ways in which the endocannabinoid levels go up, and this is something quite specific for endocannabinoids. Generally, they are present in very low amounts. They are just not there. If you take a mouse and put it in a very low temperature (around one hundred degrees below zero) the mouse dies, the brain stops functioning immediately, and you'll find essentially no anandamide. The anandamide is formed on demand when needed, and in only those areas that need that particular compound at the moment.

For example, during pain, it will be produced in certain areas. The endocannabinoids are not produced all over, and they will not go into the bloodstream like hormones. They will stay around that particular area where they are supposed to be formed. One of the functions is neuroprotection. Now, I'm speaking about mice because I'm not sure what happens with humans. I'm not working with humans and, obviously, it's not ethical to do that. If you take a mouse and cause slight damage to the skull of the mouse, or even to the brain, and if you leave the mouse, it will recover within thirty days. But if you look at the brains of the mice, you find that at least one of the endocannabinoids goes up one thousand percent, so we thought that maybe they have a neuroprotective role.

So we took mice of this type, that had been injured, and we injected them with synthetic endocannabinoids—2-AG, the second compound—and we saw that the damage went down very significantly. And there has been a lot of work on that. There has been some excellent work in California by Greenberg, and they have found the same thing in other models. So everybody now believes that these compounds play a role in neuroprotection.

David: What are your thoughts about using cannabinoids as a treatment to help prevent cancer or retard tumor growth?

Raphael: There are several groups that have found it effective in reducing tumor growth. This is probably due to the same mechanism as before with the neuroprotection. It's probably not only neuroprotective; it's probably a protective agent in general. So, to a certain extent, the endocannabinoid system can be compared with the immune system. Now, the immune system obviously guards us against protein effects, viruses, and microbes, but not all damages. So, just as our body protects itself with the immune system against microbes or viruses, it also tries to protect itself with other systems—and the endocannabinoid system is one of them. So I believe that it certainly acts against cancer cells. There is a very important group in Spain that has done some excellent work on that, and they're actually going into human work now with some cancers found in the brain. We have also done a little bit on that, and there is an Italian group that has done a lot of work on that. So, basically, it seems that this is one of the routes that our body uses to try and protect itself with—by acting on cancers using several different mechanisms, not just one.

David: Can you talk a little about the research that's currently going on with cannabinoid analogs and the development of new pharmaceutical drugs, such as in the areas of neuroprotection and pain management?

Raphael: THC itself is approved in the U.S. by the FDA, and it is used in many other countries for the prevention of vomiting during cancer chemotherapy, and for appetite enhancement. We, and many others, have found that not only THC does that, but also the endocannabinoids. This is one of the main reasons for high endocannabinoid levels during hunger and so on. Now, THC can be used, and is being used, for these two things.

Sanofi-Aventis in France is doing some interesting work. They have a compound which is an antagonist of the cannabinoid system, and they have tested it in about eight thousand obese people. They have found that it is extremely useful. Their appetite goes down slowly, as it should, and they lose weight. They plan to introduce the compound in twelve months time, I think. They're doing a lot of work in the field, and they expect huge sales.

There are compounds that are being tried by many companies. I think that just yesterday a new mixture, THC and CBD [cannabidiol], which is made by a company in England called G.W. Pharmaceuticals as a spray under the tongue, was approved in Canada. So they will be marketing it in Canada for the prevention of all kinds of multiple sclerosis effects, and they will probably get it approved in England. Here we have several things going. There is a compound which was found to be pretty good for prevention of cognition-lowering after heart surgery. After heart surgery, in some cases, there is some cognition lowering, and we found that it certainly does something to that. Initially we found this same compound was very good in the prevention of brain trauma, but large-scale experiments have not been positive. I'm not sure why.

I'm part of the faculty at the medical school here, and at Hadassah Hospital, and we use THC for a variety of things. It has to be approved in every single case by a committee at the hospital. We have used it for a very wide variety of things. We found it effective in fighting hiccups, for example. You'd be surprised how if somebody has hiccups constantly for months, how terrible it is. And it works fine. We've used it for Tourettes syndrome, which is a very nasty neurological disease. This was based on work by some colleagues in Hannover, Germany. It works very well indeed. We've tried it in cases of multiple sclerosis. We've tried it, obviously, with appetite. We gave it four hundred times to children undergoing cancer chemotherapy in order to prevent them from vomiting, and to help with the terrible situation associated with treating children for cancer and so on. They're happier, and the families are happier, so we've been very glad about it. So we try it in various diseases, where there is sufficient literature.

David: What are some of the new drugs and treatments that you foresee being developed from cannabinoid analogs in the future?

Raphael: First of all, there are those things that have been approved already, such as for improvement of appetite. That's good for cancer and AIDS, and is widely used. The other one of course is vomiting. The new drugs, I'm sure, will have to do with neuroprotection, and with certain kinds of pain—neuropathic pain, not acute pain. It doesn't work with acute pain. It works mostly with neuropathic pain, long-term pain.

It may also work in the suppression of memory. This is a something that I hope we'll be able to start shortly. There's something called post-traumatic stress disorder (PTSD), which is due to upsetting memories that stay around too long. Normally, when there is trauma people slowly forget it. This is true for humans and it's true for animals. But if the animals do not have an endocannabinoid system, they do not forget bad memories, and this was shown in a paper by a German-Italian group. In collaboration with the Canadian group, we have done some work on that, and in a different model we have seen the same thing. So I expect that the endocannabinoid system is not in good shape in those post-traumatic patients, and chances are that it will work in treating them. We are just about to develop a treatment. People that have PTSD claim that the only thing that helps them is smoking marijuana, so chances are that cannabinoid treatment may help them.

David: They just started studies here in America treating post-traumatic stress disorder with the drug MDMA.

Raphael: Yes, I know that. There is a group that is pushing MDMA quite a bit. They've been here many times, and they're close friends of mine. I don't know whether it's useful or not, but chances are that it may be. Let's see the results.

David: You once said that "Whatever THC does, anandamide does as well." What is the reason that synthetic anandamide isn't used therapeutically as an alternative THC?

Raphael: That's a very touchy subject. Many years ago when insulin was discovered—I think it was in the early twenties—it was in the clinic within six months. When cortisone was discovered fifty years ago, it was in the clinic within two years, and it became a very successful drug. We discovered anandamide twelve years ago, and it still has never been officially administered to a human. Neither has 2-AG.

David: Why is that?

Raphael: The laws have changed. I can not give anandamide to a human because the toxicology research is not there, and the toxicology research is millions of dollars to do. So somebody has to pay for that. I've asked the National Institute of Drug Abuse (NIDA) many times.

David: But it's an endogenous substance.

Raphael: Yes, but the law is that even a human endogenous substance has to be tested for toxicology and all these things. So I have asked them, I begged them actually, please do it—because a company will not, and obviously an academic person cannot do it. It's a technical thing. It's something that's quite obvious that should be done, yet it has not been done, either with anandamide or with 2-AG. So nobody has ever given anandamide or 2-AG to a human, period.

David: Why do you think that there has been so much political resistance to the notion of cannabinoids as medicine?

Raphael: I'm not sure that there is that much nowadays. It used to be much more. No company would ever touch anything like that many years ago. If they did, they did it kind of quietly. This is not so now. Sanofi-Aventis is going to introduce that antagonist on a very wide scale in the states. Actually, most of the major U.S. companies have cannabinoid programs. I know that Smith, Klyne & Beecham has one, and so do Pfizer and Merck. So possibly the other companies are actually waiting for people to come on the market, so they won't be the first ones. Now that Sanofi-Aventis is going to be on the market, and THC is already on the market, chances are that the other companies will come too. After all, most of the drugs on the market—the new drugs over the last twenty years let's say—are based on being agonists or antagonists of receptors of endogenous compounds like dopamine and so on.

David: Besides weight loss, what other uses would there be for a cannabinoid antagonist?

Raphael: One of them is nicotine withdrawal, which has some nasty symptoms. Mark Twain once said "It's easy to stop smoking; I've done it many times." (*Laughter*) So apparently this antagonist may help with that. That's one thing, and I'm not sure that there are many others. Possibly, it may help with some of the withdrawal symptoms for other drug abuse agents, like heroin perhaps, or maybe cocaine. I'm not sure, because not enough work has been done. But those are the two major things that I can see.

Another big field will be agonists specific to the CB-2 receptor. The CB-2 receptor is in the periphery. We synthesized a CB-2 specific agonists that has nothing to do with the CB-1, which is present in the brain. It is very good for all kinds of digestive system disorders. THC is excellent for treating Crohn's disease and things of that sort. It's not on the market yet, but quite a few groups are working on it. So it will definitely be very useful in those cases.

There are other things. For example, many years ago we elucidated the structure of a compound called cannabidiol, which is present in very large amounts in cannabis. It's more than THC, and it is anti-inflammatory. It is excellent against rheumatoid arthritis, at least in animals. We worked together with a London group—real top of the field people in rheumatoid arthritis—and they have never seen anything as good as that. So chances are that this particular compound, cannabidiol, can be used in rheumatoid arthritis. And it has no psychotropic effects, as a matter of fact, because it does not bind to the receptors. Maybe it has something to do with the metabolism of anandamide. Maybe it blocks the anandamide breakdown. Maybe.

This is something we saw, but whether it's relevant to its activity, frankly, I don't know. So this compound possibly will be used for rheumatoid arthritis. A company is already working on that, so it is not only the endocannabinoids as such, but also other compounds which are in the vicinity. There is also another receptor that we haven't fully identified yet. People are working on a third receptor, and we have a compound which binds to this questionable receptor actually. It has to do with peripheral action and vasodilatation. It causes vasodilatation. We have not published that yet, but I have talked about it at meetings. So vasodilatation is important, and the story is actually just starting. I hope that more and more people will join in elucidating these things.

David: Some people have suggested that the shift in consciousness that a THC intoxication causes may in and of itself have some healing potential—by shifting one's perspective of the illness, or possibly enhancing the placebo effect. What are your thoughts on this idea?

Raphael: People have been talking about this idea quite a lot. I have discussed it several times in connection with something slightly different. I thought that maybe the endocannabinoids have something to do with the conversion of objective perceptions into subjective effects. If I see something nice happening, I smile. So I convert an objective perception into a subjective feeling—happiness. But there has been no proof of that. We've been trying to find out whether we can find something and it is very difficult. The placebo effect is there. Nobody has tested this in animals, let's say, because nobody does tests for placebo effects in animals. Nobody has really tested whether the placebo effect is not some kind of an endocannabinoid effect of a sort. It is due to the doctor being nice to you, and then it is due to the actual feeling of being injected with something which you know will help you, even though it doesn't have anything active in it. But nobody, to the best of my knowledge, has shown that it has to do directly with endocannabinoids.

David: People have suggested that it enhances the placebo effect.

Raphael: Yeah, and this is what I'm saying. It seems quite plausible that it is so, but we have certainly not done that and, to the best of my knowledge, nobody has evaluated the relationship between a placebo effect and an endocannabinoid. Chances are that it's there. It makes a lot of sense, but until it has been tested, you can't say.

David: What do you think should be done to help improve medical research in general?

Raphael: Quite a few things. Maybe the rules are becoming more and more rigid, and now with several compounds being taken off the market, and the FDA being under a lot of pressure, chances are that it will be even more difficult to develop new drugs because a drug has to have side-effects. There is no possibility of a drug not having a side-effect. Aspirin would not be approved today. So chances are that we'll see a slump in new compounds coming out. I hope I'm wrong, but I'm afraid I'm not. It is not a question of money so much. I believe there is enough money. Well, there is never enough money, but there is a reasonable amount of money for medical research.

My group has had enough support for over thirty odd years, even more. We have been supported by the U.S. National Institute of Health (initially Mental Health) and then the National Institute of Drug Abuse for a long period of time. And, although we are not an American group, obviously, they have decided it's okay, we should be supported. I had to reapply for it, but I was supported for that period of time, and they have never pushed me into any direction. They have been very liberal. I've known most of the directors, and they are frequently very good scientists. The present director is an excellent scientist. Actually, she was not born in the U.S.; she's Mexican and she's an excellent scientist by any standard. So, in this respect, I can't say that I've been pushed towards proving that it's terribly bad, and that it will kill everyone. I think nothing of that sort. I've been doing my science and they've been, I hope, happy with it.

David: What are you currently working on?

Raphael: In collaboration with a group at N.I.H., we're working on a new transmitter which binds to a recently discovered receptor. Whether this particular transmitter is a neurotransmitter, a transmitter of another sort, or only a vasodilator, it's an important new compound. Actually, there are quite a few other compounds in the brain which are closely related, so we're working on that. We also have some new anticancer cannabinoid compounds which seem to be pretty good. The person working on this is Natalya Kogan, a Ph.D. student, who is exceptionally bright and deserves a lot of credit.

We recently published something about this research. These new compounds work on an enzyme called topoisomerase, and these are compounds which are very close in action to some of the known anticancer compounds. But the known compounds of this sort cause damage to the heart, and with our compounds, so far, we have seen no such damage in animals. So hopefully this new type of cannabinoid will come out on the market. There is also a possibility that cannabinoids can be used to reduce temperature, and sometimes it's important to reduce temperature because that prevents brain damage during a heat wave or heatstroke.

David: Is there anything that we haven't discussed that you would like to add?

Raphael: We've been lucky to work in a field where originally there wasn't anyone else, so we could work on our research slowly, without any major competition. Now it's a field in which there is a large group of very good people working. In the States, there are several excellent groups. There are also some excellent groups working on this in the U.K., Germany, Spain, and Italy. Though one always hears about competition between scientists, I haven't seen it that much in this field. We are a large group that is working without really competing, and we are exchanging information all the time. So it's a pleasure to be working in such a field. Maybe it has something to do with ananda.

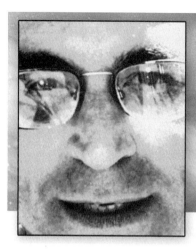

EXPLORING THE THEREAPUTIC BENEFITS OF DMT

An Interview with Dr. Rick Strassman

Rick Strassman, M.D. is a medical researcher who conducted the first U.S.-government-approved-and-funded clinical research with psychedelic drugs in over twenty years. These studies, which took place between 1990 and 1995, investigated the effects of DMT (N,N-dimethyltryptamine), a powerful naturally-occurring hallucinogen. During the project's five years, Dr. Strassman administered approximately four hundred doses of DMT to 60 human volunteers. This research took place at the University of New Mexico's School of Medicine in Albuquerque, where he was tenured Associate Professor of Psychiatry.

Dr. Strassman holds degrees from Stanford University, where he received Department Honors in Biology, and Albert Einstein College of Medicine of Yeshiva University, where he was a member of the Davidoff Honor Society. He took his internship and general psychiatry residency at the University of California, Davis Medical Center in Sacramento, and received the Sandoz Award for outstanding graduating resident in 1981. He spent ten years as a tenured professor at the University of New Mexico, performing clinical research investigating the function of the pineal hormone melatonin, in which his research group documented the first known role of melatonin in humans.

Dr. Strassman has published thirty peer-reviewed scientific papers and serves as a reviewer for several medical and psychiatric research journals. He has been a consultant to the U.S. Food and Drug Administration, National Institute on Drug Abuse, Veterans' Administration Hospitals, Social Security Administration, and other state and local agencies.

In 1984, Dr. Strassman received lay ordination in a Western Buddhist order. He co-founded, and for several years administered, a lay Buddhist meditation group associated with the same order. Dr. Strassman currently practices psychiatry in Gallup, New Mexico and is Clinical Associate Professor of Psychiatry in the University of New Mexico School of Medicine.

Dr. Strassman is also the author of the book DMT: The Spirit Molecule, *which is a compelling and fascinating account of his research with psychedelics. In the book, he discusses how DMT may be involved in near-death experiences, alien abduction encounters, and mystical experiences. As the book unfolds, what begins as a study to explore the pharmacology and phenomenology of DMT, becomes a science fiction-like journey into a hyper-dimensional reality inhabited by intelligent alien creatures. To find out more about Dr. Strassman's work, visit his Web site: www.rickstrassman. com*

I interviewed Dr. Strassman on September 28, 2004. We discussed how Buddhism helped to guide his medical research, the potential therapeutic value of psychedelic drugs, and models for understanding the DMT experience.

David: How did you become interested in medicine, and what lead you to study psychiatry?

Rick: In college, I actually didn't quite know what I wanted to do. I began as a chemistry major, because of my keen interest in fireworks, which I indulged more or less safely in high school. I had hoped to start my own fireworks business. Funny, in retrospect, how I switched from an interest in "outside world" fireworks, to ones more internal.

Nobody I knew really was that encouraging about the fireworks idea, so I switched to a zoology/biology major, but didn't think much about medical school at the time. During the summer between my 3rd and 4th year of college at Stanford, I read much of the material for the upcoming year's classes: Early Buddhism, Sleep and Dreams, The Psychology of Consciousness, Physiological Psychology. I had an epiphany of sorts that summer, deciding I'd like to combine my interest in psychedelics with Eastern religions, psychoanalytic theory and practice—all in a sort of unified theory of consciousness, that related to integrating what I saw as a biological basis for spiritual experience (the pineal, endogenous DMT, etc), with what I believed was the most comprehensive system of psychological defenses (psychoanalysis), with what I thought was the most sophisticated view of human mental "mechanics" (Buddhism).

This was a little ambitious for my medical school applications, and I had a hard time toning it down enough to fit into the format required for those applications. And, my mentor at Stanford thought I had lost my mind, telling me to keep my mouth shut. Most medical school interviews ended badly when they asked why I wanted to go to medical school. The only ones I got into were those where the interviews were short, and I didn't have a chance to launch into my reasons. Right before starting medical school, I was offered a research position in an outstanding physiological psychology laboratory at Stanford with Karl Pribram and arranged to delay entrance into medical school for a year. However, when it turned out there was no funding for the research position, I decided to start medical school on schedule.

I maintained this idealistic (somewhat manic) view during my first year of medical school, and was sorely disappointed. I got depressed, dropped out, ended up at the Zen monastery with which I was ultimately to have a 20 plus year relationship. There, at the monastery, I learned to get back to basics, and returned to medical school, got into my own psychoanalytic psychotherapy, and put the whole psychedelic research idea on the back burner.

When it came time to decide what specialty to pursue, I chose psychiatry for several reasons: the hours were good, I liked the patients, I liked the reading material, I liked other psychiatrists, and I admired my psychiatrist who had helped me a lot. Last but not least, I thought if ever I were to do psychedelic research, psychiatry would be the field in which to do it.

David: What inspired your interest in altered states of consciousness in general, and what lead you to study the effects of DMT and psilocybin?

Rick: I was very curious about how similar were states of consciousness brought on by psychedelics, and those described by mystics and seasoned meditators throughout the ages, across all cultures, as well as descriptions by those having the recently "discovered" near-death experiences. Later, I saw some of the overlap between psychedelic consciousness and psychosis. And, against my better judgment, I began seeing some overlap between the "abduction" experience and the psychedelic one, at least with respect to those of our DMT volunteers.

Once I was finally positioned to begin psychedelic research, almost 20 years after the original epiphany, DMT was a natural choice to begin such research anew. It had been used in humans in previously published research, was endogenous (that is, naturally produced) which made it a great candidate for eliciting "spontaneous psychedelic experience," it was short-acting (which I knew would be helpful on an aversive research unit), and was relatively obscure (thus less likely to draw the sort of attention that a LSD study might).

Psilocybin is chemically very similar to DMT, but is orally active, and longer-acting. I thought it might produce a more easily studied and managed state, both for phenomenological research, as well as for therapeutic work, than did DMT, which was so mind-shatteringly short-acting.

David: How has your interest in Buddhism helped to guide your medical research?

Rick: I was first drawn to Buddhism because of its unabashed manner of describing rather exotic and lofty states of consciousness in a relatively objective manner. The techniques and concepts of the mind, as defined and affected by meditation, appealed to me—it seemed that even the most outrageous states of consciousness could be held, described, even "objectified." Particularly, the Buddhist Abhidharma (the canon of psychology in Buddhism) approach to mind as a composite of a small number of mental functions, appealed to me as a facile means of developing a rating scale, a tool, for measuring the states of consciousness I anticipated finding in our psychedelic research.

This rating scale has been a legacy of the DMT research, and has been translated into several languages, used to measure effects of several different drugs, and has held up well in comparison to some of the other more traditional ways of measuring drug effects.

Later on, when I actually started practicing Zen meditation, I found it very grounding and powerful, and the state of active passivity, so to speak, or alert quietness, was useful as a means of holding the DMT sessions themselves, on my end. I also saw that some of the principles I had learned about meditation, and from teaching it, were useful in coaching the volunteers on how to deal with the things they encountered, or might encounter, during their sessions.

David: One of the most fascinating things about DMT is that it is found naturally in the brain. What function do you think endogenous DMT plays in the human brain?

Rick: I think it plays several roles. It may help mediate some of the more profound mental experiences people undergo: near-death, mystical states, psychosis. This was one of my hypotheses beginning the research: that endogenous DMT mediated these states of consciousness. Thus, if by giving exogenous DMT, we saw features found in those states, that would support our theory that elevated levels of endogenous DMT were involved.

Also, the brain brings endogenous DMT into its confines, across the blood brain barrier, using energy; something that it does for very few compounds, such as glucose, certain amino acids. Thus, it seems as if endogenous DMT is necessary for normal brain (read perceptual) function. Something like the internally generated "Matrix."

David: Do you think that DMT experiences can have therapeutic value? What about other psychedelics?

Rick: Intravenous DMT is so overwhelming that the most one can hope for is to hold on and try to remember as much as one can, at least for a single, isolated session. We found that people could work through things much more, though, psychologically, spiritually, when given repeated doses in the course of a morning, which we did in our attempt to develop tolerance to closely-spaced, repeated DMT injections. This is probably somewhat akin to what happens with ayahuasca, which is an orally active preparation of DMT (two plants: one contains DMT, and one contains an inhibitor of the enzyme that normally breaks DMT down in the gut), which lasts about 4-6 hours, and is much more workable.

Other psychedelics may be therapeutic to the extent that they elicit processes that are known to be useful in a therapeutic context: transference reactions and working through them; enhanced symbolism and imagery; increased suggestibility; increased contact between emotions and ideations; controlled regression, etc.

This all depends, though, on set and setting. These same properties could also be turned to very negative experiences, if the support and expectation for a beneficial experience aren't there.

David: In your book you expressed some doubt as to whether DMT use might have any spiritual value. What are your thoughts on this now? Do you think that DMT has any entheogenic potential?

Rick: I still don't think psychedelics, including DMT, have intrinsically good or bad values. It all depends upon how they're used and taken. Sort of like the very trite and overused analogy of a hammer: it can be used to break things apart or build things up.

David: Do you think that there is an objective reality to the worlds visited by people when they're under the influence of DMT, and do you think that the entities that so many people have encountered on DMT actually have an independent existence?

Rick: I myself think so. My colleagues think I've gone woolly-brained over this, but I think it's as good a working hypothesis as any other. I tried all other hypotheses with our volunteers, and with myself. The "this is your brain on drugs" model; the Freudian "this is your unconscious playing out repressed wishes and fears;" the Jungian "these are archetypal images symbolizing your unmet potential;" the "this is a dream;" etc. Volunteers had powerful objections to all of these explanatory models—and they were a very sophisticated group of volunteers, with decades of psychotherapy, spiritual practice, and previous psychedelic experiences.

I tried a thought-experiment, asking myself, "What if these were real worlds, and real entities? Where would they reside, and why would they care to interact with us?" This led me to some interesting speculations about parallel universes, dark matter, etc. All because we can't prove these ideas right now (lacking the proper technology) doesn't mean they should be dismissed out of hand as incorrect.

David: How do you think the DMT experience is related to the near-death experience and the alien abduction experience?

Rick: I hypothesize that DMT levels rise with the stress associated with near-death experiences, and mediate some of the more "psychedelic" features of this state.

I think that, based upon what many of our volunteers experienced via entity-contact, high levels of DMT could break down the subjective/objective membrane separating us from other levels of reality, in which perhaps some of these entities "reside." I've been criticized by the abduction "community" because of the lack of "objective" evidence of "encounters" in our volunteers. E.g., stigmata, metal objects, etc. In response to these concerns, it might be worth considering a "spectrum" of encounters—from the purely material (about which I withhold all judgment), to the purely consciousness-to-consciousness "contact" experience that may usefully describe what our volunteers underwent.

David: Where there any times during your DMT research where you witnessed something that you couldn't explain in terms of conventional science, such as a form of psychic phenomena?

Rick: I didn't see much in the way of psychic phenomena. The reports people came back with, though, were the things I had a difficult time conceptualizing, such as the entity-contact thing.

David: Do you think that the study of psychedelics might provide us with some insight into paranormal phenomena?

Rick: I'm not sure what you mean by paranormal. And, I'm not too interested in say, psi, or clairvoyance, or telepathy. Those don't seem necessarily a more enlightened way of viewing our lives and our society. However, the concept of consciousness existing without a body, and the implications this might have on our behavior, ethics, ecology, interpersonal relationships—these hold more interest to me.

David: How has your study of DMT affected your understanding of the nature of consciousness?

Rick: I think we're mighty small. But, I think what we're connected to is mighty big, and through our connection, can affect "it."

David: What kind of an influence did Terence McKenna's explorations and ideas have on your DMT research?

Rick: He introduced me to DMT. He and I had some long conversations about how to formulate a research agenda that would both fly with the traditional scientific community, and would address our deeper questions about consciousness. He was a friend, too.

David: My friend Cliff Pickover, the popular science writer, told me that he once corresponded with you about his hypothesis that DMT in the pineal glands of Biblical prophets may have "given God to humanity, and let ordinary humans perceive parallel universes." His idea is that if our human ancestors produced more endogenous DMT than we do today, then certain states of consciousness, or certain kinds of visions, would have been more likely. He suggests that many of the ancient Bible stories describe prophets who seem to have had DMT-like experiences. Cliff told me that you said to him, "If indeed we made more DMT in the past, this may have to do with the increase in artificial light that has come upon us in the past 1,000 years or so." Do you think this is a possibility?

Rick: Well, this relates to my theory about the pineal and DMT, which is basically that the pineal is a source of endogenous DMT production. I marshal a lot of circumstantial evidence for this, but there are no hard data yet. Nevertheless, the "stress" model of increased DMT production is established in humans and lower animals, as it is well established that brain, lung, and blood all make DMT, and that in lower animals and humans, endogenous levels rise with stress.

With respect to the pineal; pineal activity increases in darkness (and during winter), and decreases in increased light (and in summer). Even relatively dim artificial light (indoors) has a suppressive effect on pineal function, and it may be that if generic pineal activity were related to DMT production, decreased activity through the aegis of increased ambient light during hours which were previously dark, may have something to do with decreased normative DMT levels.

David: What kind of potential do you see for future research with psychedelics?

Rick: I don't think organized religion can handle them, because of the threat to their turf. I also don't think science can handle them because of the nature of what they reveal—at least mainstream science. Any mainstream scientist doing research into the true, real, hardcore, psychedelic experience is so hamstrung by political correctness, that they cannot discuss what they really have seen in their research, and what they think and feel about it.

Thus, for the next foreseeable future, psychedelics will exist in some sort of limbo, waiting for the proper discipline to be developed that can approach the experience through the relatively objective tools of the scientific method, and the context and wisdom of perennial religious teachings. In some ways, this is unfortunate, because much of this work is now going on underground, with no "peer-review" and general above-board forum for discussion, quality control, and the like, which occurs in the non-underground world.

David: What has your own personal experience with DMT been like, and how have psychedelics affected you?

Rick: I don't answer anything about my use or non-use of psychedelics. If I say I've used them, people accuse me of being a drug-addled zealot. If I say I've never used them, people accuse me of not knowing what I'm talking about.

David: What do you think happens to consciousness after death?

Rick: I think it continues, but in some unknown form. I think a lot depends upon the nature of our consciousness during our lives—how attached to various levels of consensus reality it is. My late/former Zen teacher used to use the analogy of a light bulb, with electric current passing through it. The light bulb goes out, but the current continues, "changed" in a way, for its experience in the bulb. He also referred to "like gravitating toward like" in terms of the idea of the need for certain aspects of consciousness to develop further, before it can return to its source. That is, dog-like aspects of our consciousness end up in a dog, human-like aspects get worked through in another human, plant-like aspects into plants, and so on.

David: What is your perspective on the concept of God?

Rick: I'm working on it. Put simply, I think God is the creator and sustainer of this whole scene. And, the creator and sustainer of cause-and-effect, which for many Buddhists, is equivalent to God, but by not "believing" in God, they get to sidestep the whole issue of a beginning or an end—which I believe, is extraordinarily important.

David: What are you currently working on?

Rick: I spend much of my time studying Jewish scripture and commentary from as conservative and medieval approach as I can. I'm interested in the Jewish conception of God (as that's my own biological/genetic/social background), and also in the Jewish mystics'/sages' ideas about non-corporeal existences. They draw from those ideas (God and spiritual realities) a very profound ethical-moral system. And such a system must be incorporated into any truly psychedelic view of reality, consciousness, and society.

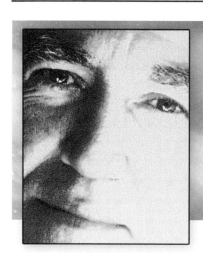

MEDICINE AND SPIRITUALITY

An Interview with Dr. Larry Dossey

Larry Dossey, M.D., is considered one of the world's experts on mind-body medicine, and is one of the leading spokespeople for integrating spirituality with medicine. He is the author of ten books on the role of consciousness and spirituality in medicine, including Space, Time & Medicine, *and* The New York Times *bestseller* Healing Words: The Power of Prayer and the Practice of Medicine.

Dr. Dossey graduated in 1967 from Southwestern Medical School in Dallas. He then served as a battalion surgeon in Vietnam and spent hundreds of hours in helicopters, rushing around with—paradoxically enough—a medical aid bag and a rifle. He says that these daily close encounters with death profoundly affected him, and they gave him an immense sense of gratitude toward life.

In the 1970s, after completing his residency in internal medicine at the Veterans Administration Hospital and Parkland Hospital in Dallas, he helped to establish the Dallas Diagnostic Association—the largest group of internal medicine practitioners in the city—and served as Chief of Staff at the Medical City Dallas Hospital. While there, he became intrigued by patients who experienced remissions that conventional medicine could not adequately explain, and by the interactions between mind and body. These experiences lead to the development of a biofeedback department at the Dallas Diagnostic Association, and to an interest in alternative and holistic medical therapies, such as imagery, visualization, and meditation.

In 1982, Dr. Dossey wrote Space, Time & Medicine, *the first of a series of books about the implications that research into mind-body healing, parapsychology, and one's world view have on medicine. This book influenced many young physicians at the time and helped promote a greater acceptance of these ideas in mainstream medicine. Some of Dr. Dossey's other books include* Beyond Illness, Recovering the Soul, Reinventing Medicine, *and* Prayer is Good Medicine.

More than anything else, Dr. Dossey is probably best known for his work popularizing the research which demonstrates that prayer can have measurable healing effects. Although the evidence for this phenomena—known in the scientific literature as "remote healing"—is impressive, as with much of the research into psychic phenomena, the carefully controlled, double-blind studies that have been done in this area are virtually unknown to the average person, and many scientists persist in ignoring the very interesting and compelling data that has resulted from these studies.

Dr. Dossey served as co-chair of the NIH panel on Mind/ Body Interventions at the government's National Center for Complementary and Alternative Medicine. For nearly ten years he was the executive editor of the medical journal Alternative Therapies in Health and Medicine, *which he helped found in 1995. Currently, he is executive editor of* Explore: The Journal of Science and Healing. *He is a very popular public speaker, and has appeared on* Oprah Winfrey, Larry King, Good Morning America, *and NBC TV's* Dateline. *Dr. Dossey was the first physician ever invited to deliver the Annual Mahatma Gandhi Peace Foundation Memorial Lecture in New Delhi, India.*

Dr. Dossey lives in New Mexico. I interviewed him on January

30, 2006. I was instantly comfortable with Larry. He's very kind and gracious. I was particularly struck by Larry's strong sense of optimism and his contagious sense of hope. We spoke about mind-body medicine, research into remote healing, the problems with conventional Western medical treatments, and the future of medicine.

David: What originally inspired your interest in medicine?

Larry: I'm still trying to figure that out. There's no tradition in my family of medicine, and there have never been any other doctors in my family, as far as I know. I seem to have an innate fascination with science. I went away to the University of Texas at Austin, and fell in love with biology and chemistry. I got a degree in pharmacy, with almost a major in chemistry, and studied pre-med as well. I actually worked my way through medical school on weekends as a registered pharmacist. So I don't know how to explain my fascination and obsession with medicine—but it's certainly very deep, and it's been a commitment all my life.

David: How did your experience in Vietnam affect your perspective on medicine?

Larry: I had one of the strangest assignments possible for a physician in Vietnam. I functioned basically as a high-powered medic, beyond anything that would resemble a M.A.S.H. unit, carrying basically an aid bag and a rifle around. I actually went on patrols, spent hundreds of hours in helicopters, and fortunately got back alive—which took some doing. It was a daily confrontation with one's own mortality. I was in combat for the entire time, and this experience certainly makes one humble about the blessings one has in this culture. I can assure you that, and I've reflected on that every day since I came back from Vietnam. It's been a kind of indwelling presence really—the fact that I did remain alive—and it's filled me with gratitude. I don't think that it changed anything about my commitment to medicine, or made me see healing in any different way, but it was a confrontation with the immediacy of death, and it really was a powerful experience for me.

David: What do you think are some of the biggest problems with the way that medicine is practiced today?

Larry: Let me just name three or four. One is that it's become so complex that it's practically unmanageable. The institute of medicine several years ago began to make a national issue about the death rate in their hospitals from errors, and the side-effects of medications, and just flat out mistakes. There was a survey of this published in the *Journal of the American Medical Association* three or four years ago in which these statistics were analyzed. In this paper the third leading cause of death came out to be hospital care. The death rate in American hospitals from medical mistakes, errors, and the side-effects of drugs now ranks as the third leading cause of death, behind heart disease and cancer.

Well, the objectors came forward and were able to reanalyze the data. I think they demoted it down to five or six, as if that's some great accomplishment. But many experts still say that it's number three. Even so, the fact that it's even number five or six is still a national scandal. It should be a disgrace. But somehow people just accept this as part of the way medicine is. So the lethality of medicine is one problem. Another problem with medicine is its applicability. It's been estimated that three-fourths of people who go to physicians have nothing physically wrong with them, which means that they're beyond the reach of what high-tech, complex, modern medicine has to offer.

There's also a problem with the expense. We're nearing fifty million people in this country who don't have health insurance. That's a national disgrace. We're the only western industrialized country for which this is so. There was a survey published in *The Wall Street Journal* last year which found that medical illness and medical expense was the leading cause of personal bankruptcy in the United States. Now, this didn't just apply to low income families. This applied to middle-income families. Many of them had college educations, and many of them had health insurance, but the insurance didn't pay. This is a scandal.

Another problem with modern medicine is that it is not as effective as we want it to be. For example, take longevity. Currently the United States ranks twenty-sixth in longevity in countries in the world, behind countries like Costa Rica. Take infant mortality. We're now thirty-ninth in the world, behind countries like Cuba, Slovenia, and Aruba. This is disgraceful. We spend more money on healthcare than any other country, I think by a factor of three now, so we're not getting our money's worth in many areas. You add up all of these things, and you think, well, we've lost our way here. I think we have lost our way, and so those are just a few of the problems I see.

David: What do you think can be done to help improve the situation with modern medicine and reverse those problems?

Larry: For one thing, we urgently need a government-financed, centralized healthcare plan for everybody. It's shameful that we don't have it; we're the only industrialized western country that does not. This is a tall order now, particularly when one political party controls all three branches of government and is opposed to such changes. But there are hopeful signs.

This gives me an opportunity to make a shameless advertisement for my new book I mentioned awhile ago called *The Extraordinary Healing Power of Ordinary Things*. In this book I've tried to steer the medical conversation away from costly, high-tech, complex things like stem cells, transplantation, drugs, and surgery. This is not because I'm opposed to those things; I really support them. But high-tech, expensive approaches have dominated the efforts of medicine in this country, to the exclusion of many other valuable approaches. So I singled out fourteen really simple, commonplace, freely available things that pay huge dividends in health that are hardly ever talked about.

Some of these things have to do with prevention and with mental attitude. This may sound like New Age stuff, but the statistics show that the health benefits of these things are absolutely huge. Most people in their lives are not going to need things like an organ transplant or stem cells. Ninety percent of us live ninety percent of life needing to focus on a completely different perspective. I'll just give you one example—optimism. People who are optimistic live longer and have a lower incidence of disease than people who are pessimistic. Who ever talks about this?

One could single out any number of other extraordinarily simple things that pass under the radar screen yet yield huge health benefits. So we need a greater sense of openness to the simple, the plain, the ordinary.

A part of a physician's education should focus on prevention, and we need a government that emphasizes prevention through public health measures. We need to provide some sort of safety net for people who get over their heads with horrible illnesses and can never get out again. The need is urgent. For instance, the leading cause of personal bankruptcy in America is medical costs, and most of these bankruptcies occur in middle-class families. I'm not a medical architect who sits around at high policy levels and imagines how we might work this out. But I do know we need to spend national energy and federal capital making these things happen.

The emphasis in medical technology and pharmaceutical manufacturing is on shareholder profits. Like what's the new Viagra going to be? I'm not opposed to corporate profits, but the tail has begun to wag the dog. Today we have this widespread practice of private, academic medical researchers who are in bed with corporations, getting stock options, perks, and kickbacks on products they develop. In many cases, the corporations control the design and reporting of clinical trials. We've taken our eye off the ball. The nation's medical endeavor should be about helping healthy people stay healthy, and helping sick people get well. We've lost our way in this mission, and we need to wake up.

David: How did you become interested in the mind-body connection?

Larry: As so often is the case in doctors' accounts of how they become interested in these matters, it was through a personal medical problem. From grade school onward, I had profoundly severe migraine headaches, associated, not just with pain, nausea, and vomiting, but also with partial blindness. The partial blindness was the worst thing, and this almost derailed my career as a physician before it even got started. I actually tried to drop out of medical school because of this problem. I was convinced it was an ethical issue. I was certain that sooner or later I would have an episode of partial blindness and hurt or kill someone, in surgery for example.

However, my advisor wouldn't permit me to drop out. He told me that the problem would get better and it got a lot worse. This was really stress-related, but back in those days one didn't really talk a lot about stress, and certainly the mind-body connection was a term that had yet to be invented when I was in medical school. We talked about psychosomatic disease, but we certainly didn't talk about the mind-body connection in positive ways.

In any case, back in the early 70s, biofeedback burst on the medical scene in this country quite by accident. I found out that reports were coming out of biofeedback centers that people with migraines who practiced biofeedback noticed that their symptoms got better. I was desperate because none of the medications that were in common use worked for me. I chased all over the country learning how to do this for myself, and it was a miraculous outcome. It was almost like turning a switch in my brain and my body. I learned about the mind-body connection, about the meaning of relaxation, and the use of imagery and visualization. I took up meditation because it was a short step from biofeedback learning to meditating, and I became absolutely fascinated with the mind-body research area.

I began to follow it intensely, got certified in teaching biofeedback, became something of an expert in the field, and established one of the first biofeedback labs in the state of Texas for my patients and the patients of the other physicians in my group. I taught biofeedback for years as part of my internal medicine practice.

From there it was really easy for me to begin to follow the research in remote healing and intercessory prayer that began to come out of universities and medical schools in the mid-eighties. I was really primed for that. That's really a fairly short version of how I got interested in the mind-body area, and consciousness in general. I'm not sure that I would have become interested in mind-body medicine as quickly as I did without the impetus of a personal medical problem, and sheer desperation. But I certainly had a personal incentive. My back was really against the wall professionally and personally because of the intractable migraine, for which nothing else was helpful.

David: What role do you think one's mind plays in the health of the body?

Larry: I think that 'bodily health' is practically an oxymoron. One can't talk anymore about the health of the body without bringing in the effects of consciousness—by which I mean belief systems, meanings, emotions, attitudes, feeling-states, and so on. The day is long gone when we can separate the two. It's just inconsistent with the data. When we try to do this we really come up short, even when we attempt to treat the body as just a physical system and ignore the mind. We have to acknowledge the numerous double-blind, randomized controlled studies that take into account the placebo response, which clearly is an indication that the mind cannot be ignored. The placebo response is simply an expression of expectation, suggestion, and optimism about how a treatment is going to turn out. There may have been a time when doctors could get away with focusing on the body and ignoring the mind, but those days are gone forever.

David: Can you talk a little about the research that has been done in remote healing and why you think that these studies are important?

Larry: They're important because they force a total revision of our ideas about the nature of consciousness and its relationship to the brain and body. The old idea is that consciousness was simply an epiphenomenon of the brain; the brain made consciousness sort of like the liver made bile. In any case, the effects of consciousness were confined to one's own body. They had no ability, in principle, to reach out and make a difference remotely in someone else—but that's precisely the new image that is forming on the medical horizon.

It's an image of what I call "nonlocal mind." "Nonlocal" is simply a fancy word for "infinite." Nonlocal mind is unrestricted to specific points in space, such as individual brains and bodies, and it's unrestricted to specific points in time, such as the present moment. This sounds nutty and off-the-wall to people who've bumped into this for the first time, but if one has the willingness to look at the data emerging from healing studies, I think that the picture becomes quite compelling—at least it has for me and many other researchers in the field.

So, just to summarize where we stand data-wise, Dr. Wayne Jonas, who is the former director of the National Center for Complementary and Alternative Medicine, recently did a review and came up with 2,200 papers and citations in this field of remote healing. Over two hundred of these studies were controlled clinical trials and laboratory studies. The quality of the studies is quite good. Using what are called CONSORT criteria, he was able to assign either an "A" or a "B" level of excellence to these studies in remote healing. Eighteen of these studies are major controlled studies in humans, eleven of which show statistically significant results. The laboratory studies look at the effects of people's intentions on nonhumans—rabbits, mice, rats, plants, even bacteria growing in test tubes, fungi, yeast, and so on.

Occasionally the subjects of these lab studies are inanimate objects, such as random event generators. The majority of all these studies yield statistical significance, which shows that something is going on that you can't ascribe to chance. This is just a huge area. It's infuriated skeptics, who really aren't very much inclined to look at the data or even read all the studies. All told, this data calls into question fundamental assumptions about the nature of consciousness, as I've mentioned, and it's forcing a revision of how consciousness operates or manifests in the world.

There's a paradox here, because for most of human history people believed that these things actually happen, but it's only in the past two hundred years that we've developed a tremendous level of intellectual indigestion over this idea that consciousness could function remotely. So it's ironic that we're getting back to this ancient idea. What's further ironic is that science, which has denied for two hundred years that these things are possible, is pointing the way back. So, in a sense, science is shooting itself in the foot by producing this sort of evidence that contradicts what it has claimed regarding consciousness for two centuries.

David: Why do you think that the study of consciousness and research into psychic phenomena has important relevance for medicine?

Larry: There are several reasons. One is that it has health consequences. In my judgment the studies clearly show that people's intentions, prayers, and healing efforts at a distance can make the difference between life and death. It's important also because we really do want an accurate idea of the nature of our own consciousness. It's important because honoring this information leads us to a view of consciousness which is full of hope about our origins and destiny.

If we acknowledge that consciousness is nonlocal—that it's infinite in space and time—then this really opens up all sorts of possibilities for the survival of consciousness following physical death. If you reason through this, and follow the implications of these studies, you begin to realize that consciousness that's nonlocal and unrestricted in time is immortal. It's eternal. This is as hopeful as the current view of the fate of consciousness is dismal. This totally reverses things. So we are lead to a position, I think, where we see that even though the body will certainly die, the most essential part of who we are can't die, even if it tried—because it's nonlocally distributed through time and space.

Our grim vision of the finality of death is revised. Death is no longer viewed as a gruesome annihilation or the total destruction of all that we are. So there are tremendous spiritual implications that flow from these considerations, in addition to the implications for health. In fact, I believe that the implications for health are the least of it. A lot of people who encounter this area take a practical, bare bones, utilitarian approach to it. They say, wow, now we've got a nifty new item in our black bag— a new trick to help people become healthier. Certainly these studies do suggest that this is a proper use of healing intentions and prayer, and I'm all for that, but the thing that really gets my juices flowing is the implication of this research for immortality. For me, that's the most exciting contribution of this entire field.

The fear of death has caused more pain and suffering for human beings throughout history than all the physical diseases combined. The fear of death is the big unmentionable—and this view of consciousness is a cure for that disease, that fear of death.

David: What role do you think that spirituality plays in health?

Larry: There are a lot of people who just don't want to get close to this prayer stuff because they think "it's just parapsychology" and that all parapsychology is crazy. However, they often feel a little more comfortable when they look at another set of data having to do with the impact of spirituality on health. There are over 1,200 studies which look at the connections between religious behavior, such as attending worship services, and health outcomes. Currently meta-analyses of these studies show that people who follow some sort of religious path in their life live an average of seven to thirteen years longer than people who don't. That's just a huge health benefit. There isn't a whole heck of lot that physicians can recommend to people that will add seven to thirteen years on average to their lifespan.

People who like to think materialistically can come up with some fairly naturalistic explanations for these health benefits. For example, people who follow religious paths often have pretty good health habits. They may smoke or drink less. They are part of a social network by virtue of belonging to a congregation, and rich social networks have a health payoff. Nobody argues much against that anymore. Also, these people have a sense of meaning and purpose in life that comes from their religious affiliation. So if you add up all these things then it's not hard for even skeptics to imagine how people who are religious might enjoy longer life and have a lower incidence of disease. And they do.

But it's when people go into the area that Rupert Sheldrake, I and others have ventured into, where we talk about the remote effects of consciousness, that people really get cold feet. So it's been our self-appointed, elective task to hold people's feet to the fire and say, look, this information isn't going to go away. There's too much of it. It's becoming more abundant, so wake up. This is where we're headed, like it or not.

David: How do you see spirituality and medicine becoming more integrated in the future?

Larry: That's inevitable. One of the most telling indicators is how medical schools have responded. Back in 1993, when I first began to publish in this field with a book called *Healing Words*, there were only three medical schools in the country that had any coursework exploring the role of spirituality in health, out of one hundred and twenty-five medical schools total. Now ninety schools offer such coursework. That is a historic development. Ninety medical schools have either formal courses, a lecture series, or some feature of their curriculum that honors and addresses this field. So it's kind of a done deal.

Young doctors have much less of a problem with this than my generation
has had. One major reason is that half the medical-school enrollment
these days is made up of young women. They have a lot less trouble
with these ideas than intellectually-oriented guys do. So I think that the
entry of women in medicine has really opened up things quite a bit.

In the final analysis, the evidence favoring spirituality is so impressive
that there's no way that medicine is going to be able to stand on the
sidelines and ignore it. Sooner or later, good data rises to the top and
prejudices sink to the bottom. This process may take awhile, and there
will certainly be people who will try to obstruct it, but I think that there's
no way to stop it.

I see this in my own career. I am embarking on a four-month author
book tour next week, and slotted into this tour are lecture appearances
at medical schools all over the country.

There's an old saying that's attributed to Max Planck, the physicist, who
helped create the revolution in physics in the last century. Planck said
that science changes funeral by funeral. And as Einstein once said, "It's
harder to crack a prejudice than an atom." I used to believe that it's
possible to come up with such compelling evidence that it would change
things overnight. Well, that didn't happen in physics, and it's not going
to happen in medicine. These things always take awhile. Moreover,
there are some physicians who are so resistant to these ideas about
consciousness and healing that they will never come around. They'll
simply die off, as Planck suggested. I hate to say it, but that has come as
a consolation to me, periodically through the years (*laughter*).

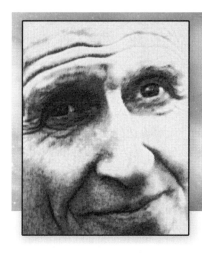

AN END TO SUFFERING

An Interview with Dr. Jack Kevorkian

Jack Kevorkian, M.D., is one of the most controversial physicians in the world. He attracted a lot of media attention in the early to mid-nineties due to his outspoken ideas about euthanasia, or "a good death," and is currently in his eighth year of prison for second degree murder because he assisted with the last wish of his patient, Thomas Youk, who was suffering from ALS.

Dr. Kevorkian graduated from the University of Michigan Medical School in 1952 with a specialty in pathology. He became Chief Pathologist at the Detroit Saratoga General Hospital in 1970. In the early 1980s, Dr. Kevorkian published a series of articles in the German journal Medicine and Law, *which outlined his ideas on euthanasia and ethics. Then, in 1987, Dr. Kevorkian began advertising in Detroit papers as a physician consultant for "death counseling." Between 1990 and 1998, Dr. Kevorkian assisted in the suicide of over one hundred terminally ill people.*

In each of these cases, Dr. Kevorkian only assisted in the suicide by attaching the person to one of the euthanasia devices that he designed. The first two deaths were assisted by means of a device called a "Thanatron," which used a needle and delivered deadly drugs mechanically through an I.V. The individual pushed a button which released a series of drugs that would end his or her own life. In 1993, after assisting in these two deaths, Dr. Kevorkian lost his medical license.

When Dr. Kevorkian could no longer obtain euthanizing drugs, some other patients were assisted by a device called a "Mercitron," which employed a gas mask fed by a canister of carbon monoxide. It's important to note that all of these cases were of voluntary euthanasia, because the individuals themselves took the final action which resulted in their own deaths. Dr. Kevorkian was tried numerous times during the 1990s for assisting in these suicides, but in every one of these cases the juries acquitted him. One juror was overheard to say the only thing Dr. Kevorkian was guilty of was being ahead of his time.

Court room conditions changed dramatically after Dr. Kevorkian appeared on 60 Minutes *with Mike Wallace. The November 22, 1998 broadcast of* 60 Minutes *featured a videotape that showed a patient in the final stages of ALS receiving a lethal injection from Dr. Kevorkian. Although Thomas Youk had provided his fully-informed consent, and this was a case of voluntary euthanasia, it was viewed differently than his previous cases because Dr. Kevorkian himself administered the lethal injection to relieve his pain and suffering.*

Although originally charged with assisted suicide, in the end Dr. Kevorkian went to trial on the charge of first-degree murder and was not allowed any witnesses. Following specific jury instructions for murder, not assisted suicide, the jury convicted him of second-degree murder and the delivery of a controlled substance on March 26, 1999. Dr. Kevorkian remains in prison in Michigan, serving a ten-to-twenty-five year sentence. The U.S. Supreme Court refused to hear his case. State and local courts denied his appeals and he has been repeatedly denied parole. He has made clear that he will no longer help patients end their lives and will now advocate legislation for this fundamental human right. He considers it a civil right of all individuals. Coincidentally, Dr. Kevorkian's access to the media was also severed the day he went to prison.

Mike Wallace, the anchor from 60 Minutes *who aired the video that was used in the trial that ultimately led to Dr. Kevorkian's imprisonment, said that he was upset with the conviction and perturbed by his lack of access to Dr. Kevorkian. In a letter to* The New York Review of Books *in 2001, Wallace wrote about the irony of Kevorkian being silenced while mass-murderer Timothy McVeigh was allowed to make all the statements he wanted to the media. In fact, the request for a lethal injection by a healthy, albeit convicted felon, Timothy McVeigh, was granted almost immediately after he declined appeals of his conviction.*

Many people believe that Dr. Kevorkian is not only being treated unfairly, but that this courageous man should be honored as a hero. Despite the U.S. government and medical establishment's opposition to euthanasia, eighty percent of the public support a patient's right to die and one in five physicians has admitted to practicing euthanasia at some point in his or her career. Many people also point out the irony in that the government rejects euthanasia but maintains the death penalty with lethal injection. Had Michigan had the death penalty, Dr. Kevorkian could have been sentenced to death for assisting someone who made a voluntary choice to end their own suffering.

Dr. Kevorkian is the author of Amendment IX: Our Cornucopia of Rights, *about how the Ninth Amendment to the Bill of Rights of the Constitution grants us rights that most people are unaware of, and are not being properly exercised. It states "The enumeration in the Constitution, of certain rights, shall not be construed to deny or disparage others retained by the people."*

Dr. Kevorkian is also the author of a unique diet book entitled Slimmeriks *and the* Demi-Diet, *and a collection of essays, color paintings, poetry, medical research proposals, sheet music, limericks, and cartoons entitled* GlimmerIQs. *To find out more about Dr. Kevorkian's books visit: www.glimmeriqs. com. Dr. Kevorkian is also an accomplished artist, whose emotionally-powerful, often surreal, and strikingly well-executed paintings have received critical acclaim. Copies of his paintings are available at Ariana Gallery in Royal Oak, Michigan. His paintings are now part of the collection of the Armenian Library and Museum of America: www.almainc. org.*

Dr. Kevorkian was awarded the Gleitsman Citizen Activist of the Year Award in 2000, and he was the subject of the 2001 documentary film Right to Exit: The Mock Trial of Dr. Jack Kevorkian. *Many prominent people have spoken out in Dr. Kevorkian's defense, and in 2002 he was nominated for the Noble Peace Prize. A major motion picture about Dr. Kevorkian's life, which will be directed by Academy Award winner Barbara Koppel, is currently in production. Kurt Vonnegut even wrote a novel entitled* God Bless You Dr. Kevorkian, *where he envisions himself as a "reporter on the afterlife," and bravely allows himself to be strapped to a gurney by Dr. Kevorkian and dispatched—round-trip—to Heaven.*

I interviewed Dr. Kevorkian in May of 2006. I was able to do this interview with the generous help of Dr. Kevorkian's attorney, Mayer Mike Morganroth, and his jury consultant and acting legal assistant, Ruth Holmes, who posed my questions to him in prison and recorded his responses. In the following interview, Dr. Kevorkian discusses his ideas about personal freedom, diet and exercise, why the practice of euthanasia is so important, and how the availability of euthanasia might actually prolong the lives of terminally-ill patients.

David: What originally inspired your interest in medicine?

Dr. Kevorkian: I was interested in a lot of things when I was young growing up in Pontiac, Michigan, with my two sisters and parents who escaped the Armenian Genocide. I considered being an engineer. I considered being a lawyer. I decided on medicine because it touches all professions. I also loved languages and taught myself to speak many of them.

David: What do you think are some of the biggest problems with modern medicine and what do you think needs to be done to help correct the situation?

Dr. Kevorkian: The biggest problem with Western medicine is that there is a need for establishing an appropriate system and structure for death with dignity. For those who are facing a terminal illness, who are in irremediable pain and suffering, and wish to exercise their right to die with dignity, a system should be available to them. We also need a more structured and reasonable organ donation and transplant systems. 18,000 people die each year waiting for organs. To help correct this situation there has to be an organized public response and outcry—which I believe is now occurring. The current system has not worked well enough to meet the medical needs.

David: Why do you think it's so important for physicians to be able to practice euthanasia without the fear of legal prosecution?

Dr. Kevorkian: Medical art and science are entirely secular and serve a dual purpose: to lengthen life and to preserve or enhance its quality. Theoretically both aims are equally important, but arbitrary (and mainly sectarian) bias fostered an obsession to prolong life, no matter how inimical to its quality.

The benefits of medicine permit its practitioners to perform acts that ordinarily are crimes. Thus we condone and even laud surgical mutilation like open heart surgery or organ transplants and tolerate for cancer treatment nearly lethal poisoning with chemotherapy. The resultant quality of life is always subordinate to the chief aim of prolonging it. Why shouldn't the ranking order sometimes be reversed? Why should we not just as readily praise and support the chief aim of relieving pain and suffering for those with terminal illnesses—humanely, expediently and with certainty—an intolerably low quality of individual life through a medical act ordinarily deemed to be homicide?

As a secular profession medicine is relevant to the full spectrum of human existence from conception through death. I think that any arbitrary legal constriction of that relevance is irrational, cruel, and barbaric.

David: How has euthanasia been viewed throughout history?

Dr. Kevorkian: Medical euthanasia was honorable and widely practiced in ancient Hippocratic Greece but later criminalized by the Church. The Renaissance philosopher-scientist Francis Bacon advocated that "the medical profession should be permitted to ease and quicken death where the end would be otherwise only delayed for a few days and at the cost of great pain."

In seventeenth-century England, Sir Edward Coke, a distinguished lawyer and judge, dismissed charges against a physician who openly performed euthanasia. It was Coke's dictum that "how long soever it hath continued, if it be against reason, it is of no force in law." Accordingly, the long-continued criminalization of euthanasia is of no force because it is flagrantly against reason.

Almost two centuries later Thomas Jefferson advocated the use of a drug to end the terminal suffering from "the inveterate cancer." In 1910, Mark Twain asked his physician to end his suffering from heart disease. Dr. Sigmund Freud's terminal agony, and also in 1936 that of England's King George V, ended with injections by their personal physicians, both vociferous advocates of the practice. The late distinguished American physician and author Dr. Walter Alvarez several decades ago published his strong endorsement of medical euthanasia.

Today more than half of all American physicians and an overwhelming majority of the public favor decriminalization of the practice, and a significant number of physicians admit to performing it furtively. The British will no longer prosecute doctors. The state of Oregon has permitted a limited form of aid in dying through ill-advised, overly restrictive legislation. It appears that the state of Maine may soon do the same. These state laws prohibit the most humane and preferable method of ending pain and suffering with a lethal injection.

The Constitutional Court in the predominantly Catholic nation Colombia in 1997 declared simply and correctly that access to medical euthanasia is a right of the people. The Netherlands has now formally decriminalized euthanasia after two or more decades of having permitted the practice within carefully set guidelines. It is also allowed in Switzerland, Germany, and Uruguay, and may soon be legalized in Catholic Belgium and France, and in Japan. One must wonder why the English-speaking countries lag in this humanitarian trend.

David: Why do you think that the U.S. government and medical establishment are so opposed to euthanasia—despite the fact that eighty percent of the public support a patient's right to die?

Dr. Kevorkian: I think that the U.S. government, medical establishment, and pharmaceutical companies are opposed to euthanasia for monetary or financial reasons. And, also, this view against PAD (physician assistance in dying) is supported by many churches and religious extremists.

David: What are your thoughts about how the availability of euthanasia might prolong the lives of terminally-ill patients?

Dr. Kevorkian: The mere availability of the euthanasia option often improves the quality of, and even prolongs, the lives of many terminal and incurably suffering patients. Having such a choice seems to dissipate the panic and helplessness by assuring a modicum of personal control. Consequently the vast majority of patients went on to die "naturally" and with few complaints despite continued excruciating suffering. This was the case with most patients who contacted me.

David: How do you envision euthanasia being put into practice by physicians?

Dr: Kevorkian: Not all physicians will want or, by temperament, be able to perform euthanasia. For them, and for patients alike, it's a matter of free choice based on personal belief, faith, or philosophy of life. The service should be a kind of medical specialty staffed by experienced and competent practitioners to whom reticent colleagues may refer inquiries. Because medical guidelines change frequently as a result of research and clinical experience, such procedural details cannot be dictated by law.

David: What do you personally think happens to consciousness after death?

Dr: Kevorkian: No living being in this world knows exactly and certainly—indeed even faintly—what absolute physical death is. One can only know that it occurred. Despite impressive philosophical and religious mythologizing, as well as the anecdotal buncombe called near-death experiences, nobody has ever survived absolute death. At present that survival would offer the only (but now inaccessible) means of gaining reliable and certain knowledge about it.

David: Many people are unaware that you wrote a diet book in 1978, which you later revised and included in your book GlimmerIQs. *What sort of suggestions would you make for improving one's diet?*

Dr: Kevorkian: It is well known that animals generally take their daily food quota by many small feedings, in contrast to a limited number of large meals for most civilized humans. Extensive research on animals has shown that the ingestion of their daily food in five separate portions had a salutary effect on blood cholesterol levels and the development of arterial atherosclerosis.

Even though the single feeders (one large meal a day) ate thirty percent less, their bodies were slightly larger and had a higher percentage of fat when compared to the slightly smaller bodies of multiple feeders (nibblers) having gained relatively heavier muscle mass. It has been estimated that fifty to seventy-five percent of daily human food intake is at the single meal called supper, which alone may account for our tendency to be fatter and flabbier.

David: What sort of recommendations would you make regarding exercise?

Dr: Kevorkian: Your chosen exercise should fit in well with your own lifestyle, one that you can do throughout life, and that is independent of weather conditions. An indoor activity of some kind would be preferable, perhaps your own individual routine not involving anyone else or any group, institution, or club. Some forms of exercise are considered to be especially beneficial to health by enhancing cardio-respiratory reserve. Exercise involving the legs is said to be more effective in that regard than is exercising the arms or trunk. Jogging, tennis, bicycling, and jumping rope are excellent ways to build up that reserve, but not all of them can be continued uninterruptedly year round without inconvenience.

David: What are your thoughts on personal freedom, and why do you think that Amendment IX to the Constitution is so important?

Dr. Kevorkian: I think that every human being is born with the lifelong, powerful, unalterable, essentially instinctual will or drive to *absolute* personal freedom. Of course, for a smoothly functioning, civilized community that absolute drive must be tempered through the judicious modulating effect of so-called relative rights essentially consisting of commonsense rules elaborated for the optimization of harmonious communal existence, and codified by means of wide-ranging, if not universal, public consensus.

The full power of natural rights is latent in Amendment IX of the Bill of Rights. Much of the bitter controversy and often bloody violence fostered by highly controversial issues throughout history could have been ameliorated or averted if responsible authorities had done their duty by tapping the trove that the Ninth offers. The point is well exemplified by the passionate battles over medical abortion (or the choice *not* to bear life) and medical euthanasia (or the choice *not* to live intolerably suffering).

David: What are your thoughts about the future of Western medicine?

Dr. Kevorkian: I'm optimistic that Western medicine will advance and start accepting newer and more progressive ideas, as well as, of course, the importance of choice on end of life issues such as death with dignity. I'm also hopeful that we'll develop more appropriate organ transplant strategies. And this is coming—slowly but surely, both medical services with proper oversights will be available in the future. The Europeans are already leading the way.

GLOSSARY

AGEs (advanced glycation end-products): Sticky unions of sugar and protein that are created in the body when excess circulating sugar molecules bind to proteins and combine with them, creating cross-linked proteins that gum up the body's vital enzymes and increase free radical damage. AGEs have been linked to numerous diseases, and are known to accelerate aging in general. Age spots on the skin and cataracts in the lens of the eye are examples of AGE formation.

Amino acids: Simple organic compounds containing nitrogen which are the building blocks of proteins.

anandamide: From the Sanskrit, ananda, which means "inner bliss". A naturally occurring brain chemical that binds to the same receptors in the brain as THC (tetrahydrocannabinol), the primary psychoactive component in marijuana. Anandamide and THC bind to the cannabinoid receptors, which are found in higher concentrations than any other receptor in the brain. Anandamide appears to help regulate emotions and plays a role in memory, the reduction of pain, and reward systems.

antioxidant: a chemical that prevents the oxidative degradation of other chemicals and helps to neutralize free radicals in the body.

ATP (adenosine triphosphate): A nucleotide, produced by the mitochondria inside cells, that is responsible for the chemical energy that drives otherwise uphill biochemical reactions in the body.

Ayurvedic medicine: The traditional medicine of India. *Ayurveda* is based on two Sanskrit terms: *ayu* meaning life, and *veda* meaning knowledge or science. The practice is said to be around 5,000 years old.

axons: A thin neuronal branch that transmits electrical impulses away from the neural cell body to other neurons (or to muscles or glands).

C-reactive protein (CRP): An acute phase protein produced by the liver that increases during systemic inflammation. Testing CRP levels in the blood may be useful as a way to assess cardiovascular disease risk, as elevated CRP levels are correlated with a higher incidence of coronary artery disease.

chelation therapy: Chelation is a natural chemical process that goes on continually in our bodies, in which a metal or mineral becomes bonded to another substance. Chelation therapy employs the synthetic amino acid and chelating agent EDTA. Used both orally and intravenously, it has been shown to help prevent arteriosclerosis, improve circulation, and remove lead and toxic heavy metals from the body.

chemokine: A type of peptide which causes specific immune cells to move toward a chemical stimulus.

cross-linking: The process of chemically joining two or more molecules by a covalent bond; i.e., when electrons are shared between atoms. This sometimes results in the formation of abnormal chemical bonds between adjacent protein strands, which deforms them and impairs their function in the body.

cryonics: The practice of preserving animals—or people who can no longer be sustained by contemporary medicine—in the extremely cold environment of liquid nitrogen (-196°C), with the hope that resuscitation may be possible in the future with nanotechnology.

dendrites: Tiny tree-like branchings at the electrical impulse-receiving end of a neuron.

differentiation: The process of acquiring individual characteristics, as occurs in the progressive diversification of cells and tissues of the embryo.

DNA: Deoxyribonucleic acid—the long complex macromolecule, consisting of two interconnected helical strands, that resides in the nucleus of every living cell and encodes the genetic instructions for building each organism.

DMT: Dimetyltryptamine—an extremely powerful, short-acting hallucinogenic tryptamine found in a number of different plant species and the South American shamanic brew Ayahuasca. Small amounts of DMT are also found naturally in the human brain, where it is secreted by the pineal gland.

double-blind: A type of scientific or clinical study in which neither the subject nor the experimenter know if the subject is receiving an experimental treatment or a placebo. This controls for the effects of expectation and belief.

endogenous: Found naturally within the body; produced within an organism. The opposite of exogenous.

endorphin: "Endogenous morphine"; the brain's naturally produced neurotransmitter which binds to the same brain receptors as opiate drugs, and helps to regulate pain and reward systems.

essential nutrient: Components of food that are required for normal body functioning which can not be synthesized by the body. Essential nutrients include vitamins, minerals, essential fatty acids, and essential amino acids.

estrogen: A group of three steroid compounds (estradiol, estriol, and estrone) that functions as the primary female sex hormone. Estrogen promotes the development of female secondary sex characteristics, such as breasts, and is involved in regulating the menstrual cycle.

exogenous: Derived or developed outside of the body or organism. The opposite of endogenous.

excitatory neurotransmitter: A type of neurotransmitter—such as dopamine—that excites, speeds up, or accelerates neural processes. The opposite of an inhibitory neurotransmitter, which slows down neural processes.

free radical: Highly reactive atoms or molecules with unpaired electrons.

Free radicals can cause substantial oxidative damage to the body and are thought to be one of the primary causes of aging. Because free radicals are necessary for normal metabolism, the body uses antioxidants to minimize free radical-induced damage.

genome: The complete set of genetic material or genes for a single organism.

genomic testing: Tests which scan an individual's DNA for gene variants, acquired mutations, and measure gene expression. Genomic testing can be helpful in predicting an individual's predisposition towards many dangerous genetic diseases. This allows people to take preventive measures, and for physicians to modify gene expression through precise, targeted, individualized interventions.

germ-line cells: The body's sex cells (sperm and ovum), whose function is to propagate the individual's DNA through sexual reproduction.

glycation: A chemical reaction between proteins and sugars, which results in toxic products that are thought to be one of the primary causes of aging.

Hayflick limit: The number of times a cell can divide and replicate itself. Every species has its own Hayflick limit which corresponds with the length of its telomeres; the end portions of chromosomes.

HDL: High-density lipoprotein, the "good" cholesterol, which removes cholesterol from the arteries before it has a chance to oxidize, and reduces the inflammatory process. Higher HDL levels are correlated with a lower incidence of cardiovascular disease.

homocysteine: Toxic metabolic byproducts formed by eating methionine, an amino acid found in animal protein foods like poultry and red meat. Elevated homocysteine levels are associated with a greater risk of cardiovascular disease.

hormone: A chemical messenger produced in one part of the body that is carried through the bloodstream to other parts of the body where it invokes a specific response. These responses vary widely, but they can include stimulating new cell growth, regulating metabolism, or preparing the body for a new phase of life, such as puberty or menopause. They may also stimulate a behavioral response, such as fleeing, fighting, or mating.

inhibitory neurotransmitter: A type of neurotransmitter—such as serotonin—that inhibits or slows down neural processes. The opposite of an excitatory neurotransmitter which accelerates neural processes.

LDL: Low-density lipoprotein, the "bad" cholesterol. The oxidation of LDL in the arteries is the first step toward vulnerable plaque formation which leads to cardiovascular disease.

MAO inhibitor: A drug that slows down the production of monoamine oxidase (MAO); an enzyme in the brain that breaks down neurotransmitters. By inhibiting the production of MAO, you increase the longevity of neurotransmitters in the synapses between neurons, and, consequently, the effects of those neurotransmitters.

MAO: Monoamine oxidase, an enzyme in the brain that breaks down neurotransmitters.

MAO-B: A type of monoamine oxidase that specifically breaks down the excitatory neurotransmitter dopamine. By inhibiting MAO-B, you enhance the effects of dopamine in the brain.

mitochondria: Structures within cells that produce energy by respiratory metabolism. Mitochondria have their own DNA and are thought to be bacteria that were captured by animal cells in the course of evolution.

MRI (Magnetic Resonance Imaging) Scan: A diagnostic technique that detects structures by their different content of atoms with certain resonances to induced magnetic fields and produces very detailed, two or three-dimensional, cross-sectional images of organs inside the body. It is especially useful for viewing soft tissue and doesn't use X-rays or any dangerous form of radiation.

nanotechnology: Atomic engineering—the ability to devise self-replicating machines, robots, and computers on a molecular level.

nanobots: Self-replicating, molecule-sized robots.

neuropeptide: Peptides that are found in the brain and nervous system. (See: peptides)

neurotransmitter: Chemicals that transmit and modulate electrical signals between neurons (brain cells) and other cells.

paradigm: A model for explaining a set of data; a belief system.

paradigm shift: A change in the perception of information.

peptides: Strings consisting of two or more amino acids linked end to end. Peptides are used as chemical messengers that communicate information between systems in the body.

PET (Positron Emission Tomography) Scan: A powerful computer-generated, imaging technique that allows physicians and researchers to see a region of the body's metabolic activity in action. PET scans rely upon the detection of gamma rays, which are emitted from tissues after the administration of radioactive glucose—which circulates throughout the body, and is more readily metabolized in those cells that are more active.

phytochemical: A naturally-occurring, plant-derived chemical substance with biological activity—such as chlorophyll, beta-carotene, or lycopene. Many phytochemicals—which give plants their color, flavor, smell, and texture—are known to improve health and prevent disease.

phytoestrogens: Estrogen-like substances found in plants, especially soy. Some isoflavones (a type of phytochemical) are classified as phytoestrogens because their chemical structure is similar to human estrogen, and they act as weak estrogens in the body. Phytoestrogens are associated with a lowered risk of many diseases, including heart disease, osteoporosis, and breast cancer.

placebo: An inactive substance, such as a sugar pill, which is tested blindly against an active substance to compensate for a possible effect created through the power of belief.

placebo effect: A measurable effect created by expectation and the power of belief.

polymerase chain reaction (PCR): A technique developed by Kary Mullis which allows biochemists to replicate minute amounts of DNA template into much larger quantities that can be used for a variety of downstream reactions and studies. PCR revolutionized the study of genetics and won Mullis the 1993 Nobel Prize in Chemistry.

remote healing: Mental influences between people which effect health in a way that isn't easily explained by conventional science.

robotics: The science and technology of designing and manufacturing robots. This combines mechanical engineering with artificial intelligence.

silent inflammation: Inflammation is a characteristic reaction of tissues to injury or disease that is marked by swelling, redness, heat, and usually pain. However, there is a common form of inflammation known as 'silent inflammation' that is painless, but extremely dangerous. Silent inflammation, which is often linked to diet, has been correlated with a higher incidence of cardiovascular disease, neurodegenerative disorders, cancer, and other illnesses.

somatic cells: The differentiated cells that constitute every part of the body, except for the germ-line cells.

stem cells: The undifferentiated cells that all other cells in the body are derived from.

telomerase: An enzyme which allows cells to divide indefinitely without the protective caps at the ends of the chromosomes shortening. The activation of telomerase in germ cells and cancer cells allows these cells to divide indefinitely because the telomerase adds telomere repeat sequences to the ends of the chromosomes every time each cell divides.

telomere: Repetitive sequences at the ends of chromosomes that serve a protective buffer. With each cell division some telomeres are lost. The length of the telomeres determines the life of the cell, because when all the telomeres are gone the cell dies. Germ cells and cancer cells avoid this fate by producing an enzyme called telomerase, which allows cells to divide indefinitely without the telomeres shortening.

testosterone: A steroid hormone from the androgen group that functions as the principal male sex hormone. Testosterone promotes the development of male secondary sex characteristics, such as facial hair, and is involved in regulating sperm production.

tocopherols: A component of vitamin E, a fat-soluble vitamin, which is composed of four tocopherols and four tocotrienols. The four tocopherols and the four tocotrienols are known as isomers because they are chemically similar, but arranged differently. Each tocopherol has an alpha, beta, gamma, and delta form, and each form has its own biological activity.

tocotrienols: A component of vitamin E, a fat-soluble vitamin, which is composed of four tocotrienols and four tocopherols. The four tocotrienols and four tocopherols are known as isomers because they are chemically similar, but arranged differently. Each tocotrienol has an alpha, beta, gamma, and delta form, and each form has its own biological activity.

vitamin: An organic compound that is essential for normal metabolism, which can not be synthesized by the body and must be supplied through diet.

IndeX

INTERNET RESOURCES

David Jay Brown
www.mavericksofthemind.com
www.sexanddrugs.info
www.animalsandearthquakes.com

Cryonics
www.alcor.org

Aubrey de Grey
www.sens.org

Larry Dossey
www.dosseydossey.com

Peter Duesberg
www.duesberg.com

Michael Fossel
http://home.earthlink.net/~mfossel/aging/id2.html

Garry Gordon
www.gordonresearch.com

John Guerin
www.agelessanimals.org

Leonard Hayflick
www.agelessanimals.org/hayflickbio.htm

Ruth Holmes:
Ruth is a handwriting examiner and forensic document expert, as well as Dr. Kevorkian's jury consultant and acting legal assistant. Dr. Kevorkian lived with Ruth's family for nearly six months before he went to prison.
www.pentec.net

Jack Kevorkian
www.glimmeriqs.com
www.almainc.org

Joseph Knoll
http://xenia.sote.hu/depts/pharmacology/staff/knoll.htm
http://en.wikipedia.org/wiki/Joseph_Knoll

Ray Kurzweil
www.KurzweilTech.com
www.KurzweilAI.net

Marios Kyriazis
www.anti-age.org.uk

Raphael Mechoulam
http://paincenter.huji.ac.il/mechoulam.htm

Kary Mullis
www.karymullis.com

Durk Pearson & Sandy Shaw
www.life-enhancement.com/ds_index.aspx

Amy E. Powers
Jack Kevorkian's photographer
www.agapeimagesinc.com

Barry Sears
www.drsears.com

Bernie Siegel
www.ecap-online.org

Rick Strassman
www.rickstrassman.com

Jacob Teitelbaum
www.endfatigue.com

Michael West
www.advancedcell.com

Andrew Weil
www.drweil.com

Jonathan Wright
www.tahoma-clinic.com

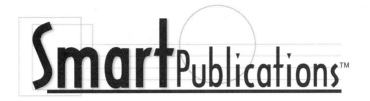

Smart Publications is happy to present you with the following information.

HOW TO FIND A KNOWLEDGEABLE AND UNDERSTANDING PHYSICIAN

The quickest and most efficient way is to visit a medical doctor or osteopath who is a member of the American College for Advancement in Medicine. All members of these professional organizations are skilled and knowledgeable in the prescription and use of natural hormones and other alternative compounds. For a referral contact:

ACAM
23121 Verdugo Dr., Ste. 204, Laguna Hills, CA 92653
1 (800) 532-3688
www.acam.org

Great Lakes College of Clinical Medicine
There are over 500 members of all disciplines that are very active in introducing therapies.
www.glccm.org

American Holistic Medical Association
Most members are versed in natural hormone replacement.
www.holisticmedicine.org

HOW TO FIND A COMPOUNDING PHARMACY

For compounds like natural testosterone or estrogen you will need to call a compounding pharmacy, and they will need a doctor's prescription (you can ask the pharmacy for a referral or consult from the list of knowledgeable physicians above).

The easiest way to locate a compounding pharmacy is to contact one of the following associations:

Professional Compounding Centers of America, Inc. (PCCA)
9901 S. Wilcrest, Houston, TX 77099
1 (800) 331-2498; FAX 1 (800) 874-5760
www.thecompounders.com

International Academy of Compounding Pharmacists (IACP)
PO BOX 1365, Sugar Land, TX 77487
1 (800) 927-4227; FAX 1 (281) 495-0602
www.iacprx.org

National Association of Compounding Pharmacists (NACP)
4015 River Road, Amarillo, TX 79108
1 (800) 687-7850; FAX 1 (800) 687-8902

HOW TO ORDER YOUR PHARMACEUTICALS FROM OVERSEAS

Thanks to AIDS activists, it has been legal for several years in the United States to order, for personal use, a 3 month supply of non-Schedule I or II drugs from overseas. Often, the overseas pharmacies have products that are unavailable in the U.S. and the quality is the same as any U.S. pharmacy. We highly recommend the following company:

International Antiaging Systems (IAS)
PO BOX 337J, Guernsey, Channel Islands, Great Britain
FAX: 011-44-870-151-4145
Email Address: ias(j)antiaging-systems.com

SOURCES FOR GHB

We regret to inform you that GHB is no longer available. GHB has been considered highly illegal and deemed the "date rape drug". There are several doctors as well as concerned citizens who are fighting these accusations. At this time, we are not able to provide any information regarding GHB and are finding other legal alternatives to supplement GHB's wonderful properties.

SOURCES FOR 5-HTP, NATURAL PROGESTERONE & TESTOSTERONE PRECURSERS

Smart Publications recommends finding a supplement company that stresses quality. It is always difficult to choose from all of the available products. We highly recommend the following company:

Health Freedom Nutrition, LLC
255 Bell St., Reno, NV 89503
1 (800) 980-8780; FAX 1 (888) 998-6889
www.hfn-usa.com

Smart Publications works hard to provide you with necessary alternatives to help maintain and sustain your health and longevity.

We hope the information provided will assist your search for knowledge and well-being.

BᴵO

David Jay Brown is the author of three previous volumes of interviews with leading-edge thinkers, *Mavericks of the Mind*, *Voices from the Edge*, and *Conversations on the Edge of the Apocalypse*. He is also the author of two science fiction novels, *Brainchild* and *Virus*. David holds a master's degree in psychobiology from New York University, and was responsible for the California-based research in two of British biologist Rupert Sheldrake's books on unexplained phenomena in science: *Dogs That Know When Their Owners Are Coming Home* and *The Sense of Being Stared At*. He lives in the Santa Cruz mountains of California. To find out more about David's work visit his award-winning Web site: www.mavericksofthemind.com

PHOTO CREDITS

David Jay Brown: *Photo by Deed DeBruno*

Aubrey de Grey: *Photo by Poppy Berry*

Larry Dossey: *Photo by Athi Mara Magadi*

Peter Duesberg: *Photo courtesy of Peter Duesberg*

Michael Fossel: *Photo by Laura Sternberg*

Garry Gordon: *Photo by Jean-Louis Husson, Feathertech.com*

John Guerin: *Photo by Larry L. Guerin, M.D.*

Leonard Hayflick: *Photo by UCSF Photo Dept.*

Jack Kevorkian: *Photo by Amy E. Powers*

Joseph Knoll: *Photo courtesy of Joseph Knoll*

Ray Kurzweil: *Photo by Michael Lutch. Courtesy of Kurzweil Technologies, Inc.*

Marios Kyriazis: *Photo courtesy of Marios Kyriazis*

Raphael Mechoulam: *Image: Boehringer Ingelheim GmbH*

Kary Mullis: *Photo by Mark Robert Halper*

Durk Pearson & Sandy Shaw: *Photo by Robert Pruzan*

Barry Sears: *Photo by Bobbie Bush Photography, 2004.*

Bernie Siegel: *Photo by Barry Bittman, M.D.*

Rick Strassman: *Photo by Stuart Abelson*

Jacob Teitelbaum: *Photo courtesy of Jacob Teitelbaum, M.D.*

Andrew Weil: *Photo by Amy Haskell, Haskell Photography, Tucson, AZ.*

Michael West: *Photo courtesy of Advanced Cell Technology, Inc.*

Jonathan Wright: *Photo courtesy of Jonathan Wright, M.D.*